MASSACHUSETTS GENERAL HOSPITAL
STUDY GUIDE FOR PSYCHIATRY EXAMS:
600 Questions and Annotated Answers

MASSACHUSETTS GENERAL HOSPITAL
STUDY GUIDE FOR PSYCHIATRY EXAMS:

600 Questions and Annotated Answers

THEODORE A. STERN, MD

Chief Emeritus, Avery D. Weisman Psychiatric Consultation Service
Director, Thomas P. Hackett Center for Scholarship in Psychosomatic Medicine
Interim Director, Center for Faculty Development
Director, Office for Clinical Careers,
Massachusetts General Hospital
Ned H. Cassem Professor of Psychiatry in the field of Psychosomatic Medicine/Consultation,
Harvard Medical School, Boston, MA
Editor-in-Chief, *Psychosomatics*

ELSEVIER

3251 Riverport Lane
St. Louis, Missouri 63043

**MASSACHUSETTS GENERAL HOSPITAL STUDY GUIDE FOR PSYCHIATRY EXAMS:
600 QUESTIONS AND ANNOTATED ANSWERS**

ISBN: 978-0-323-73296-3

Notices

Knowledge and best practice in this field are constantly changing. As new research and experience broaden our understanding, changes in research methods, professional practices, or medical treatment may become necessary.

Practitioners and researchers must always rely on their own experience and knowledge in evaluating and using any information, methods, compounds, or experiments described herein. In using such information or methods they should be mindful of their own safety and the safety of others, including parties for whom they have a professional responsibility.

With respect to any drug or pharmaceutical products identified, readers are advised to check the most current information provided (i) on procedures featured or (ii) by the manufacturer of each product to be administered, to verify the recommended dose or formula, the method and duration of administration, and contraindications. It is the responsibility of practitioners, relying on their own experience and knowledge of their patients, to make diagnoses, to determine dosages and the best treatment for each individual patient, and to take all appropriate safety precautions.

To the fullest extent of the law, neither the Publisher nor the authors, contributors, or editors, assume any liability for any injury and/or damage to persons or property as a matter of products liability, negligence or otherwise, or from any use or operation of any methods, products, instructions, or ideas contained in the material herein.

Library of Congress Control Number: 2019955461

Director, Content Development: Ellen Wurm-Cutter
Senior Content Strategist: Joslyn Chaiprasert-Paguio
Content Development Specialist: Brooke Kannady
Publishing Services Manager: Deepthi Unni
Project Manager: Bharat Narang
Design: Brian Salisbury

Printed in the United States of America

Last digit is the print number: 9 8 7 6 5 4 3 2 1

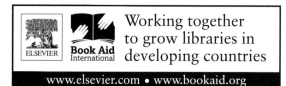

Preface

Psychiatry continues to evolve. This prompted us to create the updated version of *Massachusetts General Hospital Comprehensive Clinical Psychiatry, Second Edition*. It features 94 chapters that cover the diagnosis, pathophysiology, evaluation, and treatment of a wide range of psychiatric and neurologic conditions and states.

We understood that those studying for exams (e.g., millennials, lifelong learners) and those who are seeking to solidify their knowledge gained through layered learning (e.g., clinical experience, reading) would benefit from reviewing 600 board-style multiple-choice questions and detailed annotated answers (geared to each chapter in *Comprehensive Clinical Psychiatry, Second Edition*).

This led to the decision to create the *Massachusetts General Hospital Study Guide for Psychiatry Exams: 600 Questions and Annotated Answers*. On behalf of the patients we serve, we hope that this learning exercise distills the essence of our text, facilitates your knowledge and understanding of psychiatric problems, and brings much-needed relief.

T.A.S.

Dedication

To lifelong learners, to my mentors and colleagues (who made our textbooks possible), and to my family (who supported me at every turn).

T.A.S.

Contents

Contents

SECTION 1
APPROACH TO THE PATIENT

The Doctor–Patient Relationship

Multiple-Choice Questions

Select the appropriate answer.

Q1   Which of the following statements is LEAST accurate?

    A.   *Physician qualities have little impact on the doctor–patient relationship*

    B.   *Poor outcomes—including "noncompliance" with treatment plans, complaints to oversight boards, and malpractice actions—tend to arise when patients feel unheard, disrespected, or otherwise out of partnership with their doctors*

    C.   *Stigma is attached to mental illness in our culture*

    D.   *The relationship between doctor and patient is not merely a vehicle through which to deliver care; it is one of the most important aspects of care itself*

    E.   *The role of the physician in patient-centered care is that of an expert, who seeks to help a patient comanage his or her health to whatever extent is most comfortable for that person*

Q2   Which of the following perspectives is LEAST likely to be important in the doctor–patient relationship and to an understanding of the patient's problems?

    A.   *Biological ailments*

    B.   *Function of the P450 isoenzyme system*

    C.   *Psychological reactions*

    D.   *Social connections*

    E.   *Spirituality*

Q3   Which of the following is NOT considered a role of patient-centered physicians?

    A.   *Attempting to successfully establish common ground on the nature of the problem as the patient perceives it and attempting to synthesize these problems into workable diagnoses and problem–lists*

    B.   *Confirming and demonstrating his or her understanding through direct, nonjargonistic language to the patient*

    C.   *Deciding what is best for the patient and directing the patient to follow instructions*

    D.   *Endeavoring to create conditions of welcome, respect, and safety so that the patient can reveal his or her concerns and perspective*

    E.   *Endeavoring to understand the patient deeply, as a person, listening to both the words and the "music" of what is communicated*

Q4   Which of the following is NOT an important communication skill for enhancement of the doctor–patient relationship?

    A.   *Eliciting the patient's perspective*

    B.   *Explaining conditions and options in clear, nontechnical language*

    C.   *Generating input and consensus about paths of care*

    D.   *Helping the patient feel understood*

    E.   *Prescribing medications over the telephone*

Q5 Which of the following is LEAST likely to be considered as an overarching principle of effective clinical interviewing?

A. *An ability to engage the person in a mutual exploration of what is troubling him or her*

B. *A capacity to help patients feel at ease in telling their stories*

C. *Efficient office staff*

D. *Friendliness*

E. *Warmth*

Q6 Which of the following is LEAST likely to cause obstacles or difficulties in the doctor–patient relationship?

A. *Engaging the patient to feel heard and accurately understood*

B. *Losing sight of how intimidating, arcane, and forbidding medical practice can appear to the uninitiated*

C. *Making assumptions regarding the supposed incapacity of psychiatric patients to be full partners in their own care*

D. *Overrelying on "objective" measures (such as symptom checklists, questionnaires, tests, and other measurements that may speed diagnosis)*

E. *Using overly technical, arcane, or obtuse language*

Chapter 1

Answers

Q1 The answer is: (A) Physician qualities have little impact on the doctor–patient relationship.
Physicians' qualities have an impact on the doctor–patient relationship. These qualities support and enhance—but are not a substitute for—technical competence and cognitive mastery.

Poor outcomes—including "noncompliance" with treatment plans, complaints to oversight boards, and malpractice actions—tend to arise when patients feel unheard, disrespected, or otherwise out of partnership with their doctors.

Stigma is attached to mental illness in our culture, and it amplifies the wary sense of risk of shame and humiliation that patients may experience in any doctor–patient interaction; it makes it even more imperative that the physician work to create conditions of safety in the relationship.

The relationship between doctor and patient is not merely a vehicle through which to deliver care; it is one of the most important aspects of care itself.

In patient-centered care, there is active management of communication to avoid inadvertently hurting, shaming, or humiliating the patient through careless use of language or other slights. When such hurt or other error occurs, the practitioner apologizes clearly and in a heartfelt way to restore the relationship.

The role of the physician in patient-centered care is one of an expert who seeks to help a patient comanage his or her health to whatever extent is most comfortable for that particular person. The role is not to cede all important decisions to the patient.

Q2 The answer is: (B) Function of the P450 isoenzyme system.
Although an understanding of isoenzyme systems can facilitate selection of a given dose of a psychotropic agent, it will not directly facilitate an understanding of the patient and his or her problems or enhance the doctor–patient relationship.

An appreciation of the person from the perspective of the person's biological ailments and vulnerabilities; the person's current social connections, supports, and stressors; the person's psychological issues from the past; and how the person makes spiritual sense of a life lived with the foreknowledge of death can give us an in-depth sense of the person. In addition, knowledge of the patient's handling of existential matters can also be meaningful.

Q3 The answer is: (C) Deciding what is best for the patient and directing the patient to follow instructions.
In "relationship-centered" practice, more than patient-centered practice, the physician does not cede decision-making authority or responsibility to the patient and family, but rather enters into real dialogue about what the physician thinks is best.

The "patient-centered" physician attempts to accomplish six processes. First, the physician endeavors to create conditions of welcome, respect, and safety, so that the patient can reveal his or her concerns and perspective. Second, the physician endeavors to understand the patient deeply, as a person, listening to both the words and the "music" of what is communicated. Third, the physician confirms and demonstrates his or her understanding through direct, nonjargonistic language to the patient. Fourth, if he or she successfully establishes common ground on the nature of the problem as the patient perceives it, an attempt is made to synthesize these problems into workable diagnoses and problem–lists. Fifth, using expertise, technical mastery, and experience, a path is envisioned toward healing, and it is shared with the patient. Finally, together the physician and patient can then negotiate what path makes the most sense for this patient.

Q4 The answer is: (E) Prescribing medications over the telephone.
Although accurate documentation of data exchanged in an encounter is important for care, as is timely prescription of necessary medications, these features are not paramount in the creation and enhancement of the doctor–patient relationship. Nonetheless, timely and helpful medical and psychiatric care goes a long way in the establishment of trust that is greatly enhanced by more personal qualities.

Mindfulness helps physicians find a calm place from which to build patient relationships. Mindfulness counsels us to attend to our feelings with acceptance and compassion and to those of our patients, without a compulsion to act on these feelings. Thus the physician can be informed by the wealth of his or her inner emotional life, without being driven to act on these emotions; this can serve as a model for the relationship with the patient.

Other personal qualities in the physician that promote healthy and vibrant relationships with patients include humility, genuineness, optimism, a belief in the value of living a full life, good humor, candor, and transparency in communication.

Important communication skills include eliciting the patient's perspective; helping the patient feel understood; explaining conditions and options in clear, nontechnical language; generating input and consensus about paths of care; acknowledging difficulty in the relationship without aggravating it; welcoming input and even conflict; and working through difficulty, to mutually acceptable, win-win solutions.

Q5 The answer is: (C) Efficient office staff.

Having efficient office staff can be helpful to the satisfaction of both patients and physicians, but in and of itself efficiency of office staff does little to improve clinical interviewing.

The overarching principles of effective clinical interviewing are friendliness, warmth, a capacity to help patients feel at ease in telling their stories, and an ability to engage the person in a mutual exploration of what is troubling him or her. Demystification of the clinical encounter, by explaining what we are doing before we do it, and by making our thinking as transparent and collaborative as possible, promotes good interviews. Similarly, pausing often to ask the patient if we understand clearly, or seeking the patient's input and questions, promotes real conversation (rather than one-sided interrogation), and can yield deeper information.

Q6 The answer is: (A) Engaging the patient to feel heard and accurately understood.

The doctor–patient relationship is a key driver of clinical outcomes—both in promoting desired results and in avoiding calamities. Therefore an effective doctor–patient relationship involves both parties cocreating a working relationship that is reliable, effective, and durable. Moreover, the doctor–patient relationship accomplishes good outcomes by promoting empowered, engaged, and active partnership with patients who feel heard and accurately understood by their physicians. Successful doctor–patient relationships require physicians to practice a welcoming stance, participatory decision–making, and mindfulness about both the patient's and the physician's inner life. Especially in psychiatry, the physician must understand and relate to the patient as a person, requiring both accurate diagnosis and formulation, blending biological, social, psychological, and spiritual perspectives.

Conflict and difficulty may arise from the very nature of the physician's training, language, or office environment. Physicians who use overly technical, arcane, or obtuse language distance themselves and make communication difficult. Similarly, physicians may lose sight of how intimidating, arcane, and forbidding medical practice—perhaps especially psychiatry—can appear to the uninitiated, unless proactive steps toward demystification occur. Similarly, overreliance on "objective" measures (such as symptom checklists, questionnaires, tests, and other measurements) may speed diagnosis, but may alienate patients from effective collaboration. More insidious may be assumptions regarding the supposed incapacity of psychiatric patients to be full partners in their own care. Hurtful, dismissive language, or a lack of appreciation for the likelihood that a patient has previously experienced hurtful care, may damage the relationship. Overly brief, symptom-focused interviews that fail to address the whole person, as well as his or her preferences, questions, and concerns, are inadequate foundations for an effective relationship.

Physicians may misunderstand the patient's readiness to change and assume that once a diagnosis or problem is identified, the patient is prepared to work to change it. A patient may be unable or unwilling to acknowledge the problem that is obvious to the physician, or even if able to acknowledge it, may not be prepared to take serious action to change it. Similarly, physicians may underestimate social, psychological, or spiritual aspects of a person's suffering that complicate the person's willingness or ability to partner with the physician toward change.

Chapter 2
The Psychiatric Interview
Multiple-Choice Questions

Select the appropriate answer.

Q1   True or False. A collaborative review of the formulation and differential diagnosis can provide a platform for developing (with the patient) options and recommendations for treatment, considering the patient's amenability for therapeutic intervention.

    A. *True*

    B. *False*

Q2   True or False. Secure attachments in childhood foster emotional resilience and generate skills and habits of seeking out selected attachment figures for comfort, protection, advice, and strength.

    A. *True*

    B. *False*

Q3   Which of the following physician relationship techniques is LEAST likely to be associated with good outcomes and patient satisfaction?

    A. *Empathy*

    B. *Reaction formation*

    C. *Reflection*

    D. *Support*

    E. *Understanding*

Q4   Which of the following statements is LEAST likely to be accurate?

    A. *For higher-functioning patients, the public nature of the environment and the frantic pace of the emergency department (ED) may make it difficult for the patient to present very personal, private material in a calm fashion*

    B. *In public places (such as community health centers or schools), patients may feel worried about being recognized by neighbors or friends*

    C. *Patients are exquisitely sensitive to the environment in which they are evaluated*

    D. *There is no need to avoid the office settings in which there is an aggressive patient blocking the door, and where there is no emergency button or access to a telephone that can be used to call for help*

    E. *Whatever the setting, it is always advisable to ask the patient directly how comfortable he or she feels in the examining room, and to try to ensure privacy and a quiet environment with minimal distractions*

Q5   Which of the following statements is LEAST likely to be accurate?

    A. *A specific syndrome or symptom may have idiosyncratic significance to a patient, perhaps because a relative with a mood disorder was hospitalized for life, before the deinstitutionalization of mental disorders*

    B. *Culture rarely influences health and mental health–seeking behavior, the understanding of psychiatric symptoms, the course of psychiatric disorders, the efficacy of various treatments, or the kinds of treatments accepted*

C. *Patients generally have a poor understanding of psychiatric disorders, either from lack of information, myth, or misinformation from the media (e.g., television, radio, and the Internet)*

D. *Psychiatric disorders are commonly stigmatized, and subsequently are often accompanied by profound shame, anxiety, denial, fear, and uncertainty*

E. *Some patients (based on cognitive limitations) may not understand their symptoms*

Q6 Which of the following statements about the psychiatric interview is LEAST likely to be accurate?

A. *Psychiatric interviews should begin with a personal introduction and to establish the purpose of the interview; this helps create an alliance around the initial examination*

B. *The interviewer should indicate that the psychiatric interview is collaborative, and that any misunderstandings on the part of patient or physician should be immediately clarified*

C. *The patient should be instructed to ask questions, interrupt, and provide corrections or additions at any time*

D. *The time frame for the interview should be announced*

E. *Statements about confidentiality are unnecessary during the initial psychiatric interview*

Q7 Which of the following statements about the psychiatric interview is LEAST likely to be accurate?

A. *After the opening phases of the interview, open-ended questions may shift to more focused questions*

B. *In discussing the presenting problems, it is best to avoid a set of checklist-type questions, but one should cover the bases to create a Diagnostic and Statistical Manual of Mental Disorders, Fifth Edition–based differential diagnosis*

C. *The interviewer should begin with the presenting problem using open-ended questions*

D. *The past medical history need not be thorough as medical conditions (and their treatments) rarely cause or exacerbate psychiatric symptoms*

E. *When taking the history, it is vital to remember that the patient's primary concerns may not be the same as the physician's*

Q8 Which of the following terms is MOST closely associated with repeating the same response to stimuli (such as the same verbal response to different questions) with an inability to change the responses?

A. *Circumstantiality*

B. *Echolalia*

C. *Perseveration*

D. *Tangentiality*

E. *Thought-blocking*

Q9 Which of the following is NOT a common error in psychiatric interviewing?

A. *Defensiveness around psychiatric diagnoses and treatment, with arrogant responses to myths and complaints about psychiatry*

B. *False reassurance about the patient's condition or prognosis*

C. *Premature closure and false assumptions about symptoms*

D. *Recommendations for treatment when the diagnostic formulation is incomplete*

E. *Starting the interview with open-ended questions and development of a sense of security and attachment*

Chapter 2
Answers

Q1 The answer is: (A) True.
A collaborative review of the formulation and differential diagnosis can provide a platform for developing (with the patient) options and recommendations for treatment, considering the patient's amenability for therapeutic intervention. Few medical encounters are more intimate and potentially frightening and shameful than the psychiatric examination. As such, it is critical that the examiner create a safe space for the kind of deeply personal self-revelation required.

Q2 The answer is: (A) True.
Secure attachments in childhood foster emotional resilience and generate skills and habits of seeking out selected attachment figures for comfort, protection, advice, and strength. Relationships based on secure attachments lead to effective use of cognitive functions, emotional flexibility, enhancement of security, assignment of meaning to experiences, and effective self-regulation.

Q3 The answer is: (B) Reaction formation.
Primitive defenses (such as reaction formation) rarely enhance relationships between physician and patient.

However, the medical literature clearly indicates that good outcomes and patient satisfaction involve physician relationship techniques that involve reflection, empathy, understanding, legitimization, and support. Patients reveal more about themselves when they trust their doctors, and trust has been found to relate primarily to behavior during clinical interviews rather than to any preconceived notion of competence of the doctor or behavior outside the office.

Q4 The answer is: (D) There is no need to avoid the office settings in which there is an aggressive patient blocking the door, and where there is no emergency button or access to a telephone that can be used to call for help.
Hostile patients should be interviewed in a setting in which the doctor is protected. An office in which an aggressive patient is blocking the door, and where there is no emergency button or access to a telephone to call for help, should be avoided and alternative settings arranged. In some instances, local security may need to be called to ensure that safety is mandated.

Patients are exquisitely sensitive to the environment in which they are evaluated. There is a vast difference between being seen in an emergency department (ED), on a medical floor, on an inpatient or partial hospital unit, in a psychiatric outpatient clinic, in a private doctor's office, in a school, or in a court clinic. Each setting has its benefits and downsides. For example, in the ED or on a medical or surgical floor, space for private, undisturbed interviews is usually inadequate. Such settings are filled with action, drama, and hospital personnel who race around. ED visits may require long waits and contribute to impersonal approaches to patients and negative attitudes to psychiatric patients. For a patient with borderline traits who is in crisis, this can only create extreme frustration, and possibly exacerbation of chronic fears of deprivation, betrayal, abandonment, aloneness, and precipitation of regression. For these and higher-functioning patients, the public nature of the environment and the frantic pace of the emergency service may make it difficult for the patient to present very personal, private material in a calm fashion. In other public places (such as community health centers or schools), patients may feel worried about being recognized by neighbors or friends. Whatever the setting, it is always advisable to ask the patient directly how comfortable he or she feels in the examining room, and to try to ensure privacy and a quiet environment with minimal distractions.

Q5 The answer is: (B) Culture rarely influences health and mental health–seeking behavior, the understanding of psychiatric symptoms, the course of psychiatric disorders, the efficacy of various treatments, or the kinds of treatments accepted.

There are significant cultural differences in the way mental health and mental illness are viewed. Culture may influence health and mental health–seeking behavior, the understanding of psychiatric symptoms, the course of psychiatric disorders, the efficacy of various treatments, or the kinds of treatments accepted. Psychosis, for example, may be viewed as possession by spirits. Some cultural groups have much higher completion rates for suicide, and thus previous attempts in some individuals should be taken more seriously.

A specific syndrome or symptom may have idiosyncratic significance to a patient, perhaps because a relative with a mood disorder was hospitalized for life, before the deinstitutionalization of mental disorders.

Patients generally have a poor understanding of psychiatric disorders, either from lack of information, myth, or misinformation from the media (e.g., television, radio, and the Internet). Many patients have preconceived notions of what to expect (bad or good), based on the experience of friends or family.

Psychiatric disorders are commonly stigmatized, and subsequently are often accompanied by profound shame, anxiety, denial, fear, and uncertainty.

Some patients (based on cognitive limitations) may not understand their symptoms. These may be normal, such as the developmental stage in a school-age child, whereas others may be a function of congenital cognitive impairment, Asperger syndrome, or cerebral lacunae secondary to multiple infarcts following embolic strokes.

Q6 The answer is: (E) Statements about confidentiality are unnecessary during the initial psychiatric interview.

Confidentiality should be assured at the outset of the interview.

Psychiatric interviews should begin with a personal introduction and establish the purpose of the interview; this helps create an alliance around the initial examination. The interviewer should attempt to greet the person warmly, and use words that demonstrate care, attention, and concern.

The interviewer should indicate that this interaction is collaborative, and that any misunderstandings on the part of patient or physician should be immediately clarified. In addition, the patient should be instructed to ask questions, interrupt, and provide corrections or additions at any time. The time frame for the interview should be announced. In general, the interviewer should acknowledge that some of the issues and questions raised will be highly personal, and that if there are issues that the patient has real trouble with, he or she should let the examiner know.

These initial guidelines set the tone, quality, and style of the clinical interview.

Q7 The answer is: (D) The past medical history need not be thorough, as medical conditions (and their treatments) rarely cause or exacerbate psychiatric symptoms.

The past medical history needs to be thorough, and must include past and current medical and surgical conditions, past and current use of medications (including vitamins, herbs, and nontraditional remedies), use of substances (e.g., tobacco, alcohol, and other drugs [past and present]), an immunization and travel history, pregnancy history, menstrual history, a history of hospitalizations and day surgeries, accidents (including sequelae, if any), and a sexual history (including use of contraception, abortions, history of sexually transmitted diseases, and testing for the latter).

After the opening phases of the interview, open-ended questions may shift to more focused questions.

In discussing the presenting problems, it is best to avoid a set of checklist-type questions, but one should cover the bases to create a Diagnostic and Statistical Manual of Mental Disorders, Fifth Edition–based differential diagnosis.

The interviewer should begin with the presenting problem using open-ended questions. The patient should be encouraged to tell his or her story without interruptions. Many times the patient will turn to the doctor for elaboration, but it is best to let the patient know that he or she is the true expert and that only he or she has experienced this situation directly. It is best to use clarifying questions throughout the interview.

When taking the history, it is vital to remember that the patient's primary concerns may not be the same as the physician's.

Q8 The answer is: (C) Perseveration.

Perseveration involves repeating the same response to stimuli (such as the same verbal response to different questions) with an inability to change the responses.

Circumstantiality is a disorder of association with the inclusion of unnecessary details until one arrives at the goal of the thought. Echolalia is the persistent repetition of words or phrases of another person. Tangentiality describes the use of oblique, irrelevant, and digressive thoughts that do not convey the central idea to be communicated. Thought-blocking is an abrupt interruption in the flow of thought, in which one cannot recover what was just said. Other examples of formal thought disorder include loose associations (in which one jumps from one unconnected topic to another), clang associations (involving an association of speech without a logical connection, dictated by the sound of the words rather than by their meaning [frequently involving using rhyming or punning]), and neologisms (words made up; often a condensation of different words, which are unintelligible to the listener).

Q9 The answer is: (E) Starting the interview with open-ended questions and development of a sense of security and attachment.

A fundamental part of establishing this relationship is fostering a secure attachment between doctor and patient, to facilitate mutual and open communication, to correct misunderstandings, and to help the patient create a cohesive narrative of his or her past and present situation.

However, common errors of interviewing include: defensiveness around psychiatric diagnoses and treatment, with arrogant responses to myths and complaints about psychiatry; false reassurance about the patient's condition or prognosis; premature closure and false assumptions about symptoms; omission of significant parts of the interview owing to a theoretical bias of the interview (e.g., mind–body splitting); recommendations for treatment when the diagnostic formulation is incomplete; inadequate explanation of psychiatric disorders and their treatment, particularly not giving the patient multiple options for treatment; minimization or denial of the severity of symptoms, owing to overidentification with the patient, countertransference phenomenon (e.g., as occurs with treatment of a "very important person" in a manner inconsistent with ordinary best practice, with a resultant failure to protect the patient or others); and inadvertently shaming or embarrassing a patient, and not offering an apology.

Chapter 3
Laboratory Tests and Diagnostic Procedures
Multiple-Choice Questions

Select the appropriate answer.

Q1 In which of the following conditions will the concentration of urinary aminolevulinic acid (ALA) be increased?

    A. *Acute intermittent porphyria*

    B. *Cobalamin deficiency*

    C. *Alcohol withdrawal*

    D. *Systemic lupus erythematosus*

    E. *Wernicke-Korsakoff syndrome*

Q2 Which of the following conditions is MOST likely to cause a chronic macrocytic anemia with neurologic and psychiatric manifestations that include peripheral neuropathy, apathy, irritability, and depression?

    A. *Acute intermittent porphyria*

    B. *Alcohol withdrawal*

    C. *Cobalamin deficiency*

    D. *Systemic lupus erythematosus*

    E. *Wernicke-Korsakoff syndrome*

Q3 Which of the following conditions is BEST characterized by hirsutism, moon facies, truncal obesity, acne, and peripheral wasting?

    A. *Acute intermittent porphyria*

    B. *Cobalamin deficiency*

    C. *Hypercortisolism*

    D. *Systemic lupus erythematosus*

    E. *Thiamine deficiency*

Q4 True or False. Severe depression has been associated with nonsuppression of cortisol release.

    A. *True*

    B. *False*

Q5 In which of the following conditions is copper deposited in the cornea?

    A. *Anabolic steroid abuse*

    B. *Hemochromatosis*

    C. *Multiple sclerosis*

D. *Systemic lupus erythematosus*

E. *Wilson disease*

Q6 In which of the following conditions is Russell's sign commonly manifest?

A. *Acute intermittent porphyria*

B. *Bulimia nervosa*

C. *Cobalamin deficiency*

D. *Hypercortisolism*

E. *Thiamine deficiency*

Q7 True or False. Vitamin B$_{12}$ deficiency commonly presents with a microcytic anemia, cognitive impairment, psychosis, and fatigue.

A. *True*

B. *False*

Q8 Use of which of the following agents would be MOST apt to induce dry mouth, blurred vision, constipation, urinary hesitancy, tachycardia, and confusion?

A. *Alprazolam*

B. *Amitriptyline*

C. *Atenolol*

D. *Haloperidol*

E. *Trazodone*

Chapter 3
Answers

Q1 The answer is: (A) Acute intermittent porphyria.
Acute intermittent porphyria is an uncommon, yet important, cause of neuropsychiatric symptoms (including anxiety, mood lability, insomnia, depression, and psychosis). This diagnosis should be considered in a patient with psychiatric symptoms in conjunction with abdominal pain or neuropathy. When suggestive neurovisceral symptoms are present, the concentrations of urinary aminolevulinic acid (ALA), porphobilinogen (PBG), and porphyrin should be measured from a 24-hour urine collection. Although normal excretion of ALA is less than 7 mg per 24 hours, during an attack of acute intermittent porphyria, urinary ALA excretion is markedly elevated (sometimes to more than 10 times the upper limit of normal) as are PBG levels. In severe cases, the urine looks like port wine when exposed to sunlight, owing to a high concentration of PBG.

Q2 The answer is: (C) Cobalamin deficiency.
Cobalamin (vitamin B_{12}) deficiency is characterized by the development of a chronic macrocytic anemia with neurologic and psychiatric manifestations that include peripheral neuropathy, apathy, irritability, and depression. Encephalopathy, with associated dementia or psychosis, may also be seen.

Q3 The answer is: (C) Hypercortisolism.
Hypercortisolism may result from a variety of sources (including chronic hypersecretion of adrenocorticotropic hormone, pituitary adenoma [Cushing disease], nonpituitary neoplasm [Cushing syndrome], or from direct oversecretion of cortisol from an adrenal tumor or hyperplasia). Physical manifestations include the classic Cushingoid stigmata of hirsutism, moon facies, truncal obesity, acne, and peripheral wasting. Psychiatric symptoms often mimic both anxiety and depression; less common presentations include psychotic symptoms. Diagnostic evaluation involves measurement of adrenocorticotropic hormone (levels vary depending on the cause of the illness) and a dexamethasone suppression test (DST) to demonstrate the impaired feedback regulation of the pituitary-adrenal axis in Cushing syndrome from any etiology.

Q4 The answer is: (A) True.
Severe depression (especially melancholic depression) has been associated with nonsuppression; however, sensitivity of the DST in the detection of major depression is at best moderate, making it of little benefit as a diagnostic test for primary depression. The DST is undertaken to measure suppression of cortisol during the normal cortisol circadian rhythm, whereby dexamethasone (1 mg) is given at bedtime and cortisol levels are drawn at various times throughout the next day (generally at 08:00, 16:00, and 23:00). The normal effect is suppression of cortisol release. Nonsuppression is defined as a cortisol level greater than 5 mcg/dL, and it represents an impaired pituitary-adrenal axis feedback loop.

Q5 The answer is: (E) Wilson disease.
Wilson disease, a neurodegenerative disorder, involves the abnormal accumulation of copper, which leads to cirrhosis and to neuronal degeneration. It is an autosomal recessive disorder with the disease gene located on chromosome 13. Wilson disease should be considered in patients with manifestations that include speech impairment, extrapyramidal dysfunction, new-onset psychiatric disturbance (especially in patients younger than 30 years), and liver disease. Diagnostic workup includes analysis of a 24-hour urine for copper and plasma ceruloplasmin, as well as a slit-lamp examination for Kayser-Fleischer rings (from copper deposition in the cornea) and liver biopsy (with measurement of liver copper). Genetic testing helps confirm the diagnosis.

Q6 The answer is: (B) Bulimia nervosa.
Tooth decay or knuckle lesions (Russell's sign) typically indicate a history of self-induced vomiting, as is seen with eating disorders.

Q7 The answer is: (B) False.
Vitamin B_{12} deficiency commonly presents with a macrocytic anemia, cognitive impairment, psychosis, and fatigue; agitation and delirium may also be noted.

Q8 The answer is: (B) Amitriptyline.
Of the agents listed, amitriptyline is the most anticholinergic; this side effect accounts for dry mouth, blurred vision, constipation, urinary hesitancy, tachycardia, and confusion.

Treatment Adherence

Multiple-Choice Questions

Select the appropriate answer.

Q1   Which of the following statements about treatment adherence is MOST accurate?

A.   *Nonadherence with medical recommendations accounts for less than 2% of hospital readmissions*

B.   *Nonadherence with psychiatric treatments is remarkably low (i.e., less than 10%)*

C.   *Treatment adherence is remarkably stable with regard to the population being studied, their diagnosis, and the pharmacologic treatment employed*

D.   *Treatment compliance is defined as the degree to which a patient carries out the recommendations of the treating practitioner*

E.   *Treatment nonadherence is essentially the same for patients with psychotic disorders and anxiety disorders*

Q2   Which of the following statements related to treatment adherence is MOST accurate?

A.   *Adherence with psychiatric treatments has little impact on improvement of adherence with treatment regimens for nonpsychiatric illness*

B.   *Clinical outcomes are directly related to treatment adherence, which in turn is related to resource utilization and to the economic burden of mental illness*

C.   *Nonadherence has little impact on the risk of psychiatric hospitalization, the use of emergency services, arrests, violence, victimizations, lower mental function, lower life satisfaction, and the use of substances*

D.   *Nonadherence with treatment recommendations has little effect on the doctor–patient relationship*

E.   *Rates of suicidal ideation are unaffected by nonadherence in patients who have recently been hospitalized*

Q3   Which of the following is LEAST commonly accepted as a factor that affects treatment adherence?

A.   *Comorbid illnesses*

B.   *Cultural and religious factors*

C.   *The patient–clinician relationship*

D.   *The phase of the moon*

E.   *Socioeconomic status*

Q4   Which of the following statements regarding treatment adherence is MOST accurate?

A.   *Among patients with bipolar disorder, adherence at the time of remission fails to predict adherence at 1 year*

B.   *Having obsessive-compulsive disorder dramatically increases adherence with pharmacologic recommendations*

C.   *In patients with bipolar I disorder, less than one-third of patients are either fully or partially nonadherent with medications 4 months after an episode of mania*

D.   *Symptoms of both mania and depression directly affect treatment adherence*

E.   *With hypomania and mania comes a renewed vigor to take medications and control symptoms*

Q5 Which of the following questions would be LEAST likely to help a clinician determine if a patient is adhering with treatment recommendations?

A. *"Have you ever noticed that you occasionally forget to take your pills?"*

B. *"How often do you think about selling your medication to other people?"*

C. *"How is it going with your medication?"*

D. *"Is it time to get another refill of your medication?"*

E. *"What medications are you taking?"*

Chapter 4

Answers

Q1 The answer is: (D) Treatment compliance is defined as the degree to which a patient carries out the recommendations of the treating practitioner.

Treatment compliance is defined as the degree to which a patient carries out the recommendations of the treating practitioner; the term connotes a disappearing paternalistic model (in which the doctor determines what treatment the patient should have, and the patient faithfully and unquestioningly accepts it) and it implies that a noncompliant patient is unruly or bad. The term *adherence* has increasingly gained favor over *compliance* and represents a shift toward collaboration between the health care professional and the patient.

Studies suggest that rates of nonadherence with psychiatric treatment are alarmingly high (e.g., 24% to 90%). In a large meta-analysis, the mean rate of nonadherence was 26%.

Rates of treatment adherence vary depending on the population, the diagnosis, and the pharmacologic intervention. Particularly high rates of treatment nonadherence occur among those with psychotic disorders. This was made clear in the Clinical Antipsychotic Trials of Intervention Effectiveness investigation that reported high rates of treatment discontinuation (74%) among the intent-to-treat group within 4 months. Reasons for nonadherence are multiple, complex, and varied.

Data on nonadherence include the following: only 45% of patients referred for psychotherapy from a general hospital psychiatry outpatient department showed up for one or more appointments; nonattendance rates for patients with scheduled medical appointments are high (19% to 28%); nonadherence with medical recommendations accounts for 5% to 40% of hospital readmissions; medication doses are delayed or omitted by 30% to 50% of patients; patients with chronic diseases take their medications as prescribed only half of the time; 20% of patients stop filling their prescriptions within 1 month of their issue; and approximately one-fourth of patients do not inform their physician about having stopped their antidepressant medications.

Q2 The answer is: (B) Clinical outcomes are directly related to treatment adherence, which in turn is related to resource utilization and to the economic burden of mental illness.

Clinical outcomes are directly related to treatment adherence, which in turn is related to resource utilization and to the economic burden of mental illness. Adherence with psychiatric treatments is associated with better outcomes, a lower relapse rate, improved adherence with treatment regimens for nonpsychiatric illness, and lower rates of hospitalization. Nonadherence has been associated with a greater risk of psychiatric hospitalization, use of emergency services, arrests, violence, victimizations, lower mental function, lower life satisfaction, and more prevalent use of substances. Rates of suicidal ideation are significantly greater among patients who are treatment nonadherent following hospitalization.

Given the clinical impact of treatment nonadherence, the economic burden incurred through nonadherence is significant. Data derived from the Global Burden of Disease study conducted by the World Health Organization, the World Bank, and Harvard University revealed that mental illness, including suicide, accounts for over 15% of the burden of disease in countries such as the United States. Additionally, considering that major depression is the leading cause of disability worldwide among persons aged 5 years or older, adherence to treatment can reduce the economic burden of mental illness.

Although little studied, the negative impact (including feeling frustrated, underappreciated, helpless, ineffectual, and "burned out") of treatment nonadherence on clinicians should also be considered. Treating clinicians are affected when their patients are nonadherent with treatment. Future studies will undoubtedly measure the dispiriting impact when clinicians feel underappreciated and disaffected.

Q3 The answer is: (D) The phase of the moon.

However, the patient's maturity, resilience, and experiences affect adherence. For example, an adolescent may find his or her illness a source of embarrassment, or a middle-aged person may have concerns about how disclosure of an illness might affect their work and health insurance premiums. Negative experiences with the health care system can create mental barriers to seeking necessary treatment.

Substance abuse, medical illnesses, and dementia also adversely affect adherence.

A lack of trust in a clinician or the medical system negatively affects adherence.

Many patients are impoverished and lack health insurance; therefore they are unable to access timely and adequate care. Even small copayments can result in medication nonadherence.

Cultural beliefs affect all aspects of illness, from the patient's interpretation of symptoms to his or her beliefs about treatment. For example, some religions recommend prayer as the sole means of healing.

The structure or content of treatment itself may contribute to poor adherence. For example, a patient with paranoid schizophrenia is unlikely to continue in an unstructured psychodynamic therapy group, or a patient who does not have a car and who lives 45 miles away from a health center is unlikely to attend weekly appointments. Medication may directly cause nonadherence if it lacks efficacy or causes intolerable side effects.

Q4 The answer is: (D) Symptoms of both mania and depression directly affect treatment adherence.
Symptoms of both mania and depression directly affect treatment adherence. In depression, persistent dysphoria and hopelessness may make a patient feel that his or her condition is irreparable, and that treatment is futile. Psychomotor retardation, decreased energy, poor concentration, and diminished self-care lead to missed medications and appointments. With hypomania and mania come an elevated mood and an invigorated energy level that most patients experience as positive; this makes many unmotivated to take medications that slow them down. When insight and judgment are impaired, some patients do not believe that they have an illness that requires treatment.

Studies of treatment adherence in those with depression demonstrate that adherence is highest when the perceived need for medication is greatest and the harmfulness of medication is low. In addition, a patient's skepticism about the efficacy of antidepressant medications predicts early discontinuation of them. Reasons for nonadherence include discomfort about psychiatric diagnoses, denial of the illness, problematic side effects, fears around dependency, and the belief that medications were unhelpful following resolution of the acute phase of illness.

In a study of African American and white patients with bipolar I disorder, more than half of all patients were either fully or partially nonadherent with medications 4 months after an episode of acute mania. More than 20% denied having bipolar disorder, and they cited side effects of medications as contributing to their nonadherence. African Americans (more often than whites) cited the fear of addiction and medication use as a symbol of illness as reasons for nonadherence, which suggests that different cultures or ethnic groups may differ in their reasons for nonadherence.

Among patients with bipolar disorder, insight into treatment has been positively correlated with medication adherence, and adherence at the time of remission predicted adherence at 1 year.

Anxiety disorders are associated with hypervigilance regarding both the psychological and physical environment; this affects adherence in a number of ways. Illness may be so severe that a patient may feel unable to leave his or her home to keep appointments, or it may be difficult to titrate and to taper medications, as a patient with an anxiety disorder may attribute any physical symptom to a medication side effect. With obsessive-compulsive disorder, counting rituals and fears of contamination may make it impossible for a patient to take medications, or to comply with pharmacologic or other therapeutic recommendations.

Q5 The answer is: (B) "How often do you think about selling your medication to other people?"
Once adherence has been assessed in the initial consultation with the patient, adherence should be assessed routinely at subsequent visits. These follow-up assessments will be guided by the initial evaluation, with more or less attention paid depending on the patient's profile. For example, if a patient has few risk factors and has a demonstrated history of being conscientious and adherent with treatment, less time will be spent on the issue.

In general, questions should be asked in an empathic, nonthreatening way with a tone of genuine curiosity. For example, starting with open-ended questions (such as "How is it going with the medication?") is more likely to be received positively than starting with closed-ended ones (e.g., "Do you take your medications as prescribed?"). After beginning with an open-ended question, asking specifically about which medications the patient is taking and how the patient is taking them allows the clinician to assess the patient's understanding of the treatment recommendations. Asking questions such as "Let me confirm that my records are accurate. What medications are you taking?" to specifically address adherence, and disarming inquiries (such as, "Sometimes it is difficult to remember to take medication. Have you ever noticed that you occasionally forget to take your pills?") are less likely to be experienced as shaming or punitive. The goal is to foster a treatment relationship in which the patient feels comfortable truthfully reporting his or her behaviors.

SECTION 2
HUMAN DEVELOPMENT

Chapter 5: Child, Adolescent, and Adult Development

Child, Adolescent, and Adult Development

Multiple-Choice Questions

Select the appropriate answer.

Q1 True or False. According to Sigmund Freud's developmental theory, the oral phase precedes the anal phase.

A. *True*

B. *False*

Q2 In which of the following stages of development, according to Freud, does the child have primarily unconscious feelings of love and desire for the parent of the opposite sex, with fantasies of having sole possession of this parent and aggressive fantasies toward the same-sex parent?

A. *Anal phase*

B. *Genital phase*

C. *Latency phase*

D. *Oral phase*

E. *Phallic phase*

Q3 Which of the following individuals is MOST closely linked with a theory that involved eight developmental stages that covers an individual's entire life, and emphasizes the relationship between a person's maturing ego and both family and the larger culture in which he or she lives?

A. *John Bowlby*

B. *Erik Erikson*

C. *Sigmund Freud*

D. *Laurence Kohlberg*

E. *Jean Piaget*

Q4 Which of the following theorists maintained that there are four major stages of cognitive development (i.e., the sensorimotor intelligence period, the preoperational thought period, the concrete operations period, and the formal operations period)?

A. *John Bowlby*

B. *Erik Erikson*

C. *Sigmund Freud*

D. *Lawrence Kohlberg*

E. *Jean Piaget*

Q5   Which of the following theorists was a psychoanalyst who is MOST closely linked with the notion of attachment (i.e., the emotional bond between caregiver and infant)?

A. *John Bowlby*

B. *Erik Erikson*

C. *Sigmund Freud*

D. *Lawrence Kohlberg*

E. *Jean Piaget*

Q6   True or False. Stranger anxiety (in which the infant begins to show signs of distress at the approach of a stranger) develops earlier than does the social smile of the infant.

A. *True*

B. *False*

Q7   In which of the following ages does the child TYPICALLY demonstrate egocentricity and magical thinking?

A. *1 to 6 months*

B. *6 months to 2-1/2 years*

C. *2-1/2 to 5 years*

D. *5 to 12 years*

E. *12 to 20 years*

Q8   True or False. Preschool children tend to enjoy pretend or fantasy play more than structured games.

A. *True*

B. *False*

Chapter 5

Answers

Q1 The answer is: (A) True.

Freud's developmental theory portrayed child development as a process that unfolds across discreet, universal stages. He posited that infants are born as *polymorphously perverse,* meaning that the child has the capacity to experience libidinal pleasure from various areas of the body. Freud's stages of development were based on the area of the body (oral, anal, or phallic) that is the focus of the child's libidinal drive during that phase. According to Freud, healthy adult function requires successful resolution of the core tasks of each developmental stage. Failure to resolve the tasks of a stage leads to a specific pattern of neurosis in adult life.

The first stage of development in Freud's scheme is the *oral phase,* which begins at birth and continues through approximately 12 to 18 months of age. During this period, the infant's drives are focused on the mouth, primarily through the pleasurable sensations associated with feeding. During this phase, the infant is wholly dependent on the mother; the infant must learn to trust the mother to meet his or her basic needs. Successful resolution of the oral phase provides a basis for healthy relationships later in life and allows the individual to trust others without excessive dependency. According to Freudian theory, an infant who is orally deprived may become pessimistic, demanding, or overly dependent as an adult.

Around 18 months of age, the oral phase gives way to the *anal phase.* During this phase, the focus of the child's libidinal energy shifts to his or her increasing control of bowel function through voluntary control of the anal sphincter. Failure to successfully negotiate the tasks of the anal phase can lead to the anal-retentive character type; affected individuals are overly meticulous, miserly, stubborn, and passive-aggressive, or the anal-expulsive character type, described as reckless and messy.

Q2 The answer is: (E) Phallic phase.

Late in the phallic phase, Freud believed that the child developed primarily unconscious feelings of love and desire for the parent of the opposite sex, with fantasies of having sole possession of this parent and aggressive fantasies toward the same-sex parent. These feelings are referred to as the *Oedipal complex* after Oedipus, who unknowingly killed his father and married his mother. In boys, Freud posited that guilt about Oedipal fantasies gives rise to *castration anxiety,* which refers to the fear that the father will retaliate against the child's hostile impulses by cutting off his penis. The Oedipal complex is resolved when the child manages these conflicting fears and desires through identification with the same-sex parent. As part of this process, the child may seek out same-sex peers. Successful negotiation of the Oedipal complex provides the foundation for secure sexual identity later in life.

At the end of the phallic phase, around age 5 to 6 years, Freud believed that the child's libidinal drives entered a period of relative inactivity that continues until the onset of puberty. This period is referred to as *latency.* This period of calm between powerful drives allows the child to further develop a sense of mastery and ego-strength, while integrating the sex-role defined in the Oedipal period into this growing sense of self. With the onset of puberty, around age 11 to 13 years, the child enters the final developmental stage in Freud's model, called the *genital phase,* which continues into young adulthood. During this phase, powerful libidinal drives resurface, causing a reemergence and reworking of the conflicts experienced in earlier phases. Through this process, the adolescent develops a coherent sense of identity and is able to separate from the parents.

Q3 The answer is: (B) Erik Erikson.

Erikson, like Freud, believed that problems present in adults are largely the result of unresolved conflicts of childhood. However, Erikson's stages emphasize not the person's relationship to his or her own sexual urges and instinctual drives, but rather the relationship between a person's maturing ego and both the family and the larger social culture in which he or she lives.

Erikson proposed eight developmental stages that cover an individual's entire life; each stage is characterized by a particular challenge, or what he termed a "psychosocial crisis." The resolution of the crisis depends on the interaction between an individual's characteristics and the surrounding environment. When the developmental task at each stage has been completed, the result is a specific ego quality that a person will carry throughout the other stages. Erikson's stages describe a vital conflict or tension in which the "negative" pole is necessary for growth.

Erikson did not believe that a person could be "stuck" at any one stage; in his theory, if we live long enough, we must pass through all of the stages. The forces that push a person from stage to stage are biological maturation and social expectations. Erikson believed that success at earlier stages affected the chances of success at later ones.

Q4 The answer is: (E) Jean Piaget.

Piaget maintained that there are four major stages: the sensorimotor intelligence period, the preoperational thought period, the concrete operations period, and the formal operations period. Each period has specific features that enable a child to comprehend certain kinds of knowledge and understanding. Piaget believed that children pass through these stages at different rates, but maintained that they do so in sequence and in the same order.

Characteristics of the sensorimotor intelligence period (from birth to about 2 years) are that an infant uses senses and motor skills to obtain information and an understanding about the world around him or her. There is no conceptual or reflective thought; an object is "known" in terms of what an infant can "do" to it. A significant cognitive milestone is achieved when the infant learns the concept of object permanence, that is, that an object still exists when is it not in the child's visual field. By the end of this period a child is aware of self and others, and he or she understands that they are but one object among many.

From ages 2 to 6 years, a child uses preoperational thought, in which the child begins to develop symbolic thinking including language. The use of symbols contributes to the growth of the child's imagination. A child might use one object to represent another in play, such as a box becoming a race car. Piaget also described this period as a time when preschoolers are characterized by egocentric thinking. Egocentrism means that the child sees the world from his or her own perspective, and has difficulty seeing another person's point of view. For a child of this age, everyone thinks and feels the same way the child does. The capacity to acknowledge another's point of view develops gradually during the preschool years; whereas a 2-year-old will participate in parallel play with a peer, a 4-year-old will engage in cooperative play with another child. Toward the end of this period, a child will begin to understand and to coordinate several points of view.

Just as a child in this stage fails to consider more than one perspective in personal interactions, he or she is unable to consider more than one dimension. In his famous experiment, Piaget demonstrated that a child in a preoperational stage is unable to consider two perceptual dimensions (such as height and width). A child is shown two glasses (glass 1 and glass 2), which are filled to the same height with water. The child agrees the glasses have the same amount of liquid. Next, the child pours the liquid from glass 1 to another shorter and wider glass (glass 3) and is asked if the amount of liquid is still the same. The child in the preoperational stage will answer "No," that there is more water in glass 1 because the water is at a higher level. By age 7 years, the child will understand that there is the same amount of liquid in each glass; this is termed "conservation of liquids," and it is a concept that children master when they are entering the next stage. Children also learn conservation of number, mass, and substance as they mature.

During middle childhood (ages 7 to 11 years), Piaget described a child's cognitive style as concrete operational. The child can understand and apply logic and can interpret experiences objectively instead of intuitively. Children are able to coordinate several perspectives and are able to use concepts, such as conservation, classification (a bead can be both green and plastic, whereas a preoperational child would see the bead as either green or plastic), and seriation (blocks can be arranged in order of largest to smallest).

These "mental actions" enable the child to think systematically and with logic; however, the child's use of logic is limited to mostly that which is tangible. The final stage of Piaget's cognitive theory is formal operations, which occurs around age 11 years and continues into adulthood. In this stage, the early adolescent and then the adult can consider hypothetical and abstract thought, can consider several possibilities or outcomes, and has the capacity to understand concepts as relative rather than absolute. In formal operations, a young adult is able to discern the underlying motivations or principles of something (such as an idea, theory, or action) and can apply them to novel situations.

Q5 The answer is: (A) John Bowlby.

John Bowlby (1907–1990) was a British psychoanalyst who was interested in the role of early development in determining psychological function later in life. Bowlby particularly focused his attention on the study of *attachment,* which can be defined as the emotional bond between caregiver and infant. Bowlby's theory was grounded in his clinical work with families disrupted by World War II and with delinquent children at London's Child Guidance Clinic. Attachment theory also had its roots in evolutionary biology and studies of animal behavior, such as Harry Harlow's studies of rhesus monkeys deprived of maternal contact after birth.

Bowlby argued that human infants are born with a powerful, evolutionarily derived drive to connect with the mother. Infants exhibit *attachment behaviors* (such as smiling, sucking, and crying) that facilitate the child's connection to the mother. The child is predisposed to psychopathology if there are difficulties in forming a secure attachment (for example, in a mother with severe mental illness), or there are disruptions in attachment (such as prolonged separation from the mother). Bowlby described three stages of behavior in children who are separated from their mother for extended periods. First, the child will *protest* by calling or crying out. Then, the child will exhibit signs of *despair,* in which he or she appears to give up hope of the mother's return. Finally, the child enters a state of *detachment,* appearing to have emotionally separated himself or herself from the mother and initially appearing indifferent to her if she returns.

Q6 The answer is: (B) False.
Stranger anxiety, in which the infant begins to show signs of distress at the approach of a stranger, may begin to emerge around 6 months and is fully present by 9 months of age. Before this, infants have an accepting and even welcoming response to unfamiliar adults. However, the 9-month-old infant generally shows a strong preference for one or both parents, and may cry, stare, or cling to the parent when others attempt to interact with the child, even those who have a close relationship with the child (such as a grandparent). Stranger anxiety is often more intense when an infant has only one primary caregiver. It usually reaches its peak around age 12 to 15 months. Separation anxiety, as opposed to stranger anxiety, is defined as a child's sense of discomfort on separation from the primary caretaker and occurs when a child is between age 10 and 18 months.

The infant's early social behaviors are reflexive in nature, such as imitating the facial expressions of others that the infant may begin to do by age 4 weeks. Initially, the infant's smile is spontaneous and unrelated to external stimuli. With time, however, the infant smiles in response to stimuli in the environment (such as the appearance of a parent's face). This response is called the social smile. The social smile usually becomes distinguishable from the endogenous smile between age 6 and 8 weeks. With time and social interaction with the parents, the infant smiles in response to a growing number of stimuli (such as a favorite toy).

Q7 The answer is: (C) 2-1/2 to 5 years.
The child's thinking in the preschool years (ages 2.5 to 5 years) is primarily intuitive rather than logical. Preschool children also demonstrate egocentricity and magical thinking. They see themselves as the center of the world and have difficulty understanding the perspectives of others. For example, they may not understand that when they are pointing to a picture in a book that they are holding (facing themselves), their parent is unable to see the picture. They also blur the distinction between fantasy and reality, as evidenced by young children's belief in Santa Claus or in monsters.

Q8 The answer is: (A) True.
Cognitive skills are reflected in this age-group in the types of games children play. Preschool children tend to enjoy pretend or fantasy play more than structured games; they have not yet developed the intellectual skills to appreciate logic or strategy. By around age 7 years, however, children will engage in simple games with more complicated rules that may involve planning, such as Stratego or Guess Who?, while still reveling in the emotional pleasure of beating an opponent or having good luck in a game.

SECTION 3

PSYCHOLOGICAL AND NEUROPSYCHOLOGICAL TESTING

Diagnostic Rating Scales and Psychiatric Instruments

Multiple-Choice Questions

Select the appropriate answer.

Q1   With regard to diagnostic rating scales, which of the following terms is MOST closely associated with the answer to the question, "For a given subject, are the results consistent across different evaluators, test conditions, and test times?"

  A. *Positive predictive value*

  B. *Reliability*

  C. *Sensitivity*

  D. *Specificity*

  E. *Validity*

Q2   Which of the following diagnostic rating scales for the detection of depression is a clinician-administered instrument with several versions ranging from 6 to 31 items?

  A. *BDI*

  B. *HAM-D*

  C. *HAND*

  D. *Y-MRS*

  E. *ZUNG SDS*

Q3   Which of the following diagnostic instruments is a 30-item instrument that emphasizes three clusters of symptoms (positive symptoms [e.g., hallucinations, delusions, and disorganization], negative symptoms [e.g., apathy, blunted affect, and social withdrawal], and general psychopathology [e.g., somatic concerns, anxiety, impulse control, psychomotor retardation, mannerisms, and posturing])?

  A. *AIMS*

  B. *BARS*

  C. *BPRS*

  D. *PANSS*

  E. *SANS*

Q4   Which of the following diagnostic instruments is a clinician-administered semistructured interview designed to measure the severity of obsessive-compulsive symptoms?

  A. *BAI*

  B. *CAPS*

  C. *BSPS*

  D. *HAM-A*

  E. *Y-BOCS*

Q5   Which of the following diagnostic instruments is a clinician-administered test that covers five cognitive domains?

    A. *DAST*

    B. *DRS*

    C. *CAGE*

    D. *MAST*

    E. *MMSE*

Answers

Q1 The answer is: (B) Reliability.

Reliability refers to the extent that an instrument produces consistent measurements across different raters and testing milieus.

Positive predictive value tells us how likely the disorder is present if the test is positive.

Negative predictive value tells us how likely the disorder is absent if the test is negative.

Sensitivity tells us how likely the test will be positive if the disorder is present.

Specificity tells us how likely the test will be negative if the disorder is absent.

Validity of a rating scale conveys whether the test correctly measures what it is intended to measure, for example, detecting the true underlying condition.

Q2 The answer is: (B) HAM-D.

The Hamilton Rating Scale for Depression (HAM-D) is a clinician-administered instrument (with answers scored by the clinician from 0 to 4) that is widely used in both clinical and research settings (the 17-item HAM-D-17 is frequently used in research studies). Its questions focus on the severity of symptoms in the preceding week. A decrease of 50% or greater in the HAM-D score suggests a positive response to treatment.

The Beck Depression Inventory (BDI) is a 21-item scale on which patients must rate their symptoms on a scale from 0 to 3; the total score is tallied. The BDI tends to focus more on cognitive symptoms of depression, and it excludes atypical symptoms (such as weight gain and hypersomnia).

The Harvard Department of Psychiatry National Depression Screening Day Scale (HAND) is a self-administered scale that includes 10 questions about depression symptoms and is scored based on the experience of symptoms from 0 or "none of the time" to 3 or "all of the time."

The Young Mania Rating Scale (Y-MRS) is a clinician-rated scale of 11 items used to detect symptoms of mania, not depression.

The Zung Self-Rating Depression Scale (ZUNG SDS) is a self-administered scale with 20 items, 10 keyed positively and 10 keyed negatively; items are scored as present from 1 or "a little of the time" to 4 or "most of the time."

Q3 The answer is: (D) PANSS.

The Positive and Negative Syndrome Scale (PANSS) is a 30-item instrument that emphasizes three clusters of symptoms (positive symptoms [e.g., hallucinations, delusions, and disorganization], negative symptoms [e.g., apathy, blunted affect, and social withdrawal], and general psychopathology [e.g., somatic concerns, anxiety, impulse control, psychomotor retardation, mannerisms, and posturing]). Each item is rated on a scale from 1 (least severe) to 7 (most severe).

The Brief Psychiatric Rating Scale (BPRS) is an 18-item scale that evaluates a range of positive and negative symptoms, as well as other categories (such as depressive mood, mannerisms, posturing, hostility, and tension). Each item is rated on a 7-point scale following a clinical interview. It has been used to assess psychotic symptoms in patients with both primary psychotic disorders and secondary psychoses, such as depression with psychotic features.

More detailed inventories of positive and negative symptoms are possible with use of the 30-item Scale for the Assessment of Positive Symptoms (SAPS) and the 20-item Scale for the Assessment of Negative Symptoms (SANS). Each of these scales is rated on a scale of 0 to 5 following a semistructured clinical interview.

The Abnormal Involuntary Movement Scale (AIMS) consists of 10 items that evaluate orofacial movements, limb-trunk dyskinesias, and global severity of motor symptoms on a 5-point scale; specific instructions are provided with the scale for asking the patient certain questions or having him or her perform motor maneuvers.

Both objective measures of akathisia and subjective distress related to restlessness are assessed by the Barnes Akathisia Rating Scale (BARS), which also comes with instructions for proper rating.

Q4 The answer is: (E) Y-BOCS.

The Yale-Brown Obsessive-Compulsive Scale (Y-BOCS) is a clinician-administered semistructured interview designed to measure the severity of obsessive-compulsive symptoms. An optional checklist of 64 specific obsessive and compulsive symptoms precedes the interview. Following the interview, the examiner rates five domains in both obsessive and compulsive subscales, with a score of 0 corresponding to no symptoms and 4 corresponding to extreme symptoms. Total scores average 25 in patients with obsessive-compulsive disorder compared with less than 8 in healthy patients.

The Beck Anxiety Inventory (BAI) is a self-rated 21-item questionnaire, in which patients rate somatic and affective symptoms of anxiety on a 4-point Likert scale (0 = "not at all," 3 = "severely: I could barely stand it"). Although brief and easy to administer, it does not identify specific anxiety diagnoses or distinguish primary anxiety from comorbid psychiatric conditions.

Posttraumatic stress disorder (PTSD) can be measured with the Clinician-Administered PTSD Scale (CAPS), which is closely matched to the *Diagnostic and Statistical Manual of Mental Disorders, 4th Edition* criteria. The CAPS contains 17 items that are assessed by the clinician during a diagnostic interview; each item is rated for frequency, from 0 (never experienced) to 4 (experienced daily), and for intensity, from 0 (none) to 4 (extreme).

The Brief Social Phobia Scale (BSPS) consists of clinician-administered ratings in 11 domains related to social phobia; severity of each symptom is rated from 0 (none) to 4 (extreme), generating three subscale scores (Fear, Avoidance, and Physiological). These scores are summed and a total score greater than 20 is considered clinically significant.

The Hamilton Anxiety Rating Scale (HAM-A) is the most commonly used instrument for the evaluation of anxiety symptoms. The clinician-administered scale contains 14 items, in which specific symptoms are rated on a scale from 0 (no symptoms) to 4 (severe, grossly disabling symptoms). Administration typically requires 15 to 30 minutes; clinically significant anxiety is associated with total scores of 14 or greater.

Q5 The answer is: (B) DRS.

The Dementia Rating Scale (DRS) is a clinician-administered test that covers five cognitive domains (attention, initiation and perseveration, construction, conceptualization, and memory). Within each domain, specific items are presented in hierarchical fashion, with the most difficult items presented first. If subjects can perform the difficult items correctly, many of the remaining items in the section are skipped and scored as correct. A cutoff score of 129 or 130 has been associated with 97% sensitivity and 99% specificity in diagnosing Alzheimer disease.

The Drug Abuse Screening Test (DAST) is a self-rated survey of 28 "yes/no" questions; it also includes questions about tolerance and withdrawal.

The CAGE questionnaire is ubiquitously used to screen for alcohol abuse and dependence. It consists of four "yes/no" questions (organized by the mnemonic acronym) about alcohol consumption patterns and their psychosocial consequences. A positive answer to 2 of the 4 questions signifies a positive screen and the necessity for a more extensive workup. Questions include: "Have you ever felt you should cut down on your drinking? Have people annoyed you by criticizing your drinking? Have you ever felt bad or guilty about your drinking? Have you ever had a drink first thing in the morning to steady your nerves or to get rid of a hangover (eye-opener)?"

The Michigan Alcoholism Screening Test (MAST) is a longer self-administered instrument with 25 "yes/no" items concerning alcohol use, tolerance, and withdrawal.

Understanding and Applying Psychological Assessment

Multiple-Choice Questions

Select the appropriate answer.

Q1 Which of the following is the standard deviation for the Full-Scale IQ, the Verbal IQ, and the Performance IQ of the Wechsler Adult Intelligence Scale (for individuals aged 16 to 89 years)?

    A. *2*

    B. *5*

    C. *10*

    D. *15*

    E. *20*

Q2 Which of the following tests consists of 11 subtests (i.e., vocabulary, similarities, arithmetic, digit span, information, comprehension, picture completion, digit symbol, block design, matrix reasoning, and picture arrangement)?

    A. *MCMI*

    B. *MMPI*

    C. *PAI*

    D. *TAT*

    E. *WAIS*

Q3 Which of the following tests uses ambiguous inkblots to assess personality?

    A. *MCMI*

    B. *MMPI*

    C. *PAI*

    D. *Rorschach*

    E. *TAT*

Q4 What is the mean IQ score for those in the general population with average intelligence?

    A. *Greater than 130*

    B. *110 to 129*

    C. *90 to 109*

    D. *70 to 99*

    E. *Less than 70*

Q5 Which of the following tests has clinical scales that include (1) Hs-Hypochondriasis; (2) D-Depression; (3) Hy-Conversion Hysteria; (4) Pd-Psychopathic Deviate; (5) Mf-Masculinity-Femininity; (6) Pa-Paranoia; (7) Pt-Psychasthenia; (8) Sc-Schizophrenia; (9) Ma-Hypomania; and (10) Si-Social Introversion?

A. *MCMI*

B. *MMPI*

C. *PAI*

D. *Rorschach*

E. *TAT*

Chapter 7
Answers

Q1 The answer is: (D) 15.
This statistical feature means that a 15-point difference between a subject's Verbal and Performance IQ can be considered both statistically and clinically meaningful.

Q2 The answer is: (E) WAIS.
The Wechsler IQ tests, including the Wechsler Adult Intelligence Scale (WAIS), consists of 11 subtests (i.e., vocabulary, similarities, arithmetic, digit span, information, comprehension [to assess verbal intelligence] and picture completion, digit symbol, block design, matrix reasoning, and picture arrangement [to assess for nonverbal or performance intelligence]). All of the Wechsler subtests are constructed to have a mean score of 10 and a standard deviation of 3. Given this statistical feature, if two subtests differ by 3 or more scaled score points, the difference is clinically meaningful.

The Millon Clinical Multiaxial Inventory (MCMI-III) is a 175-item true-false self-report questionnaire designed to identify both symptom disorders (axis 1 conditions) and personality disorders; it is not an intelligence test. It consists of 3 validity scales, 10 basic personality scales, 3 severe personality scales, 6 clinical syndrome scales, and 3 severe clinical syndrome scales.

The Minnesota Multiphasic Personality Inventory-2 (MMPI-2) is a 567-item true-false self-report test of psychological function (not intelligence), with 10 clinical scales that assess major categories of psychopathology and 6 validity scales designed to assess test-taking attitudes.

The Personality Assessment Inventory (PAI) uses 344 items and a 4-point response format to make 22 scales with nonoverlapping items. It consists of 4 validity scales, 11 clinical scales, and 2 interpersonal scales. Although it is an excellent test for broadly assessing multiple domains of psychological function, it is not an intelligence test.

The Thematic Apperception Test (TAT) is a projective test (not an intelligence test) that uses a series of redrawn pictures of people of varying sex and ages engaged in some sort of activity; the respondent is instructed to tell a story about the picture that has a beginning, a middle, and end and describes what the characters in the picture are thinking and feeling.

Q3 The answer is: (D) Rorschach.
In 1921, Hermann Rorschach published his inkblot test; he died within a year of publication of his book, *Psychodiagnostik* (on his observations of responses made to inkblots by psychotic patients), without ever realizing the impact his test would have on personality assessment. The inkblots are on 10 cards or plates; the patient is required to say what the inkblot might be, and then the responses are recorded verbatim. In the second phase of the test, the examiner reviews the patient's responses and inquires as to where on the card the response was seen and what made it look that way. Scoring the Rorschach can be challenging, but thanks to the laborious efforts of Exner and his colleagues, a reliable and comprehensive scoring system is now available.

The MCMI-III is a 175-item true-false self-report questionnaire designed to identify both symptom disorders (axis 1 conditions) and personality disorders.

The MMPI-2 is a 567-item true-false self-report test of psychological function.

The PAI uses 344 items and a 4-point response format to make 22 scales with nonoverlapping items.

The TAT is a projective test (not an intelligence test) that uses a series of redrawn pictures of people of varying sex and ages engaged in some sort of activity.

Q4 The answer is: (C) 90 to 109.
IQ scores do not represent a patient's innate intelligence. Rather, IQ scores represent a patient's ordinal position or percentile ranking on the test relative to the normative sample at any given time. Full-Scale IQ scores greater than 130 are classified as Very Superior, that is, the top 2.2% of test-takers; IQ scores of 120 to 129 are Superior (accounting for 6.7% of the population); and IQ scores of 110 to 119 are called High Average (accounting for 16.1% of the population). Those with an average IQ score between 90 and 119

account for 50% of the population, whereas Low Average scores (80 to 89) account for 16.1% of people, and those with scores of 70 to 79 are termed Borderline and account for 6.7% of test-takers. Intellectual disability is categorized by an IQ score of 69 or less.

Q5 The answer is: (B) MMPI.
The MMPI-2 is a 567-item true-false self-report test of psychological function (not intelligence) with 10 clinical scales ([1] Hs-Hypochondriasis; [2] D-Depression; [3] Hy-Conversion Hysteria; [4] Pd-Psychopathic Deviate; [5] Mf-Masculinity-Femininity; [6] Pa-Paranoia; [7] Pt-Psychasthenia; [8] Sc-Schizophrenia; [9] Ma-Hypomania; and [10] Si-Social Introversion) that assess major categories of psychopathology and 6 validity scales designed to assess test-taking attitudes.

The MCMI-III consists of 3 validity scales, 10 basic personality scales (different from those listed in the question), 3 severe personality scales, 6 clinical syndrome scales, and 3 severe clinical syndrome scales.

The PAI uses 344 items and a 4-point response format to make 22 scales with nonoverlapping items. It consists of 4 validity scales, 11 clinical scales, and 2 interpersonal scales.

The Rorschach codes responses into several indexes: the Perceptual Thinking Index, the Suicide Constellation, the Depression Index, the Coping Deficit Index, the Hypervigilance Index, and the Obsessive Style Index.

The TAT is a projective test (not an intelligence test) that uses a series of redrawn pictures of people; it does not use a battery of clinical scales for scoring.

Neuropsychological Assessment
Multiple-Choice Questions

Select the appropriate answer.

Q1 Which of the following is NOT considered to be an executive function (i.e., a higher-order cognitive function)?

    A. *The ability to maintain and suddenly shift from a behavioral set*

    B. *The ability to organize information*

    C. *The ability to plan and initiate behavior*

    D. *The ability to reason abstractly*

    E. *The ability to withdraw from a painful stimulus*

Q2 Which of the following is a test of cognitive flexibility that involves the rapid alternate sequencing of numbers and letters that are randomly arranged on a page?

    A. *Tower of London Test*

    B. *Trail-Making Test Part A*

    C. *Trail-Making Test Part B*

    D. *WAIS*

    E. *Wisconsin Card Sorting Test*

Q3 Which of the following is a test of intellectual function, and determination of an intellectual quotient?

    A. *Boston Naming Test*

    B. *Functional magnetic resonance imaging scanning*

    C. *Trail-Making Test Part A*

    D. *WAIS*

    E. *Wisconsin Card Sorting Test*

Q4 Which of the following brain territories is MOST closely associated with a receptive aphasia?

    A. *Brodmann's area*

    B. *Broca's area*

    C. *The cerebellum*

    D. *The limbic system*

    E. *Wernicke's area*

Q5   In which of the following tests is the patient asked to name the color of ink in the face of a conflicting color word (e.g., respond "red" when the word "blue" is printed in red ink)?

A. *Benton Visual Form Discrimination Test*

B. *Boston Naming Test*

C. *Hooper Visual Organization Test*

D. *Rey-Osterrieth Complex Figure Test*

E. *Stroop Test*

Chapter 8

Answers

Q1 The answer is: (E) The ability to withdraw from a painful stimulus.

Executive function encompasses a group of higher-order cognitive functions (including the ability to plan and to initiate behavior, to both maintain and suddenly shift from a behavioral set, to organize information, to self-monitor one's responses, and to reason abstractly).

Withdrawal from a painful stimulus may only involve a simple reflex arc, associated with the appreciation of pain.

Q2 The answer is: (C) Trail-Making Test Part B.

One of the most commonly used and widely recognized measures of cognitive flexibility is Part B of the Trail-Making Test, which involves the rapid alternate sequencing of numbers and letters that are randomly arranged on a page.

This test differs from the simpler-to-perform Trail-Making Test Part A, which only requires the sequencing of numbers on a page.

Frontal lobe functions are also assessed by the Tower of London Test (which assesses spatial planning, rule-learning skills, and organizational strategies), by the Rey-Osterrieth Complex Figure Test (which shapes a clinical impression by determining how a person completes the task), by subtests of the Wechsler Adult Intelligence Scale ([WAIS], which identifies how a person interprets proverbs and describes similarities), and by the Wisconsin Card Sorting Test (which sees whether a person can maintain and shift the set as the rules change, needing to adapt to changes in color, shape, and number on the cards presented).

Q3 The answer is: (D) WAIS.

Intelligence can be estimated by tests that tend to correlate highly with overall intellectual function (i.e., tests of single word reading, such as the National Reading Test or the Wechsler Test of Adult Reading), or by administration of specific batteries of tests designed to assess intelligence (including the Wechsler Intelligence scales and the Stanford-Binet Intelligence Test). The WAIS is roughly divided into verbal and visual-based abilities, yielding a measure of general intellectual function.

The Boston Naming Test asks individuals to name pictured objects; abnormalities may reflect problems with primary aphasia or with degraded semantic knowledge.

The Trail-Making Test Part A, requires only the sequencing of numbers on a page; it primarily tests for attentional ability, not intelligence.

The Wisconsin Card Sorting Test (which determines whether a person can maintain and shift the set as the rules change, needing to adapt to changes in color, shape, and number on the cards presented) is a good test of executive function, not for intellectual function per se.

Functional magnetic resonance imaging scans reflect metabolic activity of the brain during a specific activity, but do not lead to quantifications of intellectual function.

Q4 The answer is: (E) Wernicke's area.

Lesions in Wernicke's area, in the superior temporal gyrus, lead to fluent aphasias, without comprehension.

Nonfluent aphasia typically results from lesions in Broca's area (in the inferior frontal gyrus); in individuals with this disorder, comprehension is intact but speech is nonfluent and telegraphic.

Brodmann's area 17 resides in the occipital cortex and its function relates to vision.

The cerebellum, although integrally related to equilibrium and balance, has also been linked to regulation of affect and cognition, but not the comprehension of spoken language.

The limbic system encompasses many integrative brain functions, but language is not one of them.

Q5 The answer is: (E) Stroop Test.

The Stroop Test is a test in which the patient is asked to name the color of ink in the face of a conflicting color word (e.g., respond "red" when the word "blue" is printed in red ink); it is a test of frontal lobe function.

The Rey-Osterrieth Complex Figure Test can provide insights into strategic learning of visual information as the extent to which an individual uses an organized approach in the encoding (copying) phase predicts subsequent incidental and delayed recall.

The Boston Naming Test involves asking a patient to name pictured objects; deficits in naming, although common in those with aphasia, are also observed in patients with degraded semantic knowledge, such as occurs in those with Alzheimer's disease.

The Benton Visual Form Discrimination Test has an individual select which of four designs is an exact match for a target design; it is a test of visuoperceptual ability.

The Hooper Visual Organization Test asks patients to identify objects based on presentation of drawings in which the object is presented in fragments that have been rearranged.

SECTION 4
THE PSYCHOTHERAPIES

Coping With Medical Illness and Psychotherapy of the Medically Ill

Multiple-Choice Questions

Select the appropriate answer.

Q1   True or False. Coping can be defined as a problem-solving behavior that is intended to bring about relief, reward, quiescence, and equilibrium.

   A.   *True*

   B.   *False*

Q2   Which of the following is NOT a characteristic of good copers?

   A.   *They are optimistic about mastering problems and, despite setbacks, generally maintain a high level of morale*

   B.   *They are inclined to excessive denial and elaborate rationalization*

   C.   *They tend to be practical and emphasize immediate problems, issues, and obstacles that must be conquered before even visualizing a remote or ideal resolution*

   D.   *They select from a wide range of potential strategies and tactics, and their policy is not to be at a loss for fallback methods*

   E.   *They heed various possible outcomes and improve coping by being aware of consequences*

Q3   Which of the following is NOT a characteristic of poor copers?

   A.   *They tend to be excessive in self-expectation, rigid in outlook, inflexible in standards, and reluctant to compromise or to ask for help*

   B.   *Their opinion of how people should behave is narrow and absolute; they allow little room for tolerance*

   C.   *They are optimistic about mastering problems and, despite setbacks, generally maintain a high level of morale*

   D.   *They are prone to firm adherence to preconceptions*

   E.   *They are inclined to excessive denial and elaborate rationalization*

Q4   True or False. In general, patients who adamantly deny difficulties tend to cope poorly.

   A.   *True*

   B.   *False*

Q5   True or False. Confidence in being able to cope can be enhanced through repeated attempts at self-appraisal, self-instruction, and self-correction.

   A.   *True*

   B.   *False*

Chapter 9

Answers

Q1 The answer is: (A) True.
Coping is perhaps best defined as a problem-solving behavior that is intended to bring about relief, reward, quiescence, and equilibrium. Nothing in this definition promises permanent resolution of problems. It does imply a combination of knowing what the problems are and how to go about reaching resolution. In ordinary language, the term *coping* is used to mean only the outcome of managing a problem, and it overlooks the intermediate process of appraisal, performance, and correction that most problem-solving entails. Coping is not a simple judgment about how some difficulty worked out. It is an extensive, recursive process of self-exploration, self-instruction, self-correction, self-rehearsal, and guidance gathered from outside sources.

Q2 The answer is: (B) They are inclined to excessive denial and elaborate rationalization.
Good copers are optimistic about mastering problems and, despite setbacks, generally maintain a high level of morale; they tend to be practical and emphasize immediate problems, issues, and obstacles that must be conquered before even visualizing a remote or ideal resolution; they select from a wide range of potential strategies and tactics, and their policy is not to be at a loss for fallback methods (in this respect, they are resourceful); they heed various possible outcomes and improve coping by being aware of consequences; they are generally flexible and open to suggestions, but they do not give up the final say in decisions; and they are quite composed, although vigilant in avoiding emotional extremes that could impair judgment.

Those who are inclined to excessive denial and elaborate rationalization tend to cope poorly.

Q3 The answer is: (C) They are optimistic about mastering problems and, despite setbacks, generally maintain a high level of morale.
Bad copers are not bad people, nor even incorrigibly ineffective people. In fact, it is too simplistic merely to indicate that bad copers have the opposite characteristics of effective copers. Each patient brings a unique set of cultural and psychological attributes to their capacity to cope. Bad copers are those who have more problems in coping with unusual, intense, and unexpected difficulties because of a variety of traits.

Bad copers tend to be excessive in self-expectation, rigid in outlook, inflexible in standards, and reluctant to compromise or to ask for help; their opinion of how people should behave is narrow and absolute; they allow little room for tolerance; they are prone to firm adherence to preconceptions; they are inclined to excessive denial and elaborate rationalization; they are unable to focus on salient problems; they tend to be more passive than usual and fail to initiate action on their own behalf; and they subject themselves to impulsive judgments or atypical behavior that fails to be effective.

Q4 The answer is: (A) True.
Patients who adamantly deny any difficulty tend to cope poorly. Sick patients have difficult lives, and the denial of adversity usually represents a relatively primitive defense that leaves such patients unprepared to accurately assess their options. Carefully timed and empathic discussion with patients of a genuine appraisal for their current condition can help them to avoid this maladaptive approach and to address their treatment more effectively.

Q5 The answer is: (A) True.
Patients can become better copers by cultivating the characteristics of effective copers. Coping is, after all, a skill that is useful in a variety of situations, although many modifications of basic principles are called for. Confidence in being able to cope can be enhanced through repeated attempts at self-appraisal, self-instruction, and self-correction. Coping well with illness— or with any problem—does not predict invariable success, but it does provide a foundation for becoming a better coper.

An Overview of the Psychotherapies

Multiple-Choice Questions

Select the appropriate answer.

Q1   Which of the following types of therapy has as its goals to recognize, interpret, and work through unconscious feelings that are problematic?

   A.   *Cognitive-behavioral therapy (CBT)*

   B.   *Dialectical behavioral therapy (DBT)*

   C.   *Interpersonal psychotherapy (IPT)*

   D.   *Psychodynamic psychotherapy*

   E.   *Supportive psychotherapy*

Q2   Which of the following is MOST closely associated with IPT?

   A.   *Aaron Beck*

   B.   *Gerald Klerman*

   C.   *Marsha Linehan*

   D.   *Peter Sifneos*

   E.   *Joseph Wolpe*

Q3   Which of the following is MOST closely associated with describing the course of life's progression through a series of developmental crises?

   A.   *Aaron Beck*

   B.   *Erik Erikson*

   C.   *Gerald Klerman*

   D.   *Marsha Linehan*

   E.   *Joseph Wolpe*

Chapter 10

Answers

Q1 The answer is: (D) Psychodynamic psychotherapy.

Psychodynamic psychotherapy has the longest organized tradition of the psychotherapies. It is also known as psychoanalytic psychotherapy or expressive psychotherapy. This psychotherapy can be brief or time-limited, but it is usually open-ended and long term. The goal of psychodynamic psychotherapy is to recognize, interpret, and work through unconscious feelings that are problematic.

Cognitive-behavioral therapy (CBT) is emerging as a widely practiced psychotherapy for depression, the anxiety disorders, and other psychiatric and medical diagnoses. In contrast to the psychodynamic model, unconscious inner conflicts and early relationships are considered less important than is here-and-now conscious awareness of thoughts, feelings, and behaviors.

Dialectical behavioral therapy (DBT) is a structured individual and group treatment that has four goals: mindfulness, interpersonal effectiveness, emotional regulation, and distress tolerance. These four goals are considered skills that are taught in carefully structured sessions with a skills training manual and handouts for each session.

Interpersonal psychotherapy (IPT) has several primary goals: the reduction of depressive symptoms and the improvement of self-esteem, and the development of more effective strategies for dealing with interpersonal relationships. IPT does not focus on transference phenomena or the unconscious.

Supportive psychotherapy is often defined by what it is not. It does not involve analysis of the transference; it does not involve challenging defenses; it does not endeavor to change the structure of personality or character; it does not involve making the unconscious conscious.

Q2 The answer is: (B) Gerald Klerman.

IPT was developed and described by Gerald Klerman and coworkers in the late 1970s. IPT is a brief therapy that is manual-driven and is generally accomplished in 12 to 16 sessions. IPT was inspired by the interpersonal focus of Adolph Meyer and Harry Stack Sullivan, and the attachment theory of John Bowlby.

Brief psychotherapy is defined as a psychotherapy with a predetermined endpoint, usually 8 to 12 visits. The theory and technique of brief psychotherapy parallels the established psychotherapy "camps." Peter Sifneos and others described time-limited psychodynamic psychotherapy.

CBT represents a merger of the pioneering work of Aaron Beck (who first developed cognitive therapy for depression in the mid-1960s) and the work of Joseph Wolpe (who in 1958 described a behavior therapy for anxiety disorders).

In the late 1980s, Marsha Linehan at the University of Washington in Seattle developed DBT for the treatment of borderline personality disorder.

Q3 The answer is: (B) Erik Erikson.

Erik Erikson observed that humans at all stages of the life cycle progress through a series of developmental crises. These crises are often discussed as a dichotomous choice between options that will either allow the individual to move forward developmentally, or conversely to get "stuck" or even regress developmentally. For example, Erikson argued that the fundamental crisis for infants was one of "trust versus mistrust." In other words, infants need to learn that they can trust their world to keep them safe and healthy, and in the absence of this experience, they will not be able to manage the inherent anxiety that is naturally part of later developmental stages, such as the challenges of "initiative versus guilt," the developmental crisis that Erikson postulated characterized school-age children. Erikson called his theory the "epigenetic model," and he characterized the stages of development from infancy through adulthood.

Gerald Klerman and coworkers developed IPT in the late 1970s.

Aaron Beck (who first developed cognitive therapy for depression in the mid-1960s) and Joseph Wolpe (who in 1958 described a behavior therapy for anxiety disorders) established the basis for CBT.

Marsha Linehan at the University of Washington in Seattle developed DBT for the treatment of borderline personality disorder.

Brief Psychotherapy: An Overview

Multiple-Choice Questions

Select the appropriate answer.

Q1 Which of the following created a dynamic existential method of brief psychotherapy?

    A. *Sigmund Freud*

    B. *Otto Kernberg*

    C. *Erich Lindemann*

    D. *James Mann*

    E. *Anton Mesmer*

Q2 Which of the following is MOST closely allied with cognitive-behavioral therapy?

    A. *Aaron Beck*

    B. *Sigmund Freud*

    C. *Gerald Klerman*

    D. *Erich Lindemann*

    E. *James Mann*

Q3 Which of the following is NOT considered to be a criterion for inclusion into brief therapy?

    A. *Active psychosis*

    B. *A real desire for relief*

    C. *A specific or circumscribed problem*

    D. *An ability to commit to treatment*

    E. *History of a positive relationship*

Q4 Which of the following practitioners prescribed a brief therapy of exactly 12 sessions?

    A. *Habib Davanloo*

    B. *Sigmund Freud*

    C. *David Malan*

    D. *James Mann*

    E. *Peter Sifneos*

Q5   Which of the following brief therapies incorporates exposure and systematic desensitization?

    A. *Behavioral therapy*

    B. *Cognitive therapy*

    C. *Electroconvulsive therapy*

    D. *Interpersonal therapy*

    E. *Pharmacotherapy*

Chapter 11

Answers

Q1 The answer is: (D) James Mann.

James Mann insisted on a treatment length of 12 sessions. For Mann, time was not just a reality, or a part of the framework; it was also a tool of treatment. During the evaluation, the therapist begins to think about the "central issue" (such as problems with separation, unresolved grief, or failure to move from one developmental stage to another). Early sessions are marked by an outpouring of data and by the formation of a positive or idealizing transference. At the midpoint, overt resistance occurs, as does negative transference. In the latter sessions comes a working through of the patient's pessimism and recollection of unconscious memories and previous bad separation events, along with an expectation of a repetition of the past. By the therapist's honest acceptance of the patient's anger and ambivalence over termination, the patient moves from a state of neurotic fear of separation and its attendant depression to the point in which the patient is ambivalent, sad, autonomous, and realistically optimistic. Sigmund Freud is often considered the father of psychoanalysis, not brief psychotherapy.

Otto Kernberg is well known for his description of, and work with, borderline psychopathology; brief psychotherapy was not at the core of his interventions.

Erich Lindemann, former Chair of the Department of Psychiatry at the Massachusetts General Hospital, is probably best known for his work with survivors of the tragic Cocoanut Grove fire in 1944; lessons learned regarding grief flowed from his clinical care and studies.

Anton Mesmer, a 19th-century practitioner in France, conducted studies on "animal magnetism"; his technique was later called "mesmerism," which was a forerunner to James Braid's hypnosis.

Q2 The answer is: (A) Aaron Beck.

The method of Aaron Beck aims at bringing the patient's automatic thoughts into awareness and demonstrating how these thoughts affect behavior and feelings. The therapist actively schedules the patient's day-to-day activity, and the patient is asked to list in some detail actual daily activities and to rate the degree of "mastery" and "pleasure" in each. These allow the therapist to review the week with the patient and to sculpt behaviors. Cognitive rehearsals are also used to help the patient foresee obstacles in the coming week. Sigmund Freud is often considered the father of psychoanalysis, not cognitive-behavioral therapy.

Gerald Klerman and his colleagues developed interpersonal psychotherapy, a highly formalized ("manualized") treatment, developed to treat patients with depression related to grief or loss, interpersonal disputes, or interpersonal deficits. This psychotherapy deemphasizes the transference and focuses not on mental content but on the process of the patient's interaction with others.

Erich Lindemann is probably best known for his work with survivors of the tragic Cocoanut Grove fire in 1944; lessons learned regarding grief flowed from his clinical care and studies

James Mann was a creator of brief psychotherapy, not cognitive-behavioral therapy.

Q3 The answer is: (A) Active psychosis.

According to practitioners of most types of brief therapy, inclusion criteria include a real desire for relief, a specific or circumscribed problem, an ability to commit to treatment, a history of a positive relationship, moderate (or less) emotional distress, and function in one or more areas of life. Exclusion criteria include active psychosis, substance abuse, and an acute risk of self-harm.

Q4 The answer is: (D) James Mann.

James Mann insisted on a treatment length of 12 sessions. For Mann, time was not just a reality, or a part of the framework; it was also a tool of treatment.

Habib Davanloo's brief therapy lasted between 1 and 40 sessions. He advised confronting resistance, especially around anger.

Sigmund Freud is often considered the father of psychoanalysis; he did not place limits on the duration of therapy.

David Malan's brief therapy lasted between 20 and 30 sessions (but ended with a fixed date). He believed insight was curative.

Peter Sifneos' brief therapy lasted 12 to 20 sessions. He interpreted transference and resistance. The focus of therapy was often narrow, for example, on Oedipal conflict, grief, and transference.

Q5 The answer is: (A) Behavioral therapy.

Behavioral therapy employs exposure, systematic desensitization, imaging, and relaxation.

Cognitive therapy deals with automatic thoughts; the therapist helps define governing rules, refutes them, assigns homework, and mandates practice of new cognitions and behaviors.

Electroconvulsive therapy is a somatic therapy that involves the application of an electrical current to the brain.

Interpersonal therapy is a manual-driven therapy that defines interpersonal deficits, role problems, and helps to reshape interpersonal behaviors.

Pharmacotherapy employs the use of psychotropic agents to modulate disturbances of affect, behavior, and cognition.

Chapter 12
Couples Therapy
Multiple-Choice Questions

Select the appropriate answer.

Q1   Which of the following problems is NOT typically considered as a focus for couples therapy?

  A.   *Disclosures of infidelity*

  B.   *Infertility*

  C.   *Malingering*

  D.   *Parenting impasses*

  E.   *Sexual dysfunction*

Q2   Which of the following terms is characterized by each member contributing a similar behavior, so that each partner compounds and exacerbates the difficulties (e.g., both members of a couple engaging in verbal abuse, so that either one's raised voice prompts an escalation of angry affect, which, in turn, triggers the other's ire)?

  A.   *Complementary relationship*

  B.   *Impulsive relationship*

  C.   *Passive-aggressive relationship*

  D.   *Platonic relationship*

  E.   *Symmetrical relationship*

Q3   Which of the following psychodynamic constructs can BEST explain the seeds of early attraction in a relationship in which "opposites attract?"

  A.   *Denial*

  B.   *Projective identification*

  C.   *Repetition compulsion*

  D.   *Splitting*

  E.   *Sublimation*

Q4   Which of the following types of theorists have delineated five stages with attendant emotional tasks?

  A.   *Behavioral theorists*

  B.   *Cognitive theorists*

  C.   *Existential theorists*

  D.   *Life-cycle theorists*

  E.   *Systemic theorists*

Q5   Which of the following is NOT one of the terms (called the "Four Horsemen of the Apocalypse") used by John Gottman to predict dissolution of a relationship?

A.   *Contempt*

B.   *Criticism*

C.   *Defensiveness*

D.   *Obsessiveness*

E.   *Stonewalling*

Q1 The answer is: (C) Malingering.

Couples therapy is often the treatment of choice for a range of problems: sexual dysfunction, alcohol and substance abuse, the disclosure of infidelity, depression and anxiety disorders, infertility, serious medical illness, and parenting impasses. In addition, couples therapy may be helpful in the resolution of polarized relational issues (e.g., the decision to marry or divorce, the choice to have a child or an abortion, or the decision to move to another city for one partner's career).

Malingering has not been viewed as a focus of couples therapy.

Q2 The answer is: (E) Symmetrical relationship.

A symmetrical relationship is characterized by each member contributing a similar behavior, so that each partner compounds and exacerbates the difficulties.

Complementarity, by contrast, refers to patterns that require each member to contribute something quite different, in a mutually interlocking manner, to maintain the relationship. A classic example of a complementary relationship is the distancer-pursuer, in which one member does most of the asking for intimacy and connection, while the other pulls back to do work, take care of the children, or be alone. The circular nature of this pattern dictates that the more one pursues, the more the other pulls back, which in turn makes the pursuer pursue more, and the distancer recoil more.

Q3 The answer is: (B) Projective identification.

One common explanation for early attraction is that "opposites attract"; this may be understood in terms of the psychodynamic construct of projective identification. This is the idea that individuals look for something in the other that is difficult for them to bear or to express, and then they act unconsciously to elicit the very behavior in the other that has been disavowed by the self. For example, a vivacious and expressive woman whose ambitions were discouraged by her family may be drawn to a cool, career-focused man, whose attempts to express his feelings were ignored growing up. She may initially find his self-confidence and drive exciting, while he finds her ability to cry and to laugh invigorating. Over time, however, she may criticize him for his self-absorption, and he may criticize her for her over-emotionality. What was the initial source of mutual attraction becomes played out as conflict between the couple.

Repetition compulsion conveys the idea that one's choice of a mate is dictated by the wish to recreate a loving relationship from childhood, or to try to master an abusive relationship by reenacting it a second time. This leads some to say that a man has "married his mother."

Denial, splitting, and sublimation do not fit the current example.

Q4 The answer is: (D) Life cycle theorists.

Life-cycle theorists have delineated five stages with attendant emotional tasks, for example, the first stage joins families through marriage, in which each couple must redefine the issues and choices of their family of origin to create room for a new marital system; the second stage is when couples become parents and in which partners make room in their relationship for new members, and redefine relationships with their extended family; the third stage is characterized by the development of the children as adolescents, when the parents must allow increased flexibility in boundaries to include adolescents' increased independence, as well as their grandparents' growing dependence; the fourth stage (the launching stage) is when young children leave home and couples reevaluate their marriage and career issues as their parenting roles diminish; and the fifth stage (often the longest stage) is when parents are on their own after the children have left home, and the couple faces aging and loss.

Systemic theorists are interested in organization and patterns of interaction, and pay attention to the rules that underlie a couple's connectedness and their decision-making. These rules are influenced by the cultural and class background of each partner, and by the unique contributions from their family of origin.

Q5 The answer is: (D) Obsessiveness.

John Gottman developed a two-pronged approach that aims to resolve conflict and improve the friendship, goodwill, and fondness in a relationship. Although the mere presence of anger is not predictive of an unstable relationship, Gottman delineated four elements whose presence during conflict is predictive of relationship dissolution. These "four horsemen" are contempt, criticism, defensiveness, and stonewalling. When all four are identified, Gottman predicts that the relationship will not last. When couples can make repair statements during a fight, the damage to the relationship is diminished.

Obsessive traits do not rise to the level of a predictor of relationship failure.

Chapter 13

Family Therapy

Multiple-Choice Questions

Select the appropriate answer.

Q1 Which of the following schools of family therapy is derived from principles of object relations and Freudian theory?

A. *Behavioral*

B. *Narrative*

C. *Psychodynamic*

D. *Structural*

E. *Systemic*

Q2 Which of the following is NOT a proponent of the psychodynamic school of family therapy?

A. *Murray Bowen*

B. *James Framo*

C. *Salvador Minuchin*

D. *Ivan Boszormenyi-Nagy*

E. *Norman Paul*

Q3 In which of the following schools of family therapy does the therapist try to make something surprising and unexpected happen, amplifying the affect in the room?

A. *Behavioral*

B. *Experiential*

C. *Psychoeducational*

D. *Structural*

E. *Systemic*

Q4 Which of the following is a MAJOR proponent of experiential family therapy?

A. *Milton Erickson*

B. *James Framo*

C. *Salvador Minuchin*

D. *Norman Paul*

E. *Virginia Satir*

Q5 In which of the following schools of family therapy does the therapist approach the family with a blueprint of what a normal family should look like, with some allowance made for cultural, ethnic, and economic variations?

A. *Behavioral*

B. *Narrative*

C. *Psychodynamic*

D. *Structural*

E. *Systemic*

Q6 In which of the following schools of family therapy does the family therapist believe that change occurs when maladaptive behavioral sequences are interrupted?

A. *Experiential*

B. *Narrative*

C. *Psychodynamic*

D. *Psychoeducational*

E. *Strategic*

Q7 In which of the following schools of family therapy might the therapist be like the detective who interviews all of the suspects about a crime, and then gathers them all in the parlor to tell them how the crime took place?

A. *Behavioral*

B. *Psychodynamic*

C. *Psychoeducational*

D. *Strategic*

E. *Systemic*

Q8 In which of the following schools of family therapy does the therapist act like a biographer who takes the family's basic stories and transforms them with a different organization, a richer grasp of language and tone, and with the addition of previously overlooked tales?

A. *Experiential*

B. *Narrative*

C. *Psychodynamic*

D. *Psychoeducational*

E. *Strategic*

Q9 Which of the following schools of family therapy employ the reflecting team, to aid in the treatment of families and the training of therapists?

A. *Experiential*

B. *Narrative*

C. *Psychodynamic*

D. *Psychoeducational*

E. *Strategic*

Q10 In which of the following schools of family therapy is the therapist like the civil engineer called on to reconfigure well-established traffic patterns in a busy city?

A. *Behavioral*

B. *Experiential*

C. *Narrative*

D. *Psychodynamic*

E. *Psychoeducational*

Chapter 13
Answers

Q1 The answer is: (C) Psychodynamic.

Psychodynamically oriented family therapy is derived from principles of object relations and Freudian theory; its goal, as is the goal of individual psychodynamic therapy, is more self-awareness, which is created by bringing unconscious material into conscious thought. At the heart of this practice is the notion that current family problems are due to unresolved issues with the previous generation. Interpersonal function is distorted by attachments to past figures, and by the handing down of secrets from one generation to the next. The psychodynamically oriented family therapist wants to free the family from excessive attachment to the previous generation and wants to help family members disclose secrets and express concomitant feelings (e.g., of anger or grief). Change is created through insight that is often revealed in one individual at a time, in a serial fashion, as others look on.

To loosen the grip of the past on the present, the therapist uses several tools (including interpretation of transferential objects in the room, interpretation of projective identification, and the use of the genogram to make sense of generational transmission of issues). In family therapy, transferential interpretations are made among family members, rather than between the patient and the therapist, as occurs in individual therapy.

Another important tool for dredging up the past is the interpretation of projective identification. Put another way, each family member behaves in such a way as to elicit the very part of the self that has been disavowed and projected onto another family member. The purpose of these mutual projections is to keep old relationships alive by the reenactment of conflicts that parents had with their families of origin.

In part, the psychodynamic family therapist gathers and analyzes multigenerational transmission of issues using a genogram, a visual representation of a family that maps at least three generations of that family's history. The genogram reveals patterns (of similarity and difference) across generations—and between the two sides of the family involving many domains: parent-child and sibling roles, symptomatic behaviors, triadic patterns, developmental milestones, repetitive stressors, and cutoffs of family members. In addition, the genogram allows the clinician to look for any resonance between a current developmental issue and a similar one in a previous generation. This intersection of past with present anxiety may heighten the meaning and valence of a current problem.

Q2 The answer is: (C) Salvador Minuchin.

Salvador Minuchin, regarded as the founding father of structural family therapy, worked extensively while head of the Philadelphia Child Guidance Clinic with inner city families and with families who faced delinquency and multiple somatic symptoms. Both populations had not previously been treated with family therapy. He delineated how to assess and to understand the existing structure of a family, and pioneered several techniques (such as the imposition of rules of communication, manipulation of space, and use of enactments to modify structure).

Each of the other practitioners listed in the following text is a proponent of psychodynamic family therapy.

James Framo invites parents and adult siblings to come to an adult child's session; this tactic allows the past to be revisited in the present. This "family of origin" work is usually brief and intensive and consists of two lengthy sessions on two consecutive days. The meetings may focus on unresolved issues or on disclosure of secrets; it allows the adult child to become less reactive to his or her parents.

Norman Paul believes that most current symptoms in a family can be connected to a previous loss that has been insufficiently mourned. In family therapy, each member mourns an important loss while other members bear witness and consequently develop new stores of empathy.

Ivan Boszormenyi-Nagy introduced the idea of the "family ledger," a multigenerational accounting system of obligations incurred and debts repaid over time. Symptoms are understood in terms of an individual's making sacrifices in his or her own life to repay an injustice from a previous generation.

Murray Bowen stressed the dual importance of the individual's differentiation of self, while maintaining a connection to the family. To promote increased independence, Bowen coached patients to return to their family of origin, and to resist the pull of triangulated relationships by insisting that interactions remain dyadic.

The psychodynamic family therapist is like a lead-testing scientist who tests for levels of lead in one's garden to assess the legacy of toxins from previous homeowners. Only when the true condition of the soil has been revealed is the current homeowner free to make decisions about whether the soil is clean enough to plant root vegetables; is somewhat contaminated, so that only fruit-bearing bushes will be safe; or is so toxic that only flowers can be grown without hauling in truckloads of clean, fresh soil. Examination of the past enables the current gardener, and, by analogy, parents, to make informed choices about how the current environment needs to be adjusted and what kind of growth is allowable.

Q3 The answer is: (B) Experiential.

In contrast to the psychodynamic family therapist's focus on the past, the experiential therapist is primarily concerned with the here and now. In this model, change occurs through growth experiences that arise in the therapy session; experiences are aimed at the disruption of familiar interactions among family members. The experiential family therapist tries to make something surprising and unexpected happen, thereby amplifying affect. In general, the expression of feeling is valued over the discovery of insight. In its embrace of experience, this model is atheoretical and it can best be understood considering its practice.

The experiential family therapist is interested in small interactions that take place during the session and uses psychodramatic, or action-oriented, techniques to create a new experience in the therapy session. He or she might "sculpt" the family, literally posing them to demonstrate the way that the family is currently organized. This therapist might hope to heighten feelings of frustration and alienation, and then to relieve those feelings with a new sculpture that places the parents together. These sculptures would serve to increase affect, to create some focus away from the identified patient, and to demonstrate the merits of the parents who are standing together to combat their child's problem.

Q4 The answer is: (E) Virginia Satir.

Virginia Satir, an early luminary in family therapy (a field that was largely founded by men), believed that good communication depends on each family member feeling self-confident and valued. She focused on what was positive in a family and used nonverbal communication to improve connections within a family. If families learned to see, to hear, and to touch more, they would have more resources available to solve problems. She is credited with the use of family sculpting as a means to demonstrate the constraining rules and roles in a family.

Another proponent of experiential family therapy is Carl Whitaker, who posited that most experience occurs outside of awareness; he practiced "therapy of the absurd," a method that accesses the unconscious by using humor, boredom, free association, metaphors, and even wrestling on the floor. Symbolic, nonverbal growth experiences followed, with an aim toward the disruption of rigid patterns of thought and behavior.

The experiential family therapist is like a folk-art artist who takes commonplace objects and transforms them into works of art. The viewer is surprised to find that a box of mismatched buttons could become the wings of a butterfly. Making the unfamiliar out of the familiar and using playful techniques to do so are key features of experiential family therapy.

Milton Erickson (whose focus on behavioral change relied on indirect suggestion through the use of stories, riddles, and metaphors) heavily influenced the strategic school of family therapy. Strategic therapists borrowed this reliance on playful storytelling techniques.

Q5 The answer is: (D) Structural.

The structural family therapist approaches a family with a blueprint of what a normal family should look like, with some allowance made for cultural, ethnic, and economic variations. Most broadly stated, a high-functioning family should have well-defined parental, marital, and sibling subsystems, clear generational boundaries (with the parents firmly in charge), and flexible relationships with outsiders.

The structural family therapist focuses on the structural properties of the family, rather than on affect or insight. Several features define structure: by the rules of the family (e.g., "What subjects can be discussed at the dinner table? What kind of affect is acceptable to express?"); by boundaries within the family (e.g., "Do the children stay clear of marital conflict? Do siblings have their own relationship?"); by boundaries between the family and the outside world (e.g., "Do parents easily request help from outsiders? Or, are they insulated?"); and by the generational hierarchy (e.g., "Who [the parents, or the adolescent, or the grandparents] is in charge of decision-making?"). In this model, change occurs when the structure shifts and when symptoms are no longer needed.

Therapists in this school support the existing rules of the family and make a relationship with each member. These individual relationships may later be used to restructure the system, for example, by empowering the parents. The therapist, assessing the formal properties of the family, would earmark the shaky alliance between the parents and the lack of well-defined marital, parental, and sibling subsystems. This family therapist might describe a family as involved in a pattern of conflict avoidance called triangulation, with each parent wanting the child to take his or her side, putting the child into an impossible loyalty bind.

As assessment becomes treatment, this therapist might challenge enmeshment by imposing a rule about communication, whereby each member should speak only for herself or himself. The therapist would try to challenge the lack of a generational hierarchy by manipulating space. For example, the therapist might ask the parents to sit side-by-side, while also instructing the children to leave the room for part of the interview. To challenge the rule that conflict should be avoided, particularly regarding disagreements about how to get one child to do something, this therapist would have the couple sit together and create a plan, while the therapist blocks any attempt to involve the child. The family might then role-play a family activity (in a session) to illustrate the child's role in their power struggle. Additionally, the children could be invited to have their own meeting to explore and to shore up their relationship.

Salvador Minuchin is regarded as the founding father of structural family therapy. The structural family therapist is like a building inspector who renders an opinion about the stability of a structure, and guides the owner to decisions regarding a large-scale renovation or merely a cosmetic touch-up. The inspector does not care about either the furnishings or the paint colors, but is concerned with whether the walls are solid, the locks are in working order, and the wiring is functional and safe. Everything else follows smoothly if the house is solidly built.

Q6 The answer is: (E) Strategic.

The strategic family therapist believes that change occurs when maladaptive behavioral sequences are interrupted. This therapist differentiates between two kinds of change: "first order," in which commonsense solutions to initial difficulties actually become unsolvable problems; and "second order," in which random events or therapeutic interventions disrupt first-order solutions. These therapists view families as fundamentally homeostatic or invested in maintaining the *status quo*, even at the expense of a symptomatic family member. Consequently, this therapist anticipates a power struggle between him or her and the family and develops strategies to destabilize the power structure in the family. One such strategy involves the use of paradox, which is used to meet the family isomorphically at the ambivalent place they present. In essence, the position taken by the family is, "Help us get rid of the symptom, but don't make us change."

This therapist then wants to introduce second-order change by use of a paradoxical strategy (e.g., prescribing a symptom that is aimed at disrupting the current behavioral sequence). This is a therapeutic double-bind, that is, an intervention that mirrors the paradoxical communication in the family.

Proponents of this school of family therapy include Milton Erickson, Jay Haley, Paul Wazlawick, John Weakland, Cloé Madanes, and Gregory Bateson.

The strategic family therapist is like a master chess player who knows from the start how he or she wants the game to turn out, and then maps out each move to get there. This therapist has a plan for each individual session, and a vision for the outcome of this problem-focused therapy. In chess, as in therapy, there is a belief that a small move will set off reverberations throughout the game. This cascade of changes can similarly be planned and mapped out by the therapist.

Q7 The answer is: (E) Systemic.

The systemic family therapist is like the detective in a British mystery who interviews all of the suspects about a crime, and then gathers them all in the parlor to tell them how the crime took place. The story he or she tells connects everyone's point of view, but is generally different from any one person's account. The experience of the reader of the story is to feel both confused and that the story makes perfect sense, although it means reevaluating each person's point of view. This mixture of confusion and resonance is what the systemic therapist aims for when he or she introduces a systemic opinion that alters meanings.

The systemic family therapist believes that change occurs when beliefs are changed, or the meaning of behavior is altered. In this view, the solutions, as well as the power to change, lie within the family. This therapist rejects the notion that the therapist holds a clear idea of what the family should look like at the end of successful treatment. The therapist does not presume to know the right truth to help a family. Instead, this therapist holds that there is no one truth, rather, some ideas are more useful than others.

The systemic therapist introduces new information in an effort to bring about systemic change. Systemic therapists use circular questions, which are aimed at surfacing differences around time, perception, ranking on a characteristic, and alliances within a family. Linear questions (e.g., "What made you depressed?") ask family members about cause and effect. Circular questions (e.g., "Who is most concerned about mother's depression? Then who? Then who?"), by contrast, take a problem and place it within the web of family relationships. Other circular questions attempt to elicit hidden comparisons and useable information.

In addition, systemic therapists employ two additional kinds of interventions: the reframe and the ritual. Reframing offers interpretations of problematic behaviors that are neutral or positive and that connect everyone in the family. The therapist uses positive connotation in redefining a problem to encourage cooperation, to introduce the idea of volition when behaviors have been regarded as outside of anyone's control, and to introduce confusion as a means to stimulate new thinking around tightly held beliefs. A ritual is introduced, not as a behavioral directive, but as an experiment. This therapist does not care if the ritual is carried out exactly as prescribed because it is the ideas contained in the ritual that contain the power to change.

Q8 The answer is: (B) Narrative.
The narrative family therapist is like a biographer who takes the family's basic stories and transforms them with a different organization, a richer grasp of language and tone, and with the addition of previously overlooked tales. The resulting story is a collaboration between therapist and family and contains story lines that hold more possibility than did the original story.

Narrative family therapists rely on the transformative power of new language to create change. They posit that families get stuck because they have become constrained by a problem-saturated story, and by constricted ways of talking among each other about their difficulties. This therapist tries to identify the dominant stories that limit the family's possibilities, and then to amplify minor or undiscovered narratives that contain more hope for change. Dominant stories include beliefs that the family holds about itself, as well as any cultural stories (such as the idea that adolescents can only become adults through rebellion and rejection of their parents) that may influence the family.

These therapists use stories in two significant ways: first, to deconstruct, or to separate, problems from the people who experience them; then to reconstruct, or to help families rewrite, the stories that they tell about their lives. These complementary processes of deconstruction and reconstruction are exemplified in the technique of externalizing the problem. With this technique, the therapist and the family create a name for the problem and attribute negative intentions to it so that the family can band together against the problem, rather than attack the individual who has the problem. The therapist subsequently asks about "unique outcomes," or times when the patient was free of the problem. The family is asked to wonder what made it possible at those times to find the strength to resist the pull of the problem. In time, these unusual moments of resistance are amplified and added to by more stories that feature the patient as competent and problem-free.

Q9 The answer is: (B) Narrative.
Narrative therapists have also developed the concept known as the reflecting team, to aid in the treatment of families and the training of therapists. With this approach, a group of clinicians observe an interview through a one-way mirror, and then speak directly to the family, offering ideas, observations, questions, and suggestions. These comments are offered tentatively and spontaneously so that the family can choose what is useful from among the team's offerings and reject the rest. Several narrative assumptions form the underpinning of the reflecting team; the abundance of ideas generated by the team will help loosen a constricted story held by the family; the relationship between the therapist and the patient should be nonhierarchical (with an emphasis placed on sharing rather than on giving information); people change under a positive connotation; and there are no right or wrong ideas, just ones that are more or less helpful to a family.

The invention of the reflecting team is credited to Tom Andersen and his colleagues at the University of Tromsø in Norway in 1985. Observing the interview from behind the mirror, Andersen found that the therapist continued to follow a pessimistic view of the family, regardless of the reframing questions that were telephoned in by the team. Finally, after several attempts to redirect the interview were thwarted, he "launched the idea to the family and the therapist that we might talk while they listened to us." With the team speaking directly to the family, presenting multiple ideas in an unrehearsed way, the concept of the reflecting team took root.

Michael White, in Australia, and David Epston, in New Zealand, are the best-known thinkers and writers of the narrative approach. In addition to their ideas of deconstructing the problem through externalizing and reauthoring, they have emphasized the political and social context in which all clinical work occurs. Relying on the work of Foucault, they critique the professional's linkage of power and knowledge. For example, they do not make diagnoses or rely on medical records kept private from their patients. Instead, they may write a letter to a patient at the end of the session and use the same letter as the clinical note for the medical record. At the close of therapy, the record may be given to the patient or, with permission, shared with other patients who are struggling with similar difficulties.

Q10 The answer is: (A) Behavioral.

The behavioral therapist is like the civil engineer called on to reconfigure well-established traffic patterns in a busy city. Congested areas must first be analyzed with respect to why drivers consistently choose these routes, despite the availability of alternatives. Next, attention should be paid to how various interests (individual, government, business) might be affected by potential changes. Concerned parties would be solicited to express their concerns. Subsequently, a reorganization can be introduced in a stepwise fashion, interrupting prior patterns to foster new ones. With each incremental change, traffic flow is measured, and adjustments are made accordingly. Ultimately, the solution seeks to serve efficiency, while maximizing the satisfaction of the individual, government, and business sectors. Behavioral family therapy relies on the ability to perform a detailed, functional behavioral analysis. The therapist begins with an assessment of the thoughts, feelings, and behaviors of each individual family member as they relate to the problem. Next, the therapist would work with the family to detail representative sequences of behaviors that mark their current distress.

By contrast, the psychoeducational therapist is like a wilderness guide leading amateur enthusiasts into a state park. Before setting foot on the trails, basic myths of the forest are dispelled through basic classroom instruction. Prospective campers might learn that no snakes indigenous to the area are poisonous, while being cautioned that some innocent-looking mushrooms are. The guide then begins to lead expeditions of increasing difficulty, pointing out examples from the classroom while gradually assigning more responsibility to the campers. Finally, before letting the group explore on their own, the guide distributes flares and radios, so that help can easily be accessed should the need arise.

Psychoeducational family therapy originated to assist families caring for a member with severe mental illness and functional impairment. The therapist understands family dysfunction as deficits in acquirable skills and knowledge. Through education and focused skills training, families and patients are empowered to effect their own change. The therapist anticipates deficiencies in several key domains. These include communication, problem-solving, coping, and knowledge of the illness. The therapist is also vigilant in identifying relationships that appear overinvolved or hypercritical, as these are associated with an increased likelihood of relapse and exacerbations of the affected member's illness. The goal of therapy is to create an environment that is more deliberate in its fostering of mastery and recovery.

Chapter 14

Group Psychotherapy

Multiple-Choice Questions

Select the appropriate answer.

Q1 In which of the following types of group therapy does the therapist generally challenge defenses, reduce shame, and interpret unconscious conflict?

A. *Cognitive-behavioral group*

B. *Inpatient group*

C. *Movement therapy group*

D. *Psychodynamic group*

E. *Supportive group*

Q2 Which of the following is LEAST likely to be a curative factor in group therapy?

A. *Diminishing shame*

B. *Evoking memories of early familial attitudes and interactions*

C. *Confronting members harshly and sadistically*

D. *Providing support*

E. *Reducing an individual's isolation*

Q3 True or False. Groups organized around medical illness have little to no impact on survival or on quality of life.

A. *True*

B. *False*

Q4 True or False. The clearer the leader is about the boundaries, the safer are the members to indulge their fantasies of wanting to corrupt the process, or to overcome the leader's authority.

A. *True*

B. *False*

Q5 True or False. The group leader is bound by the usual rules of confidentiality in the group as in any other clinical encounter with a patient.

A. *True*

B. *False*

Chapter 14

Answers

Q1 The answer is: (D) Psychodynamic group.
In a psychodynamically oriented therapy group, the group leader challenges defenses, reduces shame, and interprets unconscious conflict.

In cognitive-behavioral therapy groups, the group leader creates new options, is active, and directive.

In most inpatient groups, the group leader uses empathy and reality testing.

In movement therapy, the group leader attempts to free up inhibitions by the creation of movement.

In supportive groups, the group leader strengthens existing defenses by actively giving advice and support.

Q2 The answer is: (C) Confronting members harshly and sadistically.
Many efforts have been made to describe the curative factors in a therapy group. Summed up into the essential elements, groups help people change and grow by allowing the individual within the group to grow and develop beyond the constrictions in life that brought that person into treatment. The more common healing factors are those that act by reducing each individual's isolation, by diminishing shame (which is a major pathogenic factor in mental illness), and by evoking memories of early familial attitudes and interactions (that now can be approached differently with a new set of options and in the context of support). Another healing factor is expanding one's sublimatory options. The impulses that flourished in the context of childhood-limited defenses can now be checked by a broader emotional and behavioral repertoire that can be practiced among group members in the here-and-now. Provision of support and empathic confrontation can be curative as well. People often fear groups because they imagine they will be the target of harsh confrontation; they are unaware that the cohesive group is a marvelous source of concern and problem-solving. Finally, listening to others grieve and responding to others' awareness of our own losses can free an individual to move on.

Q3 The answer is: (B) False.
Since Joseph Hersey Pratt first offered his "classes" for tubercular patients at the Massachusetts General Hospital in 1905, people have come together to commiserate with one another around common problems, to share information, and to learn how to deal with the impact of those problems on their lives. These groups are often referred to as "symptom specific" or "population specific." Groups have been organized around medical illnesses (e.g., cancer, diabetes, and acquired immunodeficiency syndrome [AIDS]), as well as around psychological problems (e.g., bereavement), and psychosocial sequelae of trauma (e.g., war or natural disasters). The goals of such groups are to provide support and information that is embedded in a socially accepting environment, with people who are in a position to understand what the others are going through. The treatment may emerge from cognitive-behavioral principles, from psychodynamic principles, or from psychoeducational ones. Frequently, these groups tend to be time-limited; members often join at the same time and terminate together. The problems addressed in these groups are found in a broad variety of patients, from the very healthy to the more distressed, and they cut across other demographic variables (e.g., age and culture). Increasingly, research data have shown that involvement in these groups can extend the survival and the quality of life of the severely ill (e.g., women with end-stage breast cancer).

Q4 The answer is: (A) True.
The leader bears clear fiduciary responsibilities for the working of the group and the members within it. The burden is on the leader to exercise restraint and relative neutrality in the sense of nonjudgmental listening and responding to the patients' struggles. By remaining warm and neutral, the leader is able to listen nonjudgmentally to all aspects of the whole group's impulses and resistances, without taking sides or carrying the burden of policing the group, and deciding which are good feelings and interactions and which are not.

A group leader must exercise authority if the group is to be safe and containing for its members. Whether a member who is difficult in the group stays or leaves or whether a new member enters must not be left to a vote, just as such decisions are not made within a family. The privilege and burden of administrative and inclusion/exclusion matters is a serious responsibility of the group leader, as is the question of single or cotherapy leadership. It is important to remember that the leader is not a member of the group, despite the ambivalent entreaties of the members to bring the leader into the group. The clearer the leader is about the boundaries, the safer are the members to indulge their fantasies of wanting to corrupt the process, or to overcome the leader's authority.

Q5 The answer is: (A) True.

The group leader is bound by the usual rules of confidentiality in the group, as in any other clinical encounter with a patient. Except for a threat to a person or persons, this confidentiality holds and is usually elaborated on in the code of ethics of the therapist's professional organization. The same pertains to any conduct of the therapist that violates the code of ethics relative to sexual or other extraprofessional contact with a patient. Even in the most mature groups, members may inadvertently be tempted to speak to their spouses or others about an exciting moment in a therapy group. The bigger challenge is how to do this while respecting the confidentiality that is agreed on by and among members. Aside from stressing the importance of protecting the identities of patients in the group, there is little that the leader can do to ensure compliance, nor is it against the law for members to break confidentiality. Group therapists worry about whether the group can become a pool of witnesses in the case of a subpoena. Some states extend the same protection to the members that they do to the leader, namely the patient–therapist privilege, but this has not been tested and may not apply with all professionals across the disciplines.

Hypnosis

Multiple-Choice Questions

Select the appropriate answer.

Q1 Which of the following is generally considered to be the father of medical hypnosis?

    A. *James Braid*

    B. *James Esdaile*

    C. *Benjamin Franklin*

    D. *Sigmund Freud*

    E. *Anton Mesmer*

Q2 Which of the following MOST closely linked hypnosis with the use of strategic interactions (that employed use of metaphor and indirect methods of behavior-shaping)?

    A. *Hippolyte Bernheim*

    B. *Milton Erickson*

    C. *Martin Orne*

    D. *David Spiegel*

    E. *Joseph Wolpe*

Q3 Which of the following has NOT been found (through randomized clinical trials) to improve with application of hypnosis?

    A. *Cancer pain*

    B. *Hay fever*

    C. *Pain of labor and childbirth*

    D. *Postoperative wound healing*

    E. *Symptoms of irritable bowel syndrome*

Q4 Which of the following conditions or states is a contraindication to the use of hypnosis?

    A. *Conversion disorder*

    B. *Hay fever*

    C. *Obesity*

    D. *Paranoia*

    E. *Pregnancy*

Q5 True or False. Hypnotic susceptibility can be measured by use of the Stanford scales and Harvard Group scales of hypnotizability.

    A. *True*

    B. *False*

Chapter 15

Answers

Q1 The answer is: (E) Anton Mesmer.

The origin of medical hypnosis is generally attributed to Anton Mesmer, a Jesuit-trained 18th-century physician, who believed that health was determined by a proper balance of a universally present, invisible magnetic fluid. Mesmer's early method involved application of magnets. He was an important medical figure at the Austrian court, but he fell into discredit when a scandal occurred around his care of Maria Paradise, a young harpsichordist whose blindness appears to have been a form of conversion disorder.

Mesmer reestablished his practice in Paris and employed a device reminiscent of the Leyden jar, a source of significant popular interest in the Age of Enlightenment. His patients sat around a water-containing iron trough-like apparatus (*bacquet*) with a protruding iron rod. He was a colorful figure who accompanied his invocation for restored health with the passage of a wand; there was no physical contact with his patients. Susceptible individuals convulsed and were pronounced cured. An enthusiastic public greeted Mesmer's practice and theory of "animal magnetism." However, medical colleagues were less impressed.

The French Academy of Science established a committee led by Benjamin Franklin, the American Ambassador to France, who was an expert in electricity. The committee found no validation for Mesmer's magnetic theories, but determined that the effects were because of the subjects' "imagination."

James Esdaile, a 19th-century Scottish physician, was the first to take advantage of the somnambulistic state induced by Mesmerism to relieve surgical pain. Esdaile served as a military officer in the British East India Company, and took care of primarily Indian patients in and around Calcutta between 1845 and 1851. Over this period, Esdaile performed more than 3000 operations (including hundreds of major surgeries) using only Mesmerism as an anesthetic, with only a fraction of the complications and deaths that were commonplace at the time. Many of these operations were to remove scrotal tumors (scrotal hydroceles), which were endemic in India at the time, and which in extreme cases swelled to a weight greater than the rest of the body. Before Esdaile's use of Mesmeric anesthesia, surgery to remove these tumors usually resulted in death, owing to shock from massive blood loss during the operation.

Early in the 19th century, some surgeons advocated the use of this new procedure for pain reduction in the operating theater. James Braid, a British surgeon, called it "hypnosis" after the Greek root for sleep. Some questioned its apparent utility and thought it a humbug.

Although Sigmund Freud (the father of psychoanalysis) was a skilled hypnotist, he came to believe that it had an unwanted impact on transference, and it was therefore incompatible with his psychoanalytic method. Instead, Freud substituted his method of free association.

Q2 The answer is: (B) Milton Erickson.

Eriksonian hypnosis, named for its founder Milton Erikson, is a counterpoint to Freud's earlier position. Erikson advocated strategic interactions with his patients that employed use of metaphor and indirect methods of behavior-shaping. Although hypnotizability is generally considered to be an individual trait, Erikson believed that the efficacy of hypnotherapy depended on the skill of the therapist.

A prominent internist, Hippolyte Bernheim, studied hypnosis at a French school at Nancy. He worked with a country doctor known as "Pere Liebeault" for his *pro bono* work with patients who agreed to undergo hypnosis for therapeutic purposes. The Nancy School found hypnosis to be a normal phenomenon that operated through suggestion.

Martin Orne's work at the University of Pennsylvania identified the demand characteristics (that were based on a hierarchical relationship) of interaction between the hypnotist and the subject. He used sham hypnosis as an effective research tool. Orne also addressed the memory distortion that can occur with hypnosis, and exposed its lack of validity for courtroom procedures, and defined "trance logic" as a willing suspension of belief that highly hypnotizable subjects readily experience.

David Spiegel has pointed to absorption, dissociation, and automaticity as core components of the hypnotic experience. Absorption has been found to be the only personality trait related to an individual's ability to experience hypnosis.

Joseph Wolpe applied hypnosis or progressive muscle relaxation to facilitate systematic desensitization.

Q3 The answer is: (B) Hay fever.

Review of multiple randomized clinical trials shows that several conditions (e.g., cancer pain, pain of labor and childbirth, pain related to medical procedures, symptoms of irritable bowel syndrome, postoperative wound healing, and obesity) have been improved by use of hypnosis.

No evidence of efficacy (from controlled trials) has been found for use of hypnosis in schizophrenia, sufferers of hay fever, and delayed-type hypersensitivity responses.

Q4 The answer is: (D) Paranoia.

Contraindications to the use of hypnosis are limited to its use among paranoid individuals and its coercive application.

Rather than serving as a contraindication to its use, hypnosis may improve the pain of childbirth and facilitate weight loss in obesity. There is also some evidence that it may improve symptoms of conversion disorder, facilitate smoking cessation, and control tinnitus.

Q5 The answer is: (A) True.

Reliable measurement of hypnotic susceptibility is available with several scales (including the Stanford scales and Harvard Group scales of hypnotizability).

Across scales, approximately 10% to 15% of subjects fall into the "high hypnotizability" range, another 15% to 20% fall into the "low hypnotizability" range, and the remainder fall into an intermediate range.

Moderate levels of hypnotizability are important for clinical efficacy, although the level of hypnotic responsiveness does not ensure therapeutic success.

The Tellegen Absorption Scale also correlates with hypnotic responsiveness. Absorption refers to a process of concentration and a narrowing of attention. Clinical observations of absorption (for example, in competitive sports and other forms of performance) may be a clue to a patient's hypnotizability.

Cognitive-Behavioral Therapy, Behavioral Therapy, and Cognitive Therapy

Multiple-Choice Questions

Select the appropriate answer.

Q1   Which of the following types of therapy is MOST closely allied with use of exposure, relaxation, assertion training, problem-solving training, and contingency management?

A.   *Aromatherapy*

B.   *Behavioral therapy*

C.   *Hypnotherapy*

D.   *Pharmacotherapy*

E.   *Psychodynamically oriented psychotherapy*

Q2   Which of the following types of therapy is MOST closely allied with the correction of distorted thinking, and offers a means by which a patient can respond to maladaptive thoughts more adaptively?

A.   *Behavior therapy*

B.   *Cognitive therapy*

C.   *Hypnotherapy*

D.   *Pharmacotherapy*

E.   *Psychodynamically oriented psychotherapy*

Q3   Which of the following types of therapy is MOST closely allied with development of a strong, collaborative working alliance in the context of obtaining a detailed functional analysis of the patient's symptoms and the contexts in which they occur, and educating the patient about the nature of their disorder?

A.   *Aromatherapy*

B.   *Cognitive-behavioral therapy (CBT)*

C.   *Hypnotherapy*

D.   *Pharmacotherapy*

E.   *Psychodynamically oriented psychotherapy*

Q4 Which of the following types of therapy is MOST closely allied with having the patient practice interventions at home (i.e., do homework)?

A. *Aromatherapy*

B. *Cognitive-behavioral therapy (CBT)*

C. *Hypnotherapy*

D. *Pharmacotherapy*

E. *Psychodynamically oriented psychotherapy*

Q5 Which of the following terms BEST categorizes patterns that involve all-or-nothing thinking, discounting the positives, jumping to conclusions, and magnifying and minimizing?

A. *Cognitive distortions*

B. *Denial*

C. *Projection*

D. *Psychotic thinking*

E. *Splitting*

Chapter 16

Answers

Q1 The answer is: (B) Behavioral therapy.
Behavioral therapy refers to any of a large number of specific techniques that employ principles of learning to change human behavior. These techniques include exposure, relaxation, assertion training, social skills training, problem-solving training, modeling, contingency management, and behavioral activation. Many of these interventions are a direct outgrowth of principles of operant and respondent conditioning. Operant conditioning is concerned with the modification of behaviors by manipulation of the rewards and punishments, as well as the eliciting events for behavior.

Q2 The answer is: (B) Cognitive therapy.
Cognitive therapy was initially developed as a treatment for depression with the understanding that thoughts influence behavior, and it is largely maladaptive thinking styles that lead to maladaptive behavior and emotional distress, but currently includes approaches to a wide range of disorders.

Cognitive therapy provides techniques that correct distorted thinking and offers a means by which patients can respond to maladaptive thoughts more adaptively. In addition to examining cognitive distortions, cognitive therapy examines more pervasive core beliefs (e.g., "I am unlovable" or "I am incompetent") by assessing the themes that lie behind recurrent patterns of cognitive distortions. Those themes may be evaluated in regard to a patient's learning history (to assess the etiology of the beliefs with the goal of logically evaluating and altering the maladaptive beliefs).

Q3 The answer is: (B) Cognitive-behavioral therapy (CBT).
Contemporary cognitive-behavioral therapy (CBT) is a collaborative, structured, and goal-oriented intervention that often lasts 12 to 20 sessions. Treatment begins with a very detailed functional analysis of the patient's symptoms and the contexts in which they occur. Although the assessment may require some consideration of past events, such information is generally gathered if it is directly relevant to the solution of here-and-now problems. A collaborative relationship is often initiated in the context of educating the patient about the nature of the disorder, explaining the CBT model of the etiology and maintenance of the disorder, and the intervention that is derived from the model. Educating the patient serves to normalize aspects of the disorder; this can help to reduce self-blame. Psychoeducation (which includes information on the course of treatment) may also enhance patient motivation for change. The therapist and the patient also work together to develop clear, realistic treatment goals. CBT also emphasizes systematic monitoring of symptom change.

Q4 The answer is: (B) Cognitive-behavioral therapy (CBT).
CBT emphasizes home practice of interventions. Thus, review of homework is a major component of the CBT session. In reviewing the patient's homework, emphasis should be placed on what the patient learned, and what the patient wants to continue doing during the coming week for homework. The homework assignment, which is collaboratively set, should follow naturally from the problem-solving process in the treatment session. The use of homework in CBT draws from the understanding of therapy as a learning experience in which the patient acquires new skills. At the end of each CBT treatment session, a patient should be provided with an opportunity to summarize useful interventions from the session. This should also consist of asking the patient for feedback on the session, and involve efforts to enhance memories of, and the subsequent home application, for useful interventions.

Q5 The answer is: (A) Cognitive distortions.
Common examples of cognitive distortions include all-or-nothing thinking (e.g., looking at things in absolute, black-and-white categories), overgeneralization (e.g., viewing negative events as a never-ending pattern of defeat), discounting the positives (e.g., insisting that accomplishments or positive qualities "don't count"), jumping to conclusions (e.g., assuming that others are reacting negatively to you when there is

no evidence to support the assumptions or predicting that things will turn out badly), and magnifying or minimizing (e.g., blowing things out of proportion or shrinking their importance inappropriately).

These patterns of response are neither equivalent to a loss of reality testing (or psychotic thinking) nor psychological defenses.

PSYCHIATRIC DIAGNOSIS AND CONDITIONS

Chapter 17: DSM-5: A System for Psychiatric Diagnosis

DSM-5: A System for Psychiatric Diagnosis

Multiple-Choice Questions

Select the appropriate answer.

Q1   In what year was the first edition of the *Diagnostic and Statistical Manual of Mental Disorders* (DSM) published?

   A. *1949*

   B. *1952*

   C. *1955*

   D. *1958*

   E. *1961*

Q2   On which of the following DSM Axes were personality disorders and intellectual impairment located?

   A. *Axis I*

   B. *Axis II*

   C. *Axis III*

   D. *Axis IV*

   E. *Axis V*

Q3   On which of the following DSM Axes were psychosocial and environmental problems listed?

   A. *Axis I*

   B. *Axis II*

   C. *Axis III*

   D. *Axis IV*

   E. *Axis V*

Q4   Which of the following Global Assessment of Functioning (GAF) scores signifies severe symptoms?

   A. *80 to 100*

   B. *70 to 80*

   C. *60 to 70*

   D. *50 to 60*

   E. *Less than 50*

Q5   On which of the following DSM Axes would atrial fibrillation have been recorded?

    A.   *Axis I*

    B.   *Axis II*

    C.   *Axis III*

    D.   *Axis IV*

    E.   *Axis V*

Chapter 17
Answers

Q1 The answer is: (B) 1952.

From the first edition publication in 1952, to the second edition publication in 1968, and the third edition publication in 1980 (with a revised third edition in 1987), a change in emphasis took place; psychodynamic formulations were no longer intrinsic to diagnostic categorization, and the *Diagnostic and Statistical Manual of Mental Disorders* (DSM)-III was considered to be atheoretical and descriptive in its orientation (using a multiaxial system). As subsequent editions were compiled (with the DSM-IV publication in 1994 and the DSM-5 in 2013), there have been increased attempts to ensure diagnostic reliability and validity to incorporate research findings and to gather new information from field trials.

Q2 The answer is: (B) Axis II.

All psychiatric disorders included in the DSM, except for personality disorders and intellectual impairment (which were recorded on Axis II), were recorded on Axis I.

Q3 The answer is: (D) Axis IV.

Psychosocial and environmental problems were listed on Axis IV. Much of the time, Axis IV included only current problems, but in some cases past stressors are particularly relevant to diagnosis and clinical management and should be listed as well. For example, although it occurred several years previously, a contentious parental divorce that has exacerbated a teenager's anxiety disorder, and is critical to understanding the current family environment, should be included on Axis IV with the anxiety disorder listed as usual on Axis I. Sometimes, the psychosocial or environmental problem is important as a main target of treatment, rather than primarily via its effects on a separate psychiatric disorder.

Q4 The answer is: (E) Less than 50.

The Global Assessment of Functioning (GAF) is a number between 0 and 100 that summarizes the clinician's view of the patient's current degree of impairment in terms of psychosocial and occupational or educational function. Generally, normal function is coded in the 70 to 100 range, mild psychiatric symptoms fall into the 70 to 80 range, and moderate symptoms are assigned a number between 60 and 70. Severe symptoms are coded as 50 and below; higher levels of psychiatric support (such as intensive community-based treatment, residential settings, or inpatient hospitalization) are often required as function drops further down the scale. Although it may be difficult to determine in complicated cases, functional difficulty that results from "physical (or environmental) limitations" should not be considered in assigning a GAF score; the intent is to focus on the effects of mental illness. So, a patient who is no longer able to work or to live independently due to paraplegia may nonetheless receive a GAF score well above 70 if he has a wide social network, remains active in local politics, feels satisfied with life, and experiences frustration but takes effective action in the face of setbacks related to his physical problems.

The GAF score is not a static number; it changes for each patient over time. It can be used to track and succinctly communicate the course of psychiatric disorders over time and to monitor response to treatment. An increase in the GAF score from 35 to 55 during an inpatient hospitalization, for example, would suggest that the treatment plan has been at least somewhat effective, whereas a decline from 35 to 20 might suggest that it has not. Reporting the highest and lowest GAF score in the past year along with the current GAF score can also help to paint a concise picture of overall function. However, it is important to consider the limitations of the GAF scale in clinical decision-making. Neither the GAF score alone nor the entire multiaxial assessment, for that matter, can be a substitute for psychiatric clinical skill and judgment.

Q5 The answer is: (C) Axis III.

Axis III lists all relevant "general medical conditions," meaning nonpsychiatric illnesses. If the evaluator considers the medical problem and psychiatric problem to be closely interrelated, listings on both Axis I and Axis III may be appropriate. This may occur when the medical problem is thought to cause the psychiatric problem, resulting in a diagnosis of "psychiatric disorder due to a medical condition" on Axis I. It may also occur when an Axis I or II psychiatric disorder, subthreshold symptoms (e.g., anxiety or overeating), personality traits or defenses, or physiological stress responses are judged to have a negative impact on the course of a general medical condition; this scenario results in a diagnosis of "psychological factor affecting medical condition" on Axis I.

SECTION 6
DISORDERS OF COGNITION

Delirium

Multiple-Choice Questions

Select the appropriate answer.

Q1   In which of the following conditions is one MOST likely to observe dilated pupils, dry and flushed skin, elevated temperature, and disorientation?

A. *Anticholinergic excess*

B. *Hypoglycemia*

C. *Hypoxia*

D. *Meningitis*

E. *Wernicke's encephalopathy*

Q2   In which of the following conditions are myoclonic jerks in the context of delirium especially common?

A. *Anticholinergic excess*

B. *Hypoxia*

C. *Meningitis*

D. *Normeperidine toxicity*

E. *Wernicke's encephalopathy*

Q3   True or False. The electroencephalogram (EEG) of a patient with delirium is typically normal.

A. *True*

B. *False*

Q4   Which of the following agents can reverse the sedation induced by benzodiazepines?

A. *Benztropine*

B. *Flumazenil*

C. *Midazolam*

D. *Naloxone*

E. *Physostigmine*

Q5   Which of the following agents is a selective α_2-adrenergic agonist used for sedation and analgesia in the intensive care unit?

A. *Atropine*

B. *Benztropine*

C. *Dexmedetomidine*

D. *Flumazenil*

E. *Physostigmine*

Chapter 18

Answers

Q1 The answer is: (A) Anticholinergic excess.
In critical care settings, as in emergency departments, there are several (life-threatening) states that the clinician can consider routinely. These are states in which intervention needs to be especially prompt because failure to make the diagnosis may result in permanent central nervous system damage. These conditions are Wernicke's encephalopathy, withdrawal reactions, hypoxia, hypoglycemia, hypertensive encephalopathy, hyperthermia or hypothermia, intracerebral hemorrhage, meningitis/encephalitis, metabolic derangement, poisoning (whether exogenous or iatrogenic), and status epilepticus. These conditions are usefully recalled by the mnemonic device "WWHHHHIMMPS." Other, less urgent but still acute conditions that require intervention include subdural hematoma, septicemia, subacute bacterial endocarditis, hepatic or renal failure, thyrotoxicosis/myxedema, delirium tremens, anticholinergic psychosis, and complex partial seizures. If not already ruled out, when present, these conditions are easy to verify.

Anticholinergic excess typically causes dilated pupils, dry and flushed skin, elevated temperature, diminished bowel sounds, urinary retention, and disorientation. By contrast, adrenergic deliria (e.g., as from hypoglycemia) typically cause moist or clammy skin, as well as dilated pupils.

Q2 The answer is: (D) Normeperidine toxicity.
The number of drugs that can directly or indirectly (e.g., because of drug interactions) cause delirium (with its vast array of neuropsychiatric manifestations) are numerous. A common drug, such as the short-lasting meperidine, when used in doses above 300 mg/day for several days, causes central nervous system symptoms because the accumulation of its excitatory metabolite, normeperidine (which has a half-life of 30 hours), causes myoclonus (the best clue of normeperidine toxicity), anxiety, and ultimately seizures. The usual treatment for this condition is to stop the offending drug or to reduce the dose; however, at times this is not possible.

Q3 The answer is: (B) False.
Of all the diagnostic studies available, the electroencephalogram (EEG) may be the most useful tool in the diagnosis of delirium. Engel and Romano reported in 1959 their (now classic) findings on the EEG in delirium, namely generalized slowing to the theta-delta range in the patient with delirium, the consistency of this finding despite wide-ranging underlying conditions, and resolution of this slowing with effective treatment of the delirium. EEG findings may even clarify the etiology of a delirium, considering that delirium tremens is associated with low-voltage fast activity superimposed on slow waves, sedative-hypnotic toxicity produces fast beta activity (greater than 12 Hz), and hepatic encephalopathy is classically associated with triphasic waves.

Q4 The answer is: (B) Flumazenil.
Specific antidotes can reverse the delirium caused by some drugs. Flumazenil and naloxone reverse the effects of benzodiazepines and opioid analgesics, respectively. However, caution is required because use of flumazenil may precipitate seizures in a benzodiazepine-dependent patient, and naloxone can also precipitate narcotic withdrawal in a narcotic-dependent patient. Benztropine can treat extrapyramidal symptoms (e.g., dystonia) induced by antipsychotics, and physostigmine can reverse the manifestations of anticholinergic delirium. Midazolam is a benzodiazepine, not a benzodiazepine antagonist.

Q5 The answer is: (C) Dexmedetomidine
Dexmedetomidine is a selective α_2-adrenergic agonist used for sedation and analgesia in the intensive care unit setting. Its relative lack of amnestic effect may limit its use in the treatment of the patient with delirium, owing to an increased likelihood of distressing recollections persisting from the period of sedation.

Intravenous benzodiazepines (particularly diazepam, chlordiazepoxide, and lorazepam) are routinely used to treat agitated states, particularly delirium tremens and alcohol withdrawal; their effects can be reversed by use of flumazenil.

Atropine is an anticholinergic agent that is not used for either sedation or pain control.

Dementia

Multiple-Choice Questions

Select the appropriate answer.

Q1   Which of the following is considered the BEST approximation of the incidence of dementia for all individuals older than 65 years of age?

    A. *1%*

    B. *5%*

    C. *15%*

    D. *25%*

    E. *45%*

Q2   Which of the following is the MOST common cause of dementia?

    A. *Alzheimer's disease*

    B. *Creutzfeldt-Jacob disease*

    C. *Frontotemporal dementia*

    D. *Lewy body dementia*

    E. *Vascular dementia*

Q3   Which of the following is the GREATEST risk factor for Alzheimer's disease?

    A. *Genetic propensity*

    B. *Head trauma*

    C. *Longevity*

    D. *Use of NSAIDs*

    E. *Vascular pathology*

Q4   Which of the following is the neuropathological hallmark of Alzheimer's disease?

    A. *Lewy bodies*

    B. *Multifocal leukoencephalopathy*

    C. *Neurofibrillary tangles and neuritic plaques*

    D. *Subdural hemorrhages*

    E. *Unidentified bright objects*

Q5   True or False. Apolipoprotein E (*APOE*) is a susceptibility gene that increases the risk for AD without causing the disease.

    A. *True*

    B. *False*

Q6 True or False. Early-onset genes probably account for half of the cases of Alzheimer's disease (AD) that occur before age 60.

  A. *True*

  B. *False*

Q7 Which of the following terms BEST describes the class of medication to which donepezil (Aricept) belongs?

  A. *Cholinesterase inhibitor*

  B. *Glutamate antagonist*

  C. *Serotonin-norepinephrine reuptake inhibitor (SNRI)*

  D. *Selective serotonin reuptake inhibitor (SSRI)*

  E. *Tricyclic antidepressant (TCA)*

Q8 Which of the following conditions is MOST consistently manifest by progressive difficulties with balance and gait, resulting in frequent falls early in the disease, progressive loss of voluntary control of eye movements, and progressive cognitive and behavioral difficulties?

  A. *Alzheimer's disease*

  B. *Creutzfeldt-Jacob disease*

  C. *Frontotemporal dementia*

  D. *Lewy body dementia*

  E. *Progressive supranuclear palsy*

Q9 Which of the following conditions is BEST characterized by gait disturbance, frontal systems dysfunction, and urinary incontinence?

  A. *Alzheimer's disease*

  B. *Creutzfeldt-Jacob disease*

  C. *Lewy body dementia*

  D. *Normal pressure hydrocephalus*

  E. *Progressive supranuclear palsy*

Q10 Which of the following conditions is BEST characterized by a characteristic triad of dementia, myoclonus, and distinctive periodic EEG complexes?

  A. *Alzheimer's disease*

  B. *Creutzfeldt-Jacob disease*

  C. *Lewy body dementia*

  D. *Normal pressure hydrocephalus*

  E. *Progressive supranuclear palsy*

Chapter 19

Answers

Q1 The answer is: (C) 15%.

The onset of dementia is most common in the 70s and 80s, and is quite rare before age 40. Both the incidence (the number of new cases per year in the population) and the prevalence (the fraction of the population that has the disorder) rise steeply with age. This general pattern has been observed both for dementia overall and for Alzheimer's disease (AD) in particular. Estimates of the prevalence of dementia vary to some extent depending on which diagnostic criteria are used. The incidence of dementia of almost all types increases with age such that it may affect 15% of all individuals over age 65, and up to 45% of those over age 80. However, the peak age of onset varies somewhat among the dementias, with frontotemporal dementia and vascular dementia tending to begin earlier (e.g., in the 60s) and AD somewhat later.

Q2 The answer is: (A) Alzheimer's disease.

The most common type of dementia (accounting for approximately 50% to 70% of cases) is Alzheimer's disease (AD). Among the neurodegenerative dementias, Lewy body dementia is the next most common, followed by frontotemporal dementia (FTD).

Vascular dementia (formerly known as multi-infarct dementia) can have several different etiologies; it can exist separately from AD, but the two frequently co-occur. Dementias associated with Parkinson's disease and Creutzfeldt-Jacob disease (CJD) are much less common.

Q3 The answer is: (C) Longevity.

Longevity carries the greatest risk of Alzheimer's disease (AD). Vascular risk factors (except for male gender), including diabetes, atherosclerosis, hypertension, and elevated cholesterol, all increase the risk of AD, as well as of vascular dementia, although the mechanisms are unclear. A history of head trauma also increases the risk of AD.

Several pharmacological agents (notably post-menopausal estrogen supplementation, nonsteroidal antiinflammatory agents [NSAIDs], and antioxidants) are associated with a decreased risk of AD in epidemiological studies, but clinical trials of these agents have thus far been disappointing. More preliminary evidence links statins and H_2 blockers to protection against AD. Mental and physical exercise has also been associated with prevention of AD, but there is a concern that these findings may be related to the impact of prodromal symptoms at baseline. However, as part of a comprehensive vascular risk reduction program, physical exercise has many benefits that may include dementia prevention.

Q4 The answer is: (C) Neurofibrillary tangles and neuritic plaques.

In his initial 1907 case, Alois Alzheimer identified abnormal nerve cells and fiber clusters in the cerebral cortex using then new silver-staining methods at autopsy. These findings, considered to be the hallmark neuropathological lesions of AD, are known as neurofibrillary tangles (NFTs) and neuritic plaques (NPs).

Beta-amyloid protein, present in soluble form in the brain but also a major component of plaques, is thought to play a central pathophysiological role in the disease, perhaps via direct neurotoxicity. NFTs are found in neurons and are primarily composed of anomalous cytoskeletal proteins (such as hyperphosphorylated tau), which may also be toxic to neurons and contribute to AD pathophysiology.

Lewy bodies are associated with Lewy body dementia and Parkinson's disease, while progressive multifocal leukoencephalopathy is associated with infectious etiologies. Subdural hemorrhages are linked with trauma, while unidentified bright objects are radiological (not neuropathological) findings.

Q5 The answer is: (A) True.

Apolipoprotein E (*APOE*) is a susceptibility gene that increases the risk for Alzheimer's disease (AD) without causing the disease. *APOE* has three alleles, 2, 3, and 4, which have a complex relationship to risk for both AD and cardiovascular disease, with the 2 allele decreasing the risk of both disorders and increasing the longevity, and the 4 allele increasing the risk and decreasing the longevity. The effect of *APOE*-4 varies with age; it is most marked in the 60s and falls substantially beyond age 80 or 90 years. *APOE* seems to act principally by modifying the age of onset, which is lowest in those with two copies of the risk allele, and intermediate in those with one. The *APOE* effect appears to be stronger in women and in Caucasians, which may relate to their lower risk of cardiovascular disease. Investigators believe that there are more AD genes to be discovered, and one analysis predicts four to seven additional AD genes. However, these genes have been quite difficult to identify, and *APOE* remains the only documented late-onset AD gene.

Q6 The answer is: (A) True.

Four genes are recognized as being involved in AD. Three of them lead to early-onset Alzheimer's disease (AD) in an autosomal dominant fashion. Although these genes have limited public health impact, they are devastating for affected families. These early-onset genes probably account for half of the cases of AD that occur before age 60. More critically, they have made a large contribution to our understanding of the pathophysiology of AD, and to the development of promising therapeutic strategies.

Amyloid precursor protein (*APP*) on chromosome 21 was recognized first. To date, there are 26 mutations that affect 72 families. The age of onset for these *APP* mutations varies, and it is modified by *APOE* genotype.

Next discovered was presenilin 1 (*PSEN1*) on chromosome 14. There are 156 *PSEN1* mutations affecting 342 families to date; many have been found in a single family, often referred to as "genetically private." *PSEN1* mutations are associated with an age of onset in the 40s and 50s; these mutations are not modified by the *APOE* genotype. Although overall quite rare, *PSEN1* accounts for the great majority of autosomal dominant early-onset AD. *PSEN1* mutations have also been observed in nonfamilial early-onset AD cases.

The last early-onset gene is presenilin 2 (*PSEN2*) on chromosome 1. *PSEN2* has 10 reported mutations affecting 18 families to date. The age of onset is quite variable, extending into the late-onset AD range, and it is modified by *APOE* genotype.

Q7 The answer is: (A) Cholinesterase inhibitor.

Four of the five medications approved by the Food and Drug Administration (FDA) now in use for treatment of Alzheimer's disease (AD) are designed to prevent the breakdown of acetylcholine (ACh), thereby increasing concentrations of ACh in the hippocampus and the neocortex, areas of the brain important for memory and for other cognitive symptoms. These cholinesterase inhibitors include donepezil (Aricept), rivastigmine (Exelon), tacrine (Cognex), and galantamine (Razadyne). All have been shown to slow the progression of AD by stabilizing cognition and behavior, participation in activities of daily living (ADLs), and global function in mild to moderate AD, by improving cognition and behavior in moderate to severe patients with AD, by delaying nursing home placement, and by reducing both health care expenditures and caregiver burden for patients with AD. However, the effects are modest, and they are not apparent in some individuals. Tacrine is no longer widely used because of its association with hepatotoxicity.

The fifth medication, memantine (Namenda), has been proven effective in patients with more severe forms of AD. Memantine, a partial uncompetitive glutamate antagonist, normalizes glutamate receptor activity in the setting of excessive amounts of the neurotransmitter. While normal glutamate activity is thought to be essential for learning and memory, excessive quantities are thought to contribute to neurodegeneration. Memantine has been used in combination with cholinesterase inhibitors for greater effectiveness in slowing the progression of AD.

Q8 The answer is: (E) Progressive supranuclear palsy.

Progressive supranuclear palsy (PSP) is a dementia characterized by the presence of cognitive and behavioral features along with specific motor abnormalities. The classic clinical features of the disease are progressive difficulties with balance and gait, resulting in frequent falls early in the disease, progressive loss of voluntary control of eye movements, and progressive cognitive and behavioral difficulties. Patients with PSP often have difficulties with the coordination of eyelid opening and closing, dysarthria, dysphagia, and fixed facial expression akin to surprise. Symptoms similar to those of Parkinson's disease are also present, particularly akinesia and axial rigidity. The cognitive and behavioral features are usually referable to frontal lobe dysfunction and may closely resemble those of frontotemporal dementia (FTD) (such as executive dysfunction, apathy, and reduced processing speed).

Q9 The answer is: (D) Normal pressure hydrocephalus.

Normal pressure hydrocephalus (NPH) is a condition that involves enlargement of the ventricles leading to cognitive and motor difficulties. About 250,000 people in the United States suffer from this disease; it usually occurs in adults 55 years old or older. Intermittent pressure increases are thought to cause ventricular expansion over time, with damage to the adjacent white matter tracts that connect the frontal lobes. The main clinical features are gait disturbance, frontal systems dysfunction, and urinary incontinence. Patients need not have all three symptoms to have NPH. There are no clear genetic causes. The main risk factors relate to conditions that adversely affect the function of the ventricular system for cerebrospinal fluid (CSF) egress, which include history of head trauma, intracranial hemorrhage, meningitis, or any inflammatory or structural process that might damage the meninges.

Q10 The answer is: (B) Creutzfeldt-Jacob disease.

Creutzfeldt-Jacob disease (CJD) is a rare disorder that causes a characteristic triad of dementia, myoclonus, and distinctive periodic EEG complexes. The typical age of onset is around age 60 years. CJD is caused by prions, novel proteinaceous infective agents. Prion protein, PrP, an amyloid protein encoded on chromosome 20, is the major constituent of prions. PrP normally exists in a PrPc isoform; in a pathological state, it is transformed to the PrPSc isoform, which condenses in neurons and causes their death. As prion-induced changes accumulate, the cerebral cortex takes on the distinctive microscopic, vacuolar appearance of spongiform encephalopathy. The CSF in almost 90% of CJD cases contains traces of prion proteins detected by a routine lumbar puncture (LP). CJD is transmissible, and can cause pyramidal, extrapyramidal, or cerebellar impairment, as well as myoclonus. Treatment in these unfortunate cases is supportive, as it follows a characteristically rapid and fatal course over an average of 6 months.

Intellectual Disability

Multiple-Choice Questions

Select the appropriate answer.

Q1 What is the BEST estimate for the number of potential causes for intellectual disability?

A. *5*

B. *25*

C. *75*

D. *150*

E. *750*

Q2 Which of the following conditions is the MOST common inherited cause of intellectual disability?

A. *Fetal alcohol syndrome*

B. *Fragile X syndrome*

C. *Lesch-Nyhan syndrome*

D. *Prader-Willi syndrome*

E. *Williams syndrome*

Q3 Which of the following is generally considered to be the MOST common reason for psychiatric consultation and for institutionalization in those with an intellectual disability?

A. *Aggressive behavior*

B. *Communication disorders*

C. *Disordered eating*

D. *Learning disorders*

E. *Physical disabilities*

Q4 Which of the following terms BEST labels the eating of inedibles (including dirt, paper clips, and cigarette butts) that is usually seen in those with more severe intellectual disabilities?

A. *Copraxia*

B. *Pica*

C. *Rumination*

D. *Self-stimulation*

E. *Stereotypy*

Q5   Which of the following conditions typically manifests with short stature, hypogonadism, and marked obesity with hyperphagia?

A.   Down syndrome

B.   Fragile X syndrome

C.   Prader-Willi syndrome

D.   Twenty-two q-eleven (22q11) deletion syndrome

E.   Williams syndrome

Chapter 20

Answers

Q1 The answer is: (E) 750.

Currently, there are more than 750 known causes of intellectual disability; however, in up to 30% of cases, no clear etiology is found. This can be disheartening for patients, parents, families, and caregivers as they search for an understanding of a condition that will profoundly affect their lives.

Q2 The answer is: (B) Fragile X syndrome.

Fragile X syndrome is the most common inherited cause of intellectual disability, with the *FMR1* gene located on the X chromosome.

Fetal alcohol syndrome, the most common "acquired" cause of intellectual disability, has no identified chromosomal abnormality, as it is a toxin-based insult.

Down syndrome is the most common genetic cause of intellectual disability; it involves trisomy of chromosome 21.

These three etiologies account for nearly one-third of cases of intellectual disability.

Q3 The answer is: (A) Aggressive behavior.

Aggressive behavior is the main reason for psychiatric consultation and for institutionalization in those with an intellectual disability. Once a thorough assessment has been completed and no clear etiology found, the problem falls into the realm of an impulse-control disorder. Behavioral therapy is usually the first-line treatment, with subsequent psychopharmacologic intervention if behavioral therapy proves inadequate. Typically, agents used to treat impulsive aggression are tried; these include alpha-agonists, beta-blockers, lithium, other mood stabilizers/antiepileptic drugs, and antipsychotics.

Q4 The answer is: (B) Pica.

Pica involves the eating of inedibles (including dirt, paper clips, and cigarette butts). Although usually seen in those with more severe intellectual disabilities, this behavior also can be seen as a normal variant in regularly developing children. One must be aware of the potential medical hazards of ingested items; fortunately, major medical sequelae from this behavior are usually rare. Behavioral therapy (such as environmental control with limited access to preferred items and response blocking) is the mainstay of treatment. There is minimal evidence that psychopharmacologic treatments are useful, and dietary supplements have not been shown to be effective.

Copraxia involves rectal digging, feces smearing, and coprophagia. It is a rare disorder usually seen in those with profound intellectual disabilities. Once medical issues are ruled out, sensory issues can be assessed by a trained occupational therapist. Application of appropriate substitute materials can sometimes be helpful. Behavioral therapy again is a first-line treatment.

Rumination refers to repeated acts of vomiting, chewing, and reingestion of the vomitus. It is seen in those with severe to profound intellectual disabilities, and it can be associated with both gastrointestinal pathology and with behavioral issues (e.g., overfeeding).

Self-stimulation has been seen in cases of severe sensory deprivation.

Stereotypies are invariant, pathological motor behaviors or action sequences without obvious reinforcement. They often cause no real harm or dysfunction but may be upsetting to caregivers or staff who may believe they interfere with the patient's quality of life. These behaviors are often seen in institutionalized adults with severe to profound intellectual disabilities; however, they can also be a normal variant in children without cognitive delay.

First-line treatment for stereotypies is behavioral therapy.

Q5 The answer is: (C) Prader-Willi syndrome.

Individuals with Prader-Willi syndrome typically have short stature, hypogonadism, and marked obesity with hyperphagia. In approximately 70% of cases, the syndrome results from a chromosome 15 deletion. The level of intellectual disability can vary.

Individuals with Down syndrome, or trisomy 21, have the classic physical features of round face, a flat nasal bridge, and short stature. Their level of intellectual disability is variable.

Individuals with fragile X syndrome have an abnormality on the long arm of the X chromosome at the q27 site (*FMR1* gene). Common physical features include an elongated face, prominent ears, and macroorchidism. Most affected individuals are males, but females can also be affected. Their level of intellectual disability varies.

Twenty-two q-eleven (*22q11*) deletion syndrome (including velocardiofacial syndrome and DiGeorge syndrome) is an autosomal dominant condition manifested by a medical history of midline malformations (such as cleft palate, velopharyngeal insufficiency, and cardiac malformations [such as a ventricular septal defect]). Patients have small stature, a prominent tubular nose with bulbous tip, and a squared nasal root. There is often a history of speech delay with hypernasal speech. Their level of cognitive impairment varies from learning disabilities and mild intellectual impairment to more severe levels of intellectual disabilities.

Williams syndrome results from a deletion on chromosome 7. These individuals have elfin-like faces and a classic starburst (or stellate) pattern of the iris. They can have supravalvular aortic stenosis, as well as renal artery stenosis and hypertension. Their level of intellectual disability varies. Behaviorally, they can be loquacious communicators, a phenomenon referred to as "cocktail party speech" (often attributable to a higher verbal than performance IQ).

SECTION 7

MENTAL DISORDERS DUE TO ANOTHER MEDICAL CONDITION

Chapter 21: Mental Disorders Due to Another Medical Condition

Mental Disorders Due to Another Medical Condition

Multiple-Choice Questions

Select the appropriate answer.

Q1   True or False. Mental disorders due to another medical condition (DTAMC) are defined by the *Diagnostic and Statistical Manual of Mental Disorders, 5th edition* as psychiatric conditions with symptoms severe enough to merit treatment, and determined to be the direct, physiological effect of a (nonpsychiatric) medical condition.

    A. *True*

    B. *False*

Q2   True or False. The onset of psychiatric symptoms that coincides with the onset (or increased severity) of a medical condition proves causation.

    A. *True*

    B. *False*

Q3   True or False. Psychiatric manifestations uncharacteristic of primary mental disorders should raise the suspicion of a direct physiological effect of a medical condition.

    A. *True*

    B. *False*

Q4   Which of the following conditions is MOST likely to have a predilection for the temporal and inferomedial frontal lobes, and cause gustatory or olfactory hallucinations or anosmia?

    A. *Herpes simplex virus infection*

    B. *Lyme disease*

    C. *Neurosyphilis*

    D. *Rabies*

    E. *Thiamine deficiency*

Q5   In which of the following conditions are the pupils MOST likely to be small, irregular, unequal, able to accommodate but not to react to light?

    A. *Herpes simplex virus infection*

    B. *Lyme disease*

    C. *Neurosyphilis*

    D. *Rabies*

    E. *Thiamine deficiency*

Q6 Which of the following conditions is MOST likely to be induced by the administration of glucose without prior thiamine repletion?

A. *Herpes simplex virus infection*

B. *Lyme disease*

C. *Neurosyphilis*

D. *Rabies*

E. *Wernicke-Korsakoff syndrome*

Q7 Which of the following conditions is MOST likely to be manifest by psychosis, ataxia, myoclonus, and dementia and to be rapidly progressive and fatal?

A. *Creutzfeldt-Jakob disease*

B. *Herpes simplex virus infection*

C. *Lyme disease*

D. *Neurosyphilis*

E. *Wernicke-Korsakoff syndrome*

Q8 Which of the following conditions is MOST likely to be manifest by neuropathy, ataxia, paresthesias, visual field defects, depression, irritability, and psychosis?

A. *Carbon monoxide poisoning*

B. *Lead poisoning*

C. *Lyme disease*

D. *Mercury toxicity*

E. *Wernicke-Korsakoff syndrome*

Chapter 21

Answers

Q1 The answer is: (A) True.

Mental disorders due to another medical condition (DTAMC) are defined by the *Diagnostic and Statistical Manual of Mental Disorders, 5th edition* as psychiatric conditions with symptoms severe enough to merit treatment, and determined to be the direct, physiological effect of a (nonpsychiatric) medical condition. This conceptual language substitutes for previously less useful, more dichotomous terms (e.g., organic vs. functional) that minimized the psychosocial and environmental influences on physical symptoms, and implied that psychiatric symptoms were without physiological cause. General qualifiers further delineate mental disorders DTAMC from other co-occurring medical and psychiatric conditions. The mental disorder must be deemed the direct pathophysiological consequence of the medical condition, and must not be better accounted for by another, primary mental disorder. Symptoms that are only present during delirium (i.e., with fluctuations in the level of consciousness and cognitive deficits) are not considered DTAMC. Similarly, the presence of dementia (e.g., with memory impairment with aphasia, apraxia, agnosia, or disturbance of executive function) takes precedence over a diagnosis of DTAMC. Substance-induced symptoms (e.g., alcohol intoxication) do not meet criteria for DTAMC.

Q2 The answer is: (B) False.

The determination of direct physiological causality is a complex issue. The onset of psychiatric symptoms that coincides with the onset (or increased severity) of the medical condition is suggestive of, but does not prove, causation. Medical and mental disorders may merely coexist. The initial presentation of a medical condition may be psychiatric (e.g., depression that manifests before the diagnostic awareness of pancreatic carcinoma), or the psychiatric symptoms may be disproportionate to the medical severity (e.g., irritability in patients with negligible sensorimotor symptoms of multiple sclerosis). It also happens that psychiatric symptoms may occur long after the onset of medical illness (e.g., psychosis that develops after years of epilepsy). Psychiatric improvement that coincides with treatment of the medical condition supports a causal relationship, although psychiatric symptoms that do not clear with resolution of the medical condition do not rule-out causation (e.g., depression that persists beyond normalization of hypothyroidism). There are also mental disorders DTAMC that respond to, and require, direct treatment (e.g., interictal depression), which should not be interpreted as evidence of a primary mental disorder.

Q3 The answer is: (A) True.

Psychiatric manifestations uncharacteristic of primary mental disorders should raise the suspicion of a direct physiological effect of a medical condition. Features to consider include the age of onset (e.g., new-onset panic disorder in an elderly man), the usual time course (e.g., abrupt onset of depression), and exaggerated or unusual features of related symptoms (e.g., severe cognitive dysfunction with otherwise mild depressive symptoms). However, the typical manifestation of a psychiatric syndrome supports the likelihood that medical and mental disorders are comorbid but not causative. Such typical features include a history of similar episodes without the co-occurring of the medical condition, and a family history of the mental disorder.

Q4 The answer is: (A) Herpes simplex virus infection.

Herpes simplex virus is the most frequent etiology of focal encephalopathy, and may cause either simple or complex partial seizures. With a predilection for the temporal and inferomedial frontal lobes, herpes simplex virus is well known to cause gustatory or olfactory hallucinations or anosmia (loss of the sense of smell). This concentration in limbic structures may also explain the personality change, bizarre behavior, and psychotic symptoms that some affected patients exhibit. Such personality changes, cognitive difficulties, and affective lability may be persistent.

Rabies is a viral infection of the central nervous system (CNS) in mammals, generally transmitted by the infected saliva of an animal bite. The bite location, magnitude of the inoculum, and extent of host defenses are the likely determinants of the delay from contact to onset of symptoms, as the virus travels along peripheral nerves centripetally to the CNS. Paresthesias or fasciculations at the bite location are characteristic aspects that distinguish rabies from viral syndromes with otherwise similar prodromes. Physical agitation and excitation give way to episodic confusion, psychosis, and combativeness. These episodes, possibly interspersed with lucid intervals, are the harbinger of acute encephalitis, brainstem dysfunction, and coma. Autonomic dysfunction, cranial nerve involvement, upper motor neuron weakness and paralysis, and often vocal cord paralysis occur. Roughly half of rabies-infected humans experience the classic "hydrophobia" (i.e., violent and severely painful spasms of the diaphragm, laryngeal, pharyngeal, and accessory respiratory muscles, triggered by attempts to swallow liquids).

The broad range of neuropsychiatric sequelae of Lyme disease require clinicians in all areas to consider Lyme disease because the symptoms are nonspecific, highly variable, often delayed, and recurrent. The target sites for the spirochete include the heart, eyes, joints, muscles, peripheral nervous system, or CNS, where it may lie dormant for long periods (e.g., months to years) so that memory of the initial bite has long since faded.

Fatigue, irritability, confusion, labile mood, and disturbed sleep may herald Lyme encephalitis. The much less common presentation of Lyme encephalomyelitis may be confused with multiple sclerosis. Some patients go on to develop chronic encephalopathy, a broad scope of persistent disturbances in personality, behavior (e.g., disorganized, distractible, catatonic, mute, or violent), cognition (e.g., short-term memory, memory retrieval, verbal fluency, concentration, attention, orientation, and processing speed), mood (e.g., depressed, manic, or labile), thought, or perception (e.g., paranoia, hallucinations, depersonalization, hyperacusis, or photophobia). Although extremely rare, more severe sequelae may include dementia, seizures, or stroke.

The signs and symptoms of neurosyphilis can be recalled with the mnemonic PARESIS and suggest the frontal and more diffuse nature of the syndrome. Personality change may be striking, and can involve apathy, poor judgment, lack of insight, irritability, and (new onset of) poor personal hygiene and grooming. Patients may also have difficulty with calculations and short-term memory. Later signs include mood lability, delusions of grandeur, hallucinations, disorientation, and dementia.

In famine or extreme poverty, thiamine (vitamin B_1) deficiency presents as beriberi, but in the United States the alcoholism-associated Wernicke-Korsakoff syndrome is the more common presentation. Although single-system involvement occurs, the most common presentation is a blend of cerebral, neuropathic, and cardiovascular signs and symptoms. The initial symptoms tend to be nonspecific (e.g., poor concentration, apathy, mild agitation, or depressed mood), but are followed by more disabling signs (e.g., confusion, amnesia, or confabulation) of prolonged, severe deficiency.

Q5 The answer is: (C) Neurosyphilis.

Historically, less than 10% of patients with untreated syphilis develop a symptomatic form of parenchymatous neurosyphilis known as general paresis, 10 to 20 years after their initial infection. Later signs include mood lability, delusions of grandeur, hallucinations, disorientation, and dementia. It is during this late stage that the classic neurologic signs may appear (e.g., tremor, dysarthria, hyperreflexia, hypotonia, ataxia, and Argyll Robertson pupils [small, irregular, unequal, able to accommodate but not to react to light]). The diagnosis is confirmed by having a cerebrospinal fluid with elevated protein and lymphocytes and a positive (cerebrospinal fluid) Venereal Disease Research Laboratory slide test for treponemal antibodies.

Q6 The answer is: (E) Wernicke-Korsakoff syndrome.

In famine or extreme poverty, thiamine (vitamin B_1) deficiency presents as beriberi, but in the United States the alcoholism-associated Wernicke-Korsakoff syndrome is the more common presentation. Factors (such as total caloric intake and activity) seem to mediate the presentation, as most with malnutrition or alcoholism do not exhibit symptoms. Although single-system involvement occurs, the most common presentation is a blend of cerebral, neuropathic, and cardiovascular signs and symptoms. As with niacin deficiency, the initial symptoms tend to be nonspecific (e.g., poor concentration, apathy, mild agitation, or depressed mood), but are followed by more disabling signs (e.g., confusion, amnesia, or confabulation) of prolonged, severe deficiency. Iatrogenic conversion of asymptomatic thiamine deficiency to Wernicke-Korsakoff syndrome may be induced by the administration of glucose without prior thiamine repletion.

Q7 The answer is: (A) Creutzfeldt-Jakob disease.

Creutzfeldt-Jakob disease is a disease primarily of those aged 50 to 70 years. This rapidly progressive, fatal, prion disease is exceedingly rare, with most cases thought to be sporadic. Roughly 5% to 15% appear to be familial. Iatrogenic, person-to-person infection has also occurred following corneal transplantation and therapeutic use of cadaveric human growth hormone or cadaveric gonadotropins. The initial presentation may be nonspecific and include problems of cognition (memory or judgment), mood (lability), perception (illusions or distortions), or sensorimotor function (ataxic gait, vertigo, or dizziness). More ominous signs of psychosis and confusion herald the dementia and myoclonus considered the hallmarks of Creutzfeldt-Jakob disease. Patients generally die within a year, becoming spastic, mute, and finally stuporous.

Q8 The answer is: (D) Mercury toxicity.

Mercury is associated with two distinct syndromes of toxicity. If the exposure is from the organic form (e.g., from contaminated fish), then neurologic symptoms predominate (e.g., motor-sensory neuropathy, cerebellar ataxia, slurred speech, paresthesias, and visual field defects), with less dramatic psychiatric manifestations (e.g., depression, irritability, or mild dementia). Toxic inorganic mercury exposure, however, has an initial psychiatric presentation (i.e., the Mad Hatter syndrome) of depression, irritability, and psychosis, followed by less striking neurologic findings (e.g., tremor, weakness, and headache). Although occupational exposure and mercury thermometers have been largely eliminated, mercury continues to pose a threat because of its availability in folk medicines, botanical preparations, and breakable capsules (used by certain cultural or religious sects to sprinkle mercury in the home or car).

Carbon monoxide poisoning from defective heating or exhaust ventilation can present as a nondescript flu-like syndrome (e.g., malaise, cough, and nausea). Low-level exposure of a more chronic nature causes depressive symptoms and cognitive decline. More severe poisoning results in memory dysfunction, visual problems, parkinsonism, confabulation, psychosis, and delirium.

Low-level lead exposure, not solely a concern of young children, also presents with nondescript psychiatric symptoms suggestive of depression (e.g., fatigue, sleepiness, depressed mood, and apathy). Adults and adolescents are at risk for excessive lead exposure from environmental, recreational, and occupational sources. Besides the well-known risk of lead-based paint, running or biking in heavily trafficked areas, doing home repairs or remodeling, and even drinking from leaded crystal increases one's exposure. Artists of various crafts are at risk (e.g., stained glass, ceramic, and lead-figure artisans), as are art conservators. Those who use firearms for work or recreation should monitor their lead levels. Gasoline, solvents, and cleaning fluids are sources of organic lead exposure, associated with nightmares, restlessness, and psychotic symptoms. Extreme levels produce seizures and coma.

SECTION 8
SLEEP DISORDERS

Chapter 22: Sleep Disorders

Sleep Disorders

Multiple-Choice Questions

Select the appropriate answer.

Q1   In which of the following years was rapid eye movement (REM) sleep first observed on the electroencephalogram (EEG)?

   A.   *1928*

   B.   *1935*

   C.   *1953*

   D.   *1968*

   E.   *1979*

Q2   Which of the following is the interval at which REM sleep typically occurs throughout a night's sleep?

   A.   *15 minutes*

   B.   *30 minutes*

   C.   *45 minutes*

   D.   *60 minutes*

   E.   *90 minutes*

Q3   True or False. Sleepwalking tends to occur during the first third of a night's sleep.

   A.   *True*

   B.   *False*

Q4   The presence of two or more sleep-onset REM periods on a multiple sleep latency test (along with pathological sleepiness) is considered diagnostic of which of the following conditions?

   A.   *Kleine-Levin syndrome*

   B.   *Obstructive sleep apnea*

   C.   *Narcolepsy*

   D.   *Periodic limb movement disorder*

   E.   *Sleepwalking*

Q5   Which of the following agents approved for the treatment of insomnia is a melatonin receptor agonist?

   A.   *Chloral hydrate*

   B.   *Diphenhydramine*

   C.   *Mirtazapine*

   D.   *Ramelteon*

   E.   *Trazodone*

Q6 Which of the following manifestations is NOT a component of the tetrad of features of narcolepsy?

A. *Cataplexy*

B. *Hypnagogic hallucinations*

C. *Myoclonic jerking*

D. *Sleep attacks*

E. *Sleep paralysis*

Chapter 22

Answers

Q1 The answer is: (C) 1953.

The electroencephalogram (EEG), developed in 1928 by Berger, a German psychiatrist, became an important tool for understanding sleep physiology.

Rapid eye movement (REM) sleep was first observed in 1953, and the link with REM and dreaming began to emerge several years later.

Sleep apnea was first recognized in 1956, and an understanding of the prevalence and significance of this disorder continues to evolve.

Current classification of sleep stages is in great part based on all-night EEG monitoring, standardized in 1968.

New disorders, such as REM-sleep behavior disorder and nocturnal eating disorder, have been recognized within the past 15 years, confirming that this relatively young field of study is still growing.

An international classification system for sleep disorders was first published in 1979, under the chairmanship of Howard Roffwarg; the second edition of the international classification system for sleep disorders was published in 2006.

Q2 The answer is: (E) 90 minutes.

The all-night sleep EEG reveals an architecture or typical pattern of sleep that in normal humans involves the smooth 90-minute cycling between non-REM and REM sleep.

Q3 The answer is: (A) True.

Sleepwalking (somnambulism) usually occurs during slow-wave sleep (which is most common early in a night's sleep), and often occurs during the first third of the night (although it can occur during a daytime nap). Patients remain asleep during the episode, and tend to have a blank, glassy stare. They are typically unresponsive to efforts of others to communicate with them while sleepwalking, are awakened only with difficulty, and may be confused when awakened. Adults may appear to be acting out dreams during sleepwalking, and may remember fragments of dream-like experiences, but most patients are amnestic regarding the event.

Behaviors during sleepwalking may be complex, inappropriate, and at times violent or dangerous. Patients may move furniture in their house and may go outside. They may urinate in a closet or open the refrigerator and binge; they may also talk or shout. They may become violent when waking is attempted.

Episodes may terminate spontaneously, with some patients returning to bed, and others lying down and sleeping wherever they happen to be.

In most cases, the onset of sleepwalking is during childhood, with a peak in onset between ages 8 and 12 years. Many children with sleepwalking have an early history of confusional arousals.

Q4 The answer is: (C) Narcolepsy.

Patients being evaluated for narcolepsy or other forms of hypersomnolence may undergo a multiple sleep latency test. This test is also done in the sleep laboratory, after completing a polysomnogram the night before. The procedure involves giving the patient the opportunity to fall asleep during five naps spread throughout the day. Patients are awakened after napping for 20 minutes, and then remain awake for 2 hours after each nap. The average sleep latency is recorded, with values less than 5 minutes regarded as consistent with significant physiological pathological sleepiness. Also, REM latency (time from sleep onset to REM onset) is recorded; the presence of two or more sleep-onset REM periods along with pathological sleepiness is considered diagnostic of narcolepsy.

A multiple sleep latency test showing short sleep latency (less than 5 to 8 minutes on average across naps) and more than two sleep-onset REM periods is diagnostic for narcolepsy.

Q5 The answer is: (D) Ramelteon.

Ramelteon, approved by the US Food and Drug Administration for the treatment of insomnia, is a melatonin receptor agonist; it is the first hypnotic that does not act on the benzodiazepine receptor. As such, it may represent a new approach to the treatment of insomnia. Ramelteon has been efficacious for reducing sleep latency, but it does not improve sleep maintenance. Therefore it is best used in patients with complaints of trouble falling asleep. Doses of 8 mg/day are effective; higher doses provide no additional benefit. Some patients' sleep begins to improve after several weeks of nightly use, so ramelteon may be continued if there are no adverse effects, even if there is no immediate improvement in sleep.

Tryptophan and valerian root are so-called "natural" remedies for insomnia and are available as dietary supplements.

Q6 The answer is: (C) Myoclonic jerking.

The core feature of narcolepsy is an inability to maintain wakefulness during the day, and to maintain sleep at night. The intrusion of sleep into wake produces excessive daytime sleepiness and sleep attacks, the hallmark symptoms of narcolepsy. Untreated narcoleptics tend to fall asleep several times each day. The tendency to fall asleep may be highest during periods of quiet or boredom but may occur even during activity (such as driving, walking, or working, when falling asleep is highly inappropriate, or even life-threatening). The need to sleep may be irresistible. The sudden onset of irresistible sleep produces a sleep attack. Sleep attacks are usually brief (less than 1 hour), and patients typically awaken feeling refreshed. Their sleepiness, however, recurs within several hours, so planned napping may be helpful but by itself is not enough treatment.

Excessive daytime sleepiness in those with narcolepsy may be a function of their inability to sleep successfully at night. When this nocturnal sleep disruption can be resolved by medication, daytime sleepiness may improve.

Narcolepsy occurs with cataplexy (a sudden, brief decrease in or loss of muscle tone triggered by emotion) in approximately 50% to 80% of narcoleptics. Patients experience the change and may try to resist. Tone may be lost in selected muscles (producing, for example, only the droop of an eyelid), or may be widely distributed (producing collapse). Respiratory muscles are unaffected. Muscle tone begins to return after a few seconds to a few minutes, and recovery is complete and rapid. Prolonged cataplexy may occur if agents (such as antidepressants) used to manage cataplexy are suddenly withdrawn; however, this is uncommon. If an episode of cataplexy is prolonged, often an REM-onset sleep episode is experienced. The frequency of cataplexy is variable and may decrease with age. Cataplexy may occur with, or several years after, the onset of the other symptoms of narcolepsy. The emotional triggers of cataplectic attacks often involve "negative" emotions (such as anger or sadness), but attacks may also be triggered by humor and other "positive" emotions.

Patients with narcolepsy, especially those with cataplexy, often experience hypnagogic or hypnopompic hallucinations, and sleep paralysis. Hypnagogic and hypnopompic hallucinations occur, respectively, at sleep onset or while waking up, are complex, and involve visual, auditory, and somesthetic phenomena. Sleep paralysis is a brief (less than 60 seconds) period of inability to move skeletal muscles on awakening. Hypnopompic hallucinations and sleep paralysis may occur together, and are often frightening, especially during initial episodes.

Cataplexy and the other auxiliary symptoms of narcolepsy are normal concomitants of REM sleep and are only considered as abnormal if they intrude into wake or occur at sleep onset.

SECTION 9
PSYCHIATRIC DISORDERS

Impulse-Control Disorders

Multiple-Choice Questions

Select the appropriate answer.

Q1   True or False. Kleptomania is more prevalent in the general population than is pathological gambling.

    A. *True*

    B. *False*

Q2   True or False. Intermittent explosive disorder occurs more commonly in men than in women.

    A. *True*

    B. *False*

Q3   True or False. Children under the age of 18 years account for half of all arrests for arson in this country.

    A. *True*

    B. *False*

Q4   True or False. Twin studies have shown an increased incidence of pathological gambling in the twins of affected individuals.

    A. *True*

    B. *False*

Q5   True or False. Specific gene polymorphisms are more frequent in pathological gamblers.

    A. *True*

    B. *False*

Q6   True or False. Male patients with trichotillomania outnumber female patients with trichotillomania in adult treatment settings.

    A. *True*

    B. *False*

Chapter 23

Answers

Q1 The answer is: (B) False.
The prevalence of kleptomania within the general population has been estimated at six per 1000 persons; typically, there is a lag of many years between the onset of the behavior and the presentation for treatment. By contrast, a meta-analysis of epidemiologic studies of gambling has estimated a 1.1% prevalence of pathological gambling, with a 1.6% lifetime prevalence. Although 2.5 million Americans were pathological gamblers, another 3 million should be considered "problem gamblers." Pathological gambling is more likely if there is a family history of alcohol or other substance dependence, mood disorders, pathological gambling, or antisocial personality disorder.

Q2 The answer is: (A) True.
Although episodic violence is common in our society, when applying strict diagnostic criteria, intermittent explosive disorder is considered rare. Men account for approximately 80% of the cases. Intermittent explosive disorder and personality change owing to a general medical condition, aggressive types, are the diagnoses most often given to a patient with episodic violent behavior. Risk factors include physical abuse in childhood, a chaotic family environment, substance abuse, and psychiatric disorders in the patient or in his or her relatives.

Q3 The answer is: (A) True.
Pyromania is the irresistible impulse to set fires, without any motive beyond creating the fire itself; it occurs in the absence of any other condition that would impair judgment. Pyromania is rare, but fire setting comes to the attention of the psychiatrist more commonly. Much of the research in this area focuses on individuals who set fires, not on pyromania *per se*. Children under the age of 18 years account for half of all arrests for arson; much of the research on effective treatment concentrates on this age group.

Psychiatric disorders that are highly comorbid with fire-setting behavior include a high incidence of the conditions that exclude the diagnosis of pyromania, that is, intellectual disability, conduct disorder, alcohol and other substance abuse, schizophrenia, mania, and antisocial personality disorder.

Q4 The answer is: (A) True.
Pathological gambling is more likely if there is a family history of alcohol or other substance dependence, mood disorders, pathological gambling, or antisocial personality disorder. Twin studies have shown an increased incidence of pathological gambling in the twins of affected individuals. There is also an increased incidence of alcohol dependence and major depressive disorder in co-twin, suggesting a common genetic vulnerability for both disorders. Pathological gambling is highly comorbid with alcohol dependence or abuse, other substance dependence or abuse, and mood, anxiety, or personality disorders; in women, it is also highly comorbid with nicotine dependence.

Q5 The answer is: (A) True.
Some specific gene polymorphisms are more frequent in pathological gamblers. The Taq-A1 allele of the D_2 dopamine receptor, associated with other impulsive and addictive disorders, is more frequent in pathological gamblers. A less functional 7-repeat allele of the D_4 dopamine receptor has a higher incidence in female pathological gamblers. A 3-repeat allele of an MAO_A promoter with lower transcriptional activity has a higher incidence in male pathological gamblers; this gene has lower transcriptional activity. Male pathological gamblers also have a higher incidence of a short variant of a serotonin transporter with reduced promoter activity.

Q6 The answer is: (B) False.
The average age of onset of trichotillomania is between 11 and 13 years; female patients far outnumber male patients in adult treatment settings. The prevalence of trichotillomania may be underestimated due to patient shame and denial of the behavior. A survey of college students showed that 0.6% of men and

women had met full *Diagnostic and Statistical Manual of Mental Disorders, Third Edition Revised* criteria for trichotillomania at some point in their lives. In this same study, 1.5% of men and 3.4% of women reported hair pulling with visible hair loss, but without the tension and relief needed to meet diagnostic criteria. Ten percent to 13% of college freshman reported regular hair pulling, with 1% to 2% having bald patches sometime in their lifetime, and 1% to 2% reporting distress or tension related to the behavior. Trichotillomania is highly comorbid with other Axis I disorders including mood disorders, anxiety disorders, substance abuse, and eating disorders. Evaluated according to the *Diagnostic and Statistical Manual of Mental Disorders, Third Edition Revised*, two-thirds of patients in one study met criteria for anxiety or a mood disorder; one-half met criteria for an Axis II disorder. Three-quarters of first-degree relatives of the participants had an Axis I disorder, and 5% of them were hair pullers.

Chapter 24

Somatic Symptom Disorders

Multiple-Choice Questions

Select the appropriate answer.

Q1 Which of the following involves a loss or change in sensory or motor function that is suggestive of a physical disorder but that is caused by psychological factors?

    A. *Conversion disorder*

    B. *Factitious disorder*

    C. *Hypochondriasis*

    D. *Malingering*

    E. *Somatoform pain disorder*

Q2 Which of the following is a chronic syndrome of recurring multiple somatic symptoms (with at least four different pain symptoms, two gastrointestinal symptoms, one sexual symptom, and one pseudoneurologic symptom other than pain) that are NOT explainable medically and are associated with psychosocial distress and with medical help-seeking?

    A. *Conversion disorder*

    B. *Factitious disorder*

    C. *Hypochondriasis*

    D. *Malingering*

    E. *Somatization disorder*

Q3 In which of the following is there a preoccupation with the fear or belief that one has a serious, undiagnosed disease?

    A. *Conversion disorder*

    B. *Factitious disorder*

    C. *Hypochondriasis*

    D. *Malingering*

    E. *Somatization disorder*

Q4 In which of the following conditions does the afflicted patient imagine some defect or deformity in his or her appearance, most commonly of the face, the breasts, or the genitals?

    A. *Body dysmorphic disorder (BDD)*

    B. *Borderline personality disorder*

    C. *Factitious disorder*

    D. *Obsessive-compulsive disorder*

    E. *Somatization disorder*

Chapter 24
Answers

Q1 The answer is: (A) Conversion disorder.

Conversion disorder is perhaps the classic somatic symptom and related disorder; it involves a loss or change in sensory or motor function that is suggestive of a physical disorder but that is caused by psychological factors. Common symptoms include paralysis, aphonia, seizures, disturbances of gait and coordination, blindness, tunnel vision, and anesthesia. The primary evidence for the psychological cause consists of a temporal relationship between symptom-onset and psychologically meaningful environmental precipitants or stressors. A patient who developed conversion blindness, for instance, may have seen her husband with another woman before she complained of being unable to see. The conversion symptom is not under voluntary control, although the patient may be able to modulate its severity. A patient with a functional gait disturbance or a weak arm, for example, may, with intense concentration, be able to demonstrate slightly better control or strength. The *Diagnostic and Statistical Manual of Mental Disorders, Fourth Edition* (DSM-IV) eliminated pain and sexual dysfunction as conversion symptoms.

Confidence in the diagnosis is based often on the demonstration that function is normal in the symptomatic body part. Electromyograms, evoked responses of vision and hearing, slit-lamp examinations, funduscopic examinations, retinoscopic examinations, pulmonary function tests, and barium swallows are examples of tests that should be normal. This negative evidence is critical; it requires meticulous review by the clinician. Positive evidence includes not only the psychological data but also any demonstration of normal function in the supposedly disabled body part. Detective work begins with close observation of the patient, including times when the patient is unaware of the observer's presence.

The diagnosis of conversion cannot rest comfortably only on the absence of organic disease. Caution in diagnosing conversion symptoms is based on the reports that 13% to 30% of those with this diagnosis have gone on to develop an organic condition that, in retrospect, was related to the original symptom.

Functional brain imaging has added a dimension to the study of the patient with conversion disorder; there have been reports of functional neuroanatomic abnormalities in patients with conversion (i.e., sensorimotor loss).

Q2 The answer is: (E) Somatization disorder.

Originally termed *hysteria* or Briquet syndrome, the condition received the DSM-IV designation of somatization disorder; this condition has been solidly established as clinically and epidemiologically distinct. It is a chronic syndrome of recurring multiple somatic symptoms that are not explainable medically and are associated with psychosocial distress and with medical help-seeking. The disorder is much more common in women than it is in men, and it tends to occur in those of low socioeconomic status. Women with this disorder tend to have histories as children of missing, disturbed, or defective parents, and of sexual or physical abuse.

DSM-IV diagnostic criteria included at least four different pain symptoms (e.g., headache; back, joint, extremity, or chest pain; painful urination, intercourse, or menstruation); two gastrointestinal symptoms (e.g., nausea, bloating, diarrhea, and food intolerance); one sexual symptom (e.g., menstrual symptoms, erectile or ejaculatory dysfunction, or sexual indifference); and one pseudoneurologic symptom other than pain (e.g., deafness, paralysis, a lump in the throat, aphonia, fainting, anesthesia, or blindness). The symptoms must be disproportionate to demonstrable medical disease, and severe enough to result in medical attention or significant role impairment.

Q3 The answer is: (C) Hypochondriasis.

DSM-IV identified the predominant feature of hypochondriasis as a preoccupation with the fear or belief that one has a serious, undiagnosed disease. This concern was based on a misinterpretation of benign physical signs and symptoms as evidence of disease. Other diagnostic criteria include the absence of a physical disorder that accounts for the patient's symptoms or for his or her interpretation of them; persistence of the disease fear or belief despite appropriate medical reassurance; clinically significant distress or role impairment; and duration of at least 6 months. By this definition, hypochondriasis (or illness anxiety disorder) is quite prevalent. It is found in approximately 5% of medical outpatients and occurs equally between the sexes.

Fundamentally, hypochondriasis represents an overconcern about illness and a fearful attitude toward one's health. Afflicted patients are absorbed by their bodies and preoccupied with their symptoms. Their assessment of their health becomes both a way of reacting to life's stresses and demands, and a nonverbal language for communicating with others. Such inclinations and beliefs share similarities with those of the somatizer. The cognitive style of the typical hypochondriac is obsessive, however, whereas the cognitive style of the typical somatizer is histrionic.

Hypochondriasis is a chronic and disabling condition, and the prognosis is generally poor.

Q4 The answer is: (A) Body dysmorphic disorder (BDD).
Monosymptomatic hypochondriasis refers to several distinct syndromes characterized by a single, fixed, false belief that one is diseased. The disease conviction is generally delusional, and grossly disproportionate to any objective disease or deformity. This belief is tightly circumscribed, no other thought disorder is present, and the remainder of the patient's personality remains intact and unaffected. Body dysmorphic disorder (BDD), formerly termed dysmorphophobia, is one of the most common of these syndromes. Other forms of monosymptomatic hypochondriasis include the delusional belief that one is infested with a parasite or insect, and the delusion that one emits an offensive odor (olfactory reference syndrome).

The patient with BDD imagines some defect or deformity in his or her appearance, most commonly of the face, breasts, or genitals. The average age of onset for these patients is younger than age 20 years, with male and female patients equally represented. Typical male patients seek plastic surgeons with the conviction that their noses are too large or disfiguring. The typical female patient may be convinced that her facial skin is "scarred," making her appearance grotesque, and will seek a plastic surgery or dermatologic consultation. BDD is commonly accompanied by a mood disorder (including atypical depression with rejection sensitivity), social phobia, obsessive-compulsive disorder, and substance use disorders. The rate of suicide ideation, attempts, and suicide is notable.

Chapter 25

Factitious Disorders and Malingering

Multiple-Choice Questions

Select the appropriate answer.

Q1 In which of the following conditions is there a conscious production of signs and or symptoms to assume the sick role?

A. *Conversion disorder*

B. *Factitious illness*

C. *Hypochondriasis*

D. *Malingering*

E. *Somatization disorder*

Q2 In which of the following conditions is pseudologia fantastica MOST often seen?

A. *Conversion disorder*

B. *Factitious illness*

C. *Hypochondriasis*

D. *Malingering*

E. *Somatization disorder*

Q3 In which of the following conditions are approximate answers to questions MOST often provided?

A. *Conversion disorder*

B. *Dissociative identity disorder*

C. *Ganser syndrome*

D. *Hypochondriasis*

E. *Somatization disorder*

Q4 In which of the following conditions are symptoms MOST closely related to unconscious conflicts?

A. *Briquet syndrome*

B. *Factitious disorder not otherwise specified*

C. *Factitious illness*

D. *Malingering*

E. *Munchausen syndrome by proxy*

Q5   In which of the following conditions are laparotomaphilia migrans, neurologica diabolica, dermatitis autogenica, and hyperpyrexia figmentatica considered to be subtypes?

A. *Conversion disorder*

B. *Factitious illness*

C. *Hypochondriasis*

D. *Malingering*

E. *Somatization disorder*

Chapter 25

Answers

Q1 The answer is: (B) Factitious illness.

Factitious illness is a complicated disorder that is marked by the conscious production of symptoms without clear secondary gain. Unlike malingering, in which there is obvious secondary gain, those with factitious disorder are driven to feign illness without obvious direct benefit except to assume the sick role; in fact, they often put their health at considerable risk. They may fake, exaggerate, intentionally worsen, or simply create symptoms. They do not admit to self-harm, but rather hide it from their doctors; herein lies the paradox—those with factitious illness present to health care providers requesting help, but intentionally hide the self-induced cause of their illness.

In conversion disorder, hypochondriasis, and somatic symptom and related disorders, the afflicted individual does nothing to himself or herself to create, simulate, or feign illness.

Q2 The answer is: (B) Factitious illness.

In factitious disorder with predominantly physical signs and symptoms, the common presentation is that of a general medical condition. Examples of faked clinical problems run the gamut from fever, bleeding, hypoglycemia, and seizures to more elaborate productions, including cancers and infection with HIV. Although the term *Munchausen syndrome* is often used interchangeably with the physical type of factitious disorder, the classic Munchausen syndrome is reserved for the most severe and chronic form of the disorder, which is marked by the following three components: recurrent hospitalization, travel from hospital to hospital (peregrination), and pseudologia fantastica. Pseudologia fantastica refers to the production of intricate and colorful stories or fantasies associated with the patient's presentation. It is a form of pathological lying characterized by overlapping fact and fiction, with a repetitive quality and often with grandiosity or assumption of the victim role by the storyteller. In some cases, it may be difficult to determine whether these lies are actually delusions or conscious deceptions.

Q3 The answer is: (C) Ganser syndrome.

Ganser syndrome, which is characterized by providing approximate answers to questions (as well as having amnesia, disorientation, and perceptual disturbances), may be related to factitious disorder with psychological symptoms. Although it was originally described as a form of malingering (mostly by prisoners), Ganser-like syndromes may be seen in medical populations as well.

Q4 The answer is: (A) Briquet syndrome.

Somatization disorder (Briquet syndrome) and conversion disorder may be mistaken for factitious disorder. The principal difference among them is that the former is distinguished by symptoms not under one's voluntary control, but rather as a result of unconscious conflicts. Moreover, these patients are typically not as savvy about medical diagnoses, and there is no secondary gain. This contrasts with those who malinger and who intentionally feign symptoms for obvious secondary gain (often financial, legal, or drug-seeking).

Q5 The answer is: (B) Factitious illness.

Faked clinical syndromes are the hallmark of factitious illness, and any organ system can be involved in the charade. Examples include the following: the acute abdominal type (laparotomaphilia migrans) with abdominal pain (multiple surgeries may result in true adhesions and subsequent bowel obstruction); the neurologic type (neurologica diabolica) with headache, loss of consciousness, or seizures; the hematologic type with anemia from bloodletting or anticoagulant use; the endocrinologic type with hypoglycemia (from exogenous insulin), hyperthyroidism (from exogenous thyroid hormone), or hyperglycemia (from withholding of insulin); the cardiac type with chest pain or arrhythmia; the dermatologic type (dermatitis autogenica) with self-inflicted wounds or chemical abrasions; the febrile type (hyperpyrexia figmentatica) with manipulation of a thermometer to produce fever; and the infectious type, with wounds infected with multiple organisms (often from fecal material).

Chapter 26

Alcohol-Related Disorders

Multiple-Choice Questions

Select the appropriate answer.

Q1 Which of the following statements about alcohol-related problems is LEAST likely to be accurate?

A. *Excessive or risky alcohol consumption is the third leading cause of death in the United States, accounting for approximately 85,000 deaths annually*

B. *If a large quantity is consumed, and especially when rapidly consumed, alcohol-induced amnesia ("blackouts") can occur*

C. *It is estimated that alcohol causes about 70% to 80% of esophageal cancer, liver cancer, cirrhosis of the liver, homicide, epileptic seizures, and motor vehicle accidents worldwide*

D. *Some common consequences of alcohol misuse include motor vehicle and other accidents, violence and vandalism, unwanted sexual experiences, liver and cardiovascular diseases, cancers, fetal alcohol spectrum disorders, depression, panic attacks, and suicide*

E. *The economic burden attributed to alcohol-related problems in the United States approaches $200 billion annually*

Q2 True or False. A 70 kg man metabolizes approximately 10 mL of absolute ethanol (or 1.5 to 2 drink equivalents; 1 standard drink = 0.5 oz of whiskey, 4 oz of wine, or 12 oz of beer) per hour.

A. *True*

B. *False*

Q3 True or False. Symptoms of alcohol withdrawal typically emerge 2 to 3 days after discontinuation of alcohol and resolve within 3 to 5 days of their appearance.

A. *True*

B. *False*

Q4 Which of the following conditions is typically manifest by ophthalmoplegia, ataxia, and confusion?

A. *Alcohol intoxication*

B. *Alcohol withdrawal*

C. *Delirium tremens*

D. *Korsakoff syndrome*

E. *Wernicke encephalopathy*

Q5 Which of the following is the BEST treatment for a patient with Wernicke encephalopathy?

A. *Benztropine*

B. *Chlordiazepoxide*

C. *Haloperidol*

D. *Naloxone*

E. *Thiamine*

Q6 True or False. Magnetic resonance and diffusion tensor imaging studies typically reveal a loss of brain tissue, and neuropsychological tests show cognitive impairments in individuals who either have an alcohol use disorder or are heavy drinkers.

    A. *True*

    B. *False*

Q7 Which of the following is a 4-item screening test for alcohol use and abuse?

    A. *The AUDIT*

    B. *The CAGE*

    C. *The CIWA-AD*

    D. *The MAST*

    E. *The SASQ*

Chapter 26

Answers

Q1 The answer is: (C) It is estimated that alcohol causes about 70% to 80% of esophageal cancer, liver cancer, cirrhosis of the liver, homicide, epileptic seizures, and motor vehicle accidents worldwide.
It is estimated that alcohol causes approximately 20% to 30% (i.e., not 70% to 80%) of esophageal cancer, liver cancer, cirrhosis of the liver, homicide, epileptic seizures, and motor vehicle accidents worldwide.

Q2 The answer is: (A) True.
Resolution of intoxication follows steady-state kinetics, so that a 70-kg man metabolizes approximately 10 mL of absolute ethanol (or 1.5 to 2 drink equivalents; 1 standard drink = 0.5 oz of whiskey, 4 oz of wine, or 12 oz of beer) per hour.

Q3 The answer is: (B) False.
Uncomplicated withdrawal is surprisingly common and is frequently missed. The most common features of uncomplicated alcohol withdrawal emerge within hours, and resolve after 3 to 5 days.

Early features (irritability, tremor, and loss of appetite) of uncomplicated withdrawal symptoms are predictable. A hallmark of the withdrawal syndrome is generalized tremor (fast in frequency and more pronounced when the patient is under stress). This tremor may involve the tongue to such an extent that the patient cannot talk. The lower extremities may tremble so much that the patient cannot walk. The hands and arms may shake so violently that a drinking glass cannot be held without spilling the contents. The patient may be hypervigilant, have a pronounced startle response, and complain of insomnia.

Less commonly, patients experience hallucinations or seizures associated with alcohol withdrawal. These symptoms may persist for as long as 2 weeks and then clear without the development of delirium. Grand mal seizures ("rum fits") may occur, usually within the first 2 days after abstinence. More than one out of every three patients who suffer seizures develops subsequent delirium tremens.

Q4 The answer is: (E) Wernicke encephalopathy.
Wernicke encephalopathy appears suddenly and is characterized by ophthalmoplegia and ataxia followed by mental disturbance. The ocular disturbance, which occurs in only 17% of cases, consists of paresis or paralysis of the external recti, nystagmus, and a disturbance in conjugate gaze. A global confusional state consists of disorientation, unresponsiveness, and derangement of perception and memory. Exhaustion, apathy, dehydration, and profound lethargy are also part of the picture. The patient is apt to be somnolent, confused, slow to reply, and may fall asleep in midsentence.

Q5 The answer is: (E) Thiamine.
Once treatment with thiamine is started for Wernicke encephalopathy, improvement is often evident in the ocular palsies within hours. Recovery from ocular muscle paralysis is complete within days or weeks. According to Victor and coworkers, approximately one-third recovered from the state of global confusion within 6 days of treatment, another third within 1 month, and the remainder within 2 months. The state of global confusion is almost always reversible, in marked contrast to the memory impairment of Korsakoff psychosis.

Administration of the B vitamin thiamine (given intramuscularly or intravenously) should be routine for all suspected cases of alcohol intoxication and dependence. The treatment for Wernicke encephalopathy and Korsakoff psychosis is identical, and both are medical emergencies. Because subclinical cognitive impairments can occur even in apparently well-nourished patients, routine management should include thiamine, folic acid, and multivitamins with minerals, particularly zinc. Prompt use of vitamins, particularly thiamine, prevents advancement of the disease and reverses at least a portion of the lesions in which permanent damage has not yet been done. The response to treatment is therefore an important diagnostic aid. In patients who show only ocular and ataxic signs, the prompt administration of thiamine is crucial in preventing the development of an irreversible and incapacitating amnestic disorder. Treatment consists of 100 mg of thiamine and 1 mg of folic acid (given intravenously) immediately and 100 mg of intramuscular thiamine each day until a normal diet is resumed, followed by oral doses for 30 days.

Q6 The answer is: (A) True.

Magnetic resonance and diffusion tensor imaging studies typically reveal a loss of brain tissue, and neuropsychological tests show cognitive impairments in individuals who either have an alcohol use disorder or are heavy drinkers. Abnormalities on scans have been reported in 50% or more of individuals with chronic alcohol dependence. These abnormalities can occur in individuals in whom there is neither clinical nor neuropsychological test evidence of cognitive defects. In individuals with chronic alcohol dependence, magnetic resonance imaging has demonstrated accelerating gray matter loss with age, which is to some extent reversible with abstinence, suggesting that some of these changes are secondary to changes in brain tissue hydration.

Q7 The answer is: (B) The CAGE.

The National Institute on Alcohol Abuse and Alcoholism has recommended either the use of a single alcohol screening question (SASQ) or administration of the 10-question Alcohol Use Disorders Identification Test (AUDIT) self-report questionnaire as standard screening procedures for the detection of alcohol-related problems. The AUDIT with a manual is available for free (and in Spanish), and has been validated across a variety of cultural and ethnic groups. When using the SASQ, clinicians are advised to ask if an individual has consumed five or more standard drinks (for a man) on one occasion during the last year (four drinks for women). A positive response may indicate an alcohol-related problem and requires more detailed assessment.

A more traditional alternative screening interview is captured by the 4-question CAGE acronym. However, compared to the SASQ or the AUDIT the CAGE lacks sensitivity to detect hazardous/problem drinking. Similar to the CAGE interview, the TWEAK interview (i.e., "Tolerance," others "Worried" about your drinking, "Eye-opener," "Amnesia," ever wanted to/tried to "Cut down") is brief and has good psychometric properties, but similar to the CAGE lacks sensitivity to detect hazardous drinking.

The 24-question Michigan Alcoholism Screening Test (MAST) is another self-report measure with good psychometric properties, but it is longer than the AUDIT.

Medical screens may also be used. Screening for recent alcohol use can be carried out with a breathalyzer, or a sample of urine or saliva. For more chronic use, laboratory markers, such as the serum gamma-glutamyl transpeptidase, the mean corpuscular volume, and the carbohydrate-deficient transferrin, can be used. However, these measures lack sensitivity, but can be helpful if used in combination and when used with other screening measures, such as the AUDIT.

Screening for alcohol withdrawal is also critical considering that, as mentioned previously, the alcohol withdrawal syndrome can be life-threatening. The Clinical Institute Withdrawal Assessment for Alcohol Dependence (CIWA-AD) is a semistructured, 8-item, 5-minute interview used to assess and quantify severity of withdrawal from alcohol. It is easy to administer and possesses very good psychometric properties. Thus it is an efficient and reliable method that can prevent serious, life-threatening problems, and is useful to help clinicians determine levels of care.

Chapter 27

Drug Addiction

Multiple-Choice Questions

Select the appropriate answer.

Q1 The signs and symptoms of acute cocaine intoxication are MOST similar to those of intoxication with which of the following agents?

A. *Alprazolam*

B. *Amphetamine*

C. *Carbon monoxide*

D. *Haloperidol*

E. *Phenobarbital*

Q2 Withdrawal reactions (manifest by hypertension, tachycardia, hyperreflexia, and fever) are LEAST likely after abrupt discontinuation after chronic use from which of the following drugs?

A. *Alcohol*

B. *Alprazolam*

C. *Cocaine*

D. *Secobarbital*

E. *Lorazepam*

Q3 Long-term use of which of the following agents is MOST closely linked with a paranoid psychosis?

A. *Alcohol*

B. *Alprazolam*

C. *Amitriptyline*

D. *Dextroamphetamine*

E. *Lorazepam*

Q4 The cluster of signs and symptoms (i.e., dysphoric mood, nausea, vomiting, body aches, lacrimation, rhinorrhea, pupillary dilation, sweating, piloerection, diarrhea, yawning, fever, insomnia, irritability, and drug craving) are MOST closely linked with withdrawal from which of the following class of drugs?

A. *Anticholinergics*

B. *Antipsychotics*

C. *Benzodiazepines*

D. *Opiates*

E. *Tricyclic antidepressants*

Q5 Which of the following drugs has been approved for use in the office-based treatment of opiate dependence, and provides an attractive alternative to methadone treatment for higher-functioning individuals and for those with shorter histories of opiate dependence?

A. *Alprazolam*

B. *Amitriptyline*

C. *Buprenorphine*

D. *Dextroamphetamine*

E. *Duloxetine*

Q6 Which of the following is generally considered to be an alpha$_2$-adrenergic agonist?

A. *Amitriptyline*

B. *Buprenorphine*

C. *Clonazepam*

D. *Clonidine*

E. *Dextroamphetamine*

Q7 Which of the following drugs is MOST likely to counteract the effects of a benzodiazepine overdose?

A. *Benztropine*

B. *Flumazenil*

C. *Haloperidol*

D. *Naloxone*

E. *Physostigmine*

Chapter 27

Answers

Q1 The answer is: (B) Amphetamine.
The signs and symptoms of acute cocaine intoxication are similar to those of amphetamine abuse. Typical complaints associated with intoxication include anorexia, insomnia, anxiety, hyperactivity, and rapid speech and thought processes ("speeding"). Signs of adrenergic hyperactivity (such as hyperreflexia, tachycardia, diaphoresis, and dilated pupils responsive to light) may also be seen. More severe symptoms (such as hyperpyrexia, hypertension, and cocaine-induced vasospastic events [e.g., stroke or myocardial infarction]) are relatively rare among users but are common in those seen in hospital emergency departments. Patients may also manifest stereotyped movements of the mouth, face, or extremities.

The most serious psychiatric problem associated with chronic cocaine use is a cocaine-induced psychosis (manifest by visual and auditory hallucinations and paranoid delusions often associated with violent behavior). Tactile hallucinations (called "coke bugs") involve the perception that something is crawling under the skin. A cocaine psychosis may be indistinguishable from an amphetamine psychosis, but it is usually shorter in duration. High doses of stimulants can also cause a state of excitation and mental confusion. Drugs (e.g., alprazolam and phenobarbital) that work at the alcohol-benzodiazepine-barbiturate receptor tend to cause sedation, not hyperactivity; carbon monoxide in excess leads to somnolence and to coma, whereas haloperidol generally results in behavioral calm, not adrenergic excess.

Q2 The answer is: (C) Cocaine.
Chronic users of cocaine typically follow a cyclical pattern of 2 or 3 days of heavy binge use, followed by a withdrawal "crash." Detoxification is accomplished by the abrupt cessation of all cocaine use, usually through restricted access (e.g., a loss of funds or contacts, or incarceration). The major complication of withdrawal is a severe depression with suicidal ideation. A less severe anhedonic state may persist for 2 to 3 months and is thought to reflect a more persistent state of dopamine depletion.

By contrast, withdrawal from drugs that work at the alcohol-benzodiazepine-barbiturate receptor are closely linked with physiological symptoms (manifest by hypertension, tachycardia, hyperreflexia, and fever).

Q3 The answer is: (D) Dextroamphetamine.
The signs and symptoms of acute amphetamine intoxication are similar to those of cocaine abuse. Long-term effects also include depression, brain dysfunction, and weight loss. The other classic syndrome seen in either acute or chronic amphetamine intoxication is a paranoid psychosis without delirium. Although typically seen in young people who use intravenous methamphetamine hydrochloride, it can also occur in chronic users of dextroamphetamine or other amphetamines.

A paranoid psychosis may also occur with or without other manifestations of amphetamine intoxication. The absence of disorientation distinguishes this condition from most other toxic psychoses. This syndrome is clinically indistinguishable from an acute episode of schizophrenia of the paranoid type, and the correct diagnosis is often made in retrospect based on a history of amphetamine use and with a urine test that is positive for amphetamines. Use of haloperidol or low-dose atypical antipsychotics are often effective in the acute management of this type of substance-induced psychosis.

Other distinctive features of chronic stimulant abuse include dental problems (e.g., caries, missing teeth, bleeding and infected gums), muscle cramps (related to dehydration and low levels of magnesium and potassium), constipation (due to dehydration), nasal perforations, and excoriated skin lesions (speed bumps). The urine may have a stale smell due to ammonia constituents used in the illicit manufacture of methamphetamine.

Q4 The answer is: (D) Opiates.
The classic signs of opiate withdrawal are easily recognized, and usually begin 8 to 12 hours after the last dose (of a short-lasting agent). The patient generally admits to the need for drugs and shows sweating, yawning, lacrimation, tremor, rhinorrhea, marked irritability, dilated pupils, piloerection ("gooseflesh"),

and an increased respiratory rate. More severe signs of withdrawal occur 24 to 36 hours after the last dose and include tachycardia, hypertension, insomnia, nausea, vomiting, and abdominal cramps. Untreated, the syndrome subsides in 3 to 7 days. Withdrawal symptoms are similar in patients addicted to methadone, but they may not appear until 24 to 36 hours after the last dose (because of methadone's longer half-life) and abate over 2 to 4 weeks. Patients addicted to oxycodone may present with a particularly severe and prolonged withdrawal syndrome and may require high doses of opiates for adequate control.

Q5 The answer is: (C) Buprenorphine.

Buprenorphine has been approved for use in the office-based treatment of opiate dependence and provides an attractive alternative to methadone treatment for higher-functioning individuals and for those with shorter histories of opiate dependence. To initiate buprenorphine treatment, a patient should be instructed to refrain from the use of heroin, or any other opiate, for at least 24 hours. Once opiate withdrawal is documented (and monitored with an opiate withdrawal scale, such as the Clinical Opiate Withdrawal Scale), treatment should begin with 4 mg/1 mg of sublingual buprenorphine/naloxone. The patient should be observed for 1 to 4 hours after the initial dose for any signs of precipitated withdrawal. Additional doses of 4 mg/1 mg can be given every 2 to 4 hours as needed to stabilize the patient. Most clinicians do not prescribe more than 12 mg/3 mg on the first day. Should precipitated withdrawal occur, more aggressive dosing is recommended to manage the withdrawal symptoms. Most patients can be maintained on sublingual doses in the range of 12 to 16 mg/day; an adequate stabilizing dose can usually be achieved within 2 to 3 days.

Q6 The answer is: (D) Clonidine.

Clonidine, an alpha$_2$-adrenergic agonist, suppresses the noradrenergic symptoms of withdrawal and can be used as an alternative medication for withdrawal. Clonidine should not be substituted for methadone until the methadone dose has been reduced to 20 mg/day. After an initial oral dose of 0.2 mg of clonidine, patients usually require doses in the range of 0.1 to 0.2 mg every 4 to 6 hours. The total dose should not exceed 1.2 mg/day. Patients on clonidine should be monitored closely for side effects (particularly hypotension and sedation). Clonidine doses should be withheld for a systolic blood pressure below 90 mm Hg, or diastolic blood pressure below 60 mm Hg. In an inpatient setting, clonidine can be tapered and discontinued over 3 to 4 days. A transdermal clonidine patch is often applied on the third day. Because clonidine does not adequately suppress the subjective symptoms of withdrawal, as does methadone and buprenorphine, and is relatively ineffective for the treatment of muscle aches and insomnia, it is not acceptable for many addicts.

Q7 The answer is: (B) Flumazenil.

Flumazenil, a specific benzodiazepine antagonist, reverses the life-threatening effects of a benzodiazepine overdose. An initial intravenous dose of 0.2 mg should be given over 30 seconds, followed by a second 0.2 mg intravenous dose if there is no response after 45 seconds. This procedure can be repeated at 1-minute intervals (up to a cumulative dose of 5 mg). This treatment is contraindicated in individuals dependent on benzodiazepines or those taking tricyclic antidepressants because flumazenil may precipitate seizures in these patients. When flumazenil is contraindicated, benzodiazepine overdoses should be handled similarly to other sedative-hypnotic overdoses.

Benztropine may reverse extrapyramidal side effects of dopamine blockers, naloxone may reverse opiate intoxication, physostigmine may reverse anticholinergic excess, and haloperidol may reduce the manifestations of psychosis.

Psychosis and Schizophrenia

Multiple-Choice Questions

Select the appropriate answer.

Q1   Which of the following statements is LEAST accurate?

A.   *Even if schizophrenia is successfully treated, function often remains impaired; moreover, there is a high risk of recurrence of psychotic symptoms*

B.   *In addition to psychosis, patients with schizophrenia experience cognitive and negative symptoms that adversely affect function*

C.   *Psychosocial treatment is the mainstay of treatment for schizophrenia; it is most effective in the treatment of acute psychosis and the prevention of relapse*

D.   *Schizophrenia is a clinical diagnosis based on a combination of characteristic symptoms of sufficient severity (in the absence of other factors that would account for them) that typically begins in adolescence or early adulthood*

E.   *Schizophrenia is a complex genetic disease; its expression depends on multiple susceptibility genes that interact with environmental insults. Some of these insults may occur during in utero brain development*

Q2   Which of the following statements is LEAST accurate?

A.   *For most patients, having schizophrenia means living in the community with some degree of residual symptoms*

B.   *Prevention of suicide and prevention of morbidity and mortality associated with antipsychotics are important goals of management*

C.   *Psychosis is a specific term that is synonymous with schizophrenia*

D.   *Considering that schizophrenia is a chronic illness, rehabilitation that focuses on optimization of work and social function is as important as symptom control*

E.   *The prognosis of schizophrenia varies from complete recovery (after a period of acute illness) to severe, ongoing symptoms that require institutionalization*

Q3   Which of the following first called the chronic psychotic condition (that had been named dementia praecox) schizophrenia?

A.   *Francine Benes*

B.   *Eugen Bleuler*

C.   *Sigmund Freud*

D.   *Stephan Heckers*

E.   *Emil Kraepelin*

Q4   Which of the following is the MOST likely lifetime morbidity risk of schizophrenia?

A.   *1%*

B.   *3%*

C.   *5%*

D.   *7%*

E.   *10%*

Q5   Which of the following statements is LEAST likely to be accurate?

    A. *Paternal age increases the risk for schizophrenia in a linear fashion*

    B. *Several susceptibility genes have been tentatively linked to schizophrenia*

    C. *The dopamine hypothesis was built on two pillars of evidence: (1) amphetamines, known dopamine receptor agonists, can produce a schizophrenia-like state in healthy adults; and (2) the discovery that the antipsychotic effect of the phenothiazines was associated with their ability to block the D_2 dopamine receptor*

    D. *The cellular hallmarks of schizophrenia are neurofibrillary plaques and tangles in the brain*

    E. *Most patients with schizophrenia lack a family history of the disorder*

Q6   In schizophrenia, which is the MOST common type of hallucination?

    A. *Auditory*

    B. *Gustatory*

    C. *Olfactory*

    D. *Tactile*

    E. *Visual*

Q7   True or False. Only antipsychotics are US Food and Drug Administration–approved for the treatment of schizophrenia.

    A. *True*

    B. *False*

Chapter 28

Answers

Q1 The answer is: (C) Psychosocial treatment is the mainstay of treatment for schizophrenia; it is most effective in the treatment of acute psychosis and the prevention of relapse.
Antipsychotic medications are the mainstay of treatment for schizophrenia; they are most effective in the treatment of acute psychosis and the prevention of relapse.

Schizophrenia is a clinical diagnosis based on a combination of characteristic symptoms of sufficient severity (in the absence of other factors that would account for them) that typically begins in adolescence or early adulthood.

Schizophrenia is a complex genetic disease; its expression depends on multiple susceptibility genes that interact with environmental insults. Some of these insults may occur during *in utero* brain development.

In addition to psychosis, patients with schizophrenia experience cognitive and negative symptoms that adversely affect function.

Even if schizophrenia is successfully treated, function often remains impaired; moreover, there is a high risk of recurrence of psychotic symptoms.

Q2 The answer is: (C) Psychosis is a specific term that is synonymous with schizophrenia.
Psychosis is not a specific diagnosis, as it can occur in a wide variety of clinical contexts. Of the psychotic disorders, the prototypical condition is schizophrenia. In schizophrenia, psychotic symptoms occur chronically, without gross organic abnormalities of the brain (hence, the term "functional" psychosis) or a severe medical disturbance (as in a delirium). Moreover, psychosis may occur when the mood is normal, thus differentiating it from bipolar disorder or from psychotic depression. Although psychosis is a defining (and often the most apparent) clinical feature of schizophrenia, other symptom clusters (e.g., negative symptoms and cognitive symptoms) are largely responsible for the psychosocial disability that usually accompanies this disorder.

Q3 The answer is: (B) Eugen Bleuler.
Although it was Emil Kraepelin who originally described schizophrenia and categorized madness into episodic mood disorders and chronic psychotic illnesses (and labeled it with the term *dementia praecox*) at the close of the 19th century, the condition was later renamed schizophrenia by Eugen Bleuler. In the 100 years since the condition was identified, much progress has been made (in large part the result of the discovery of the first antipsychotic, chlorpromazine), turning schizophrenia from an illness treated in asylums (state hospitals) to one treated in community settings. However, the fundamental Kraepelinian dichotomy between schizophrenia (and related psychotic disorders) and manic-depressive illness has remained unchanged.

Neuroanatomic studies of the brain conducted by a variety of modern investigators (including Francine Benes and Stephan Heckers) have furthered our understanding of this condition.

Q4 The answer is: (A) 1%.
Schizophrenia is a syndrome that occurs in all cultures and in all parts of the world. Epidemiologic studies have found incidence rates between 7.7 and 43.0 (median 15.2) new cases per 100,000. The point-prevalence is about 5 per 1000, whereas the lifetime morbidity risk is around 1%. Sex differences exist; men have a 30% to 40% higher lifetime risk for schizophrenia than women, and the age of onset is roughly 3 to 4 years later for women.

The old dogma that cited the identical incidence and prevalence rates of schizophrenia around the globe is not quite correct. Clear geographic differences exist, albeit within a fairly narrow range of two- to threefold differences. The fact that these modest variations in rates exist between cultures, and within subgroups in cultures, likely reflects different risk factors for schizophrenia in different populations.

Q5 The answer is: (D) The cellular hallmarks of schizophrenia are neurofibrillary plaques and tangles in the brain.

Neurofibrillary plaques and tangles are pathognomonic of Alzheimer disease, not schizophrenia. In schizophrenia, there is no clear loss of cortical neurons; instead there is subtle disarray in cortical cytoarchitecture and a decreased volume of neuropil (comprised of axodendritic processes, glia, and cerebral vasculature).

Paternal age increases the risk for schizophrenia in a linear fashion. Compared with the children of fathers who are less than age 25 years, the relative risk for children increases steadily with paternal age to about 2.0 for fathers in the 45 to 49 year age group, and to almost 3.0 for fathers older than age 50 years. This increase in risk with paternal age is consistent with the hypothesis that *de novo* mutations contribute to the genetic risk in schizophrenia. New mutations could explain why a disorder with lower fertility rates has not disappeared; in men as opposed to women, the germ-line cells, spermatogonia, continue to divide throughout life, allowing replication errors to accumulate and to be transmitted to offspring.

Several susceptibility genes have been tentatively linked to schizophrenia. The most promising candidate genes are involved in brain development, frontal lobe function, myelination, synaptic function, and glutamate transmission. It is likely that most genes are not specific for schizophrenia; instead, they confer risk for neuropsychiatric disorders that cut across current clinical diagnoses. Several genetic disorders, such as 22q11 deletion syndrome (velocardiofacial syndrome or DiGeorge syndrome) or Klinefelter syndrome (XXY syndrome), increase the risk for psychosis in affected individuals.

An interaction between susceptibility genes and environment forms the basis for the neurodevelopmental hypothesis of schizophrenia in which a clinically silent, latent propensity toward schizophrenia (e.g., a genetic vulnerability or insult during brain development, such as intrauterine infections or maternal starvation) gets uncovered when the brain matures (e.g., during the naturally occurring pruning of dendritic arborization) or additional insults (e.g., cannabis use) push a vulnerable brain toward psychosis.

The dopamine hypothesis was built on two pillars of evidence: (1) amphetamines, known dopamine receptor agonists, can produce a schizophrenia-like state in healthy adults; and (2) the discovery that the antipsychotic effect of the phenothiazines was associated with their ability to block the D_2 dopamine receptor.

The majority of patients with schizophrenia lack a family history of the disorder. Nevertheless, the fact that genes matter was shown in now classic twin and adoption studies of the 1960s. For monozygotic twins, the risk of developing schizophrenia approaches 50% for the unaffected twin if the co-twin has schizophrenia. Having siblings or parents (i.e., first-degree relatives) with schizophrenia increases an individual's risk to approximately 10-fold above that seen in the general population. With greater genetic distance, the risk for schizophrenia decreases to a twofold risk over the population risk for second-degree relatives.

Q6 The answer is: (A) Auditory.

The hallmarks of acute schizophrenia are hallucinations and delusions, sometimes grouped together as positive symptoms. Hallucinations are perceptions without an external stimulus, and they can occur in any sensory modality. However, by far the most common type of hallucination is auditory, occurring in at least two-thirds of patients over the course of their illness. Certain types of third-person (Schneiderian) hallucinations are frequently encountered: several voices talking about the patient, often in a derogatory way; a voice giving a running commentary on what the patient is doing; or a voice repeating what the patient is thinking. Although hallucinations in other modalities are possible, visual or olfactory hallucinations should raise the suspicion for an organic etiology of the hallucinations.

Q7 The answer is: (A) True.

Only antipsychotics are US Food and Drug Administration–approved for the treatment of schizophrenia. In clinical practice, many patients receive medications other than antipsychotics (particularly antidepressants for depression and anxiolytics for anxiety) for the symptomatic treatment of residual psychopathology. The role of mood stabilizers for narrowly defined schizophrenia is limited. Valproate is useful as an adjunct in acute psychotic exacerbations to hasten response, and lamotrigine may augment the therapeutic effects of clozapine. Partial and full agonists at the glycine site of the N-methyl-D-aspartate receptor (e.g., D-cycloserine, glycine, or D-serine) have shown some efficacy for negative symptoms. Improving cognition with alpha-amino-3-hydroxy-5-methyl-4-isoxazolepropionic acid modulators or nicotinic agonists is an area of active research, but to date these medications are not available clinically.

Mood Disorders: Depressive Disorders (Major Depressive Disorder)

Multiple-Choice Questions

Select the appropriate answer.

Q1   Which of the following conditions is diagnosed when a patient reports either depressed mood (it can be irritable mood in children and adolescents) or reduced interest/pleasure, or both, and five or more of the following symptoms (insomnia or hypersomnia, reduced interest or pleasure, excessive guilt/feelings of worthlessness, reduced energy or fatigue, diminished ability to concentrate or make decisions, loss or increase of either appetite or weight, psychomotor agitation or retardation, thoughts of suicide or death/suicidal behavior)?

A.   *Adjustment disorder with depressed mood*

B.   *Bipolar disorder*

C.   *Cyclothymic disorder*

D.   *Dysthymic disorder*

E.   *Major depressive disorder (MDD)*

Q2   Which of the following disorders is diagnosed when depressed mood (although it can be irritable mood in children/ adolescents for more than 1 year) is present for more days than not, for at least 2 years in addition to three or fewer of the following symptoms (insomnia or hypersomnia, reduced interest or pleasure, excessive guilt/feelings of worthlessness, reduced energy or fatigue, diminished ability to concentrate or make decisions, loss or increase of either appetite or weight, psychomotor agitation or retardation, thoughts of suicide or death/suicidal behavior)?

A.   *Adjustment disorder with depressed mood*

B.   *Bipolar disorder*

C.   *Cyclothymic disorder*

D.   *Dysthymic disorder*

E.   *Major depressive disorder (MDD)*

Q3   Which of the following terms BEST defines an inability to experience pleasure?

A.   *Abulia*

B.   *Alexithymia*

C.   *Anhedonia*

D.   *Apathy*

E.   *Aphasia*

Q4 Approximately what percentage of outpatients with MDD are predominantly irritable when depressed and manifest intermittent outbursts of anger, termed anger attacks?

A. *Less than 2%*

B. *5% to 10%*

C. *15% to 25%*

D. *30% to 40%*

E. *More than 50%*

Q5 According to both the Epidemiological Catchment Area Study and the National Comorbidity Survey Study, what is the BEST approximation of the cross-sectional prevalence rates for major depression?

A. *Less than 2%*

B. *2% to 5%*

C. *5% to 10%*

D. *10% to 20%*

E. *More than 25%*

Chapter 29

Answers

Q1 The answer is: (E) Major depressive disorder (MDD).

Major depressive disorder (MDD) is diagnosed when a patient reports either depressed mood (it can be irritable mood in children and adolescents) or reduced interest/pleasure, or both, and four or more of the following symptoms (insomnia or hypersomnia, reduced interest or pleasure, excessive guilt/feelings of worthlessness, reduced energy or fatigue, diminished ability to concentrate or make decisions, loss or increase of either appetite or weight, psychomotor agitation or retardation, thoughts of suicide or death/ suicidal behavior).

Q2 The answer is: (D) Dysthymic disorder.

When a depressive syndrome persists for at least 2 years, it is called chronic depression. However, when depressed mood or lack of interest/pleasure are associated with only a few of the neurovegetative symptoms (not exceeding three), then that mild syndrome lasting at least 2 weeks is called minor depression or depressive disorder not otherwise specified. The persistence of this syndrome for at least 2 years is called dysthymic disorder. In dysthymic disorder, the presence of a chronically (or at least intermittent) depressed mood for at least 2 years is heterogeneous clinically and etiologically, although it is clearly related to MDD. More than 70% of the patients with dysthymic disorder go on to develop MDD and to have recurrent major depressive episodes that are superimposed on the dysthymic disorder (i.e., double depression). As in the case of MDD, most dysthymic patients have comorbid medical or psychiatric disorders. Although milder than MDD, dysthymic disorder may have profound consequences on quality of life and effective function in multiple life-roles; this degree of morbidity is more reflective of the duration of dysthymic disorder than is the number of symptoms experienced.

Q3 The answer is: (C) Anhedonia.

The term melancholic depression is used to describe severely depressed patients who are unable to experience pleasure (i.e., anhedonia) and/or who lose normal emotional responsiveness to positive experiences.

Abulia is the loss or impairment of willpower (often seen in frontal lobe dysfunction). Alexithymia is the inability to put feelings into words. Apathy is indifference or the absence of emotion. Aphasia is a weakening or loss of the faculty of transmission of ideas by language in any of its forms (reading, writing, speaking), or failure in the appreciation of the written, printed, or spoken word.

Q4 The answer is: (D) 30% to 40%.

A significant proportion (30% to 40%) of outpatients with MDD are predominantly irritable when depressed, and they manifest intermittent outbursts of anger, termed anger attacks. Anger attacks emerge abruptly with minimal interpersonal provocation and are associated with a paroxysm of autonomic arousal reminiscent of panic attacks, but featuring explosive verbal or physical anger, usually directed at close companions or family members. These patients have distinctive clinical features associated with the anger attacks, and they also appear to have decreased central serotonergic activity compared with patients without anger attacks.

Q5 The answer is: (B) 2% to 5%.

Both the Epidemiological Catchment Area Study and the National Comorbidity Survey Study have found that major depression is a prevalent disorder in the general population, with cross-sectional rates ranging from 2.3% to 4.9%, respectively.

Lifetime prevalence of MDD in both the United States and Western Europe has hovered around 13.3% to 17.1% in the general population. A more recent study found that the 6-month prevalence of MDD was 17% among Western European populations.

Bipolar Disorder

Multiple-Choice Questions

Select the appropriate answer.

Q1   According to the National Comorbidity Survey–Replication study, the lifetime prevalence of bipolar disorder (BPD) is closest to what percentage?

A.   *2%*

B.   *7%*

C.   *12%*

D.   *18%*

E.   *25%*

Q2   Which of the following is the STRONGEST established risk factor for BPD?

A.   *A family history of bipolar disorder (BPD)*

B.   *Pregnancy*

C.   *Season of birth*

D.   *Stressful life events*

E.   *Traumatic brain injuries*

Q3   True or False. The key feature for the diagnosis of BPD is the presence of at LEAST one period of mood elevation or significant irritability meeting criteria for a manic, mixed, or hypomanic episode.

A.   *True*

B.   *False*

Q4   True or False. Psychosis is NOT represented in the diagnostic features for BPD.

A.   *True*

B.   *False*

Q5   True or False. Less than 25% of patients with bipolar I experience a mixed state at some point in the disease course.

A.   *True*

B.   *False*

Q6   Which of the following MOST closely represents the switch rate from depression to mania or hypomania after initiation of an antidepressant?

A.   *1%*

B.   *5%*

C.   *10%*

D.   *15%*

E.   *25%*

Q7 Which of the following agents is LEAST likely to be efficacious for the treatment of mania?

A. *Clonazepam*

B. *Lamotrigine*

C. *Lithium*

D. *Olanzapine*

E. *Valproate*

Answers

Q1 The answer is: (A) 2%.

The National Comorbidity Survey–Replication study, in which a random population-based sample of about 9000 adults was contacted and screened using *Diagnostic and Statistical Manual of Mental Disorders, Fourth Edition* (DSM-IV)–based questions, estimated a lifetime prevalence of 1% for bipolar I disorder and 1.1% for bipolar II disorder. A previous population-based survey using a validated self-report questionnaire estimated the prevalence of bipolar disorder (BPD) at 3.4% to 3.7%. In the National Comorbidity Survey–Replication study, the prevalence of "subthreshold" BPD—that is, two or more core features of hypomania, without meeting criteria for BPD—was estimated at 2.4%. With this broader definition, the prevalence of all "bipolar spectrum" disorders reaches 4.4%.

Q2 The answer is: (A) A family history of bipolar disorder (BPD).

The strongest established risk factor for BPD is a family history of BPD. Individuals with a first-degree relative (a parent or sibling) with BPD have a risk approximately 5 to 10 times that of those in the general population. Importantly, however, their risk for major depressive disorder (MDD) is also increased two-fold; given the greater prevalence of MDD, this means that family members of bipolar individuals are at greater risk for MDD than BPD, although some authors argue that many of those diagnosed with MDD simply have unrecognized BPD.

A number of putative environmental risks have been described for BPD; these include pregnancy and obstetric complications, season of birth (winter or spring birth, perhaps indicating maternal exposure to infection), stressful life events, traumatic brain injuries, and multiple sclerosis. In multiple sclerosis, for example, the prevalence of BPD is roughly doubled; this increase does not appear to result from adverse effects of pharmacotherapy. The prevalence may also be increased among individuals with certain neurologic disorders, including epilepsy. Another intriguing finding is the association between dietary omega-3 fatty acid consumption and risk of mood disorders. Most such studies focus broadly on depressed mood, although one study reporting on data from 18 countries found greater seafood consumption to be associated with a lower risk for BPD.

Q3 The answer is: (A) True.

The key feature for the diagnosis of BPD is the presence of at least one period of mood elevation or significant irritability meeting criteria for a manic, mixed, or hypomanic episode.

A manic episode is identified when a patient experiences an elevated or irritable mood for at least 1 week, along with at least three associated symptoms. If the predominant affect is irritable, four rather than three associated symptoms are required. If the symptoms result in hospitalization at any point, the 1-week criterion is not required—for example, a patient hospitalized after 3 days of manic symptoms is still considered to have experienced a manic episode. As with episodes of major depression, DSM-IV criteria also require that symptoms be sufficient to markedly impair occupational or social function or be associated with psychotic symptoms. Interrater reliability of the DSM-IV mania criteria have been shown to be quite high.

Hypomanic symptoms are generally similar to, but less severe and impairing than, manic symptoms. DSM-IV criteria require at least 4 days of mood elevation or irritability, along with associated symptoms. There are three important, but often overlooked, aspects of these criteria that bear highlighting. First, symptoms must be observable by others—that is, a purely subjective report of hypomania is not sufficient for a diagnosis. Second, symptoms represent a change from the individual's baseline; those who are "always" cheerful, impulsive, and talkative are "not" considered chronically hypomanic. Third, symptoms by definition do not cause significant functional impairment—hypomanic-like symptoms that lead to loss of a job, for example, could be considered mania. As these criteria may be difficult to operationalize, it is not surprising that interrater reliability of hypomania criteria is somewhat lower. Some diagnostic systems propose that 1 to 3 days of hypomanic symptoms are required to identify hypomania; this approach trades specificity for sensitivity.

Q4 The answer is: (A) True.

Of note, psychosis is not represented in the diagnostic features for BPD. However, psychotic symptoms are common during both manic/mixed and depressive episodes. One Finnish population-based study found a prevalence of 0.24% for psychotic bipolar I disorder. The lifetime prevalence of psychotic symptoms in another cohort of patients who were bipolar was approximately 40%. So-called "mood-congruent" psychotic symptoms are often seen—for example, grandiose delusions during mania or delusions of decay and doom during depression. Psychosis typically resolves along with the mood symptoms, although diagnostic criteria acknowledge that psychotic symptoms may linger beyond the end of the mood episode.

Q5 The answer is: (B) False.

Up to 40% of patients with bipolar I experience a mixed state at some point in their disease course. Recently, the concept of subthreshold mixed states has received increasing attention: patients who do not meet the stringent criteria for a mixed state (who do not meet full criteria for both a manic and a depressive episode simultaneously) but nonetheless have some degree of both types of symptoms. Depressive symptoms are common during manic or hypomanic episodes, underscoring the importance of inquiring about both poles. Conversely, during depressive episodes, patients may experience some degree of hypomanic symptoms, such as racing thoughts. The prognostic implications, if any, of these subthreshold mixed states has not been well studied.

Q6 The answer is: (A) 1%.

A small number of patients experience the onset of mania or hypomania after initiation of antidepressants. Some authors refer to this phenomenon as "bipolar III." The true prevalence and time course of this phenomenon are difficult to estimate, particularly for a switch to hypomania, because in clinical practice, as well as in randomized controlled trials (RCTs), such symptoms of elevated mood may not be aggressively investigated. A patient who presents 2 weeks after beginning an antidepressant feeling "great" and congratulating the clinician on his or her excellent skills requires careful questioning about manic/hypomanic symptoms, but more often is congratulated in turn on his or her excellent antidepressant response. In one of the largest prospective antidepressant treatment studies to date in MDD, there was little or no evidence of antidepressant-induced mood elevation. Likewise, most randomized trials in MDD report switch-rates of less than 1%.

Such switches are typically described as early (often within 2 weeks) and abrupt (in some cases overnight) with the onset of mood elevation, although the time course has not been well established and it is possible that patients "switch" after prolonged antidepressant exposure, and perhaps even after antidepressant discontinuation. Some patients describe colors being more vivid, or having an abrupt urge to undertake new projects. Importantly, the switch must be discriminated from the immense relief many patients experience with resolution of their depressive symptoms. It does not represent simply the absence of depressive symptoms, but the presence of hypomanic/manic symptoms. Close longitudinal follow-up may be required to clarify the diagnosis.

Q7 The answer is: (B) Lamotrigine.

Multiple first-line agents have been established for mania. Those with greatest evidence of efficacy include lithium, valproate, and second-generation antipsychotics, for example, olanzapine. Among the second-generation antipsychotics, there appears to be little difference in efficacy. Whether they are used alone or in combination typically depends on the severity of illness—combination therapy may have modestly greater efficacy. If a single pharmacotherapy does not achieve improvement within a short period, a second one may be added, or the patient may be switched to an alternative first-line agent.

A number of other pharmacotherapies have been studied in mania; RCTs suggest that gabapentin, topiramate, and lamotrigine are not efficacious in acute treatment.

Benzodiazepines are commonly used as adjunctive treatments among manic patients, specifically to reduce agitation and to promote sleep; they have shown greater efficacy than placebo in RCTs for agitation.

A question of substantial clinical interest has been whether combining multiple antimanic agents achieves better response than monotherapy. Haloperidol plus valproate was superior to haloperidol alone in one RCT. Meta-analyses likewise suggest modest advantage in efficacy for combination therapy, although this must be weighed against an increase in adverse effects. Generally, monotherapy is preferred for less ill patients, whereas combination therapy is used for those who are more ill (e.g., hospitalized).

Chapter 31

Psychiatric Illness during Pregnancy and the Postpartum Period

Multiple-Choice Questions

Select the appropriate answer.

Q1 Which of the following categories in the classification of risk (derived from human and animal studies) is designated as safe for use during pregnancy?

A. A

B. B

C. C

D. D

E. X

Q2 Which of the following agents should be avoided when possible given the increased risk of cardiac malformations with first-trimester exposure to this medication?

A. Bupropion

B. Citalopram

C. Desipramine

D. Fluoxetine

E. Paroxetine

Q3 True or False. Severely depressed patients who are acutely suicidal or psychotic and who require hospitalization can be safely and effectively treated with electroconvulsive therapy (ECT).

A. True

B. False

Q4 Which of the following agents is MOST closely associated with the development of Ebstein anomaly following exposure during the first trimester of pregnancy?

A. Bupropion

B. Citalopram

C. Desipramine

D. Fluoxetine

E. Lithium

Q5 Which of the following agents is MOST closely associated with prenatal exposure and the development of neural tube defects and spina bifida?

A. *Citalopram*

B. *Fluoxetine*

C. *Lamotrigine*

D. *Lithium*

E. *Valproic acid*

Q6 True or False. For breastfeeding women taking psychotropics, the risks to their nursing infants is roughly the same for use of lithium and fluoxetine.

A. *True*

B. *False*

Q7 Which of the following is the rate at which a recurrence of postpartum depression will occur given a history of postpartum depression?

A. *2%*

B. *10%*

C. *20%*

D. *50%*

E. *70%*

Q8 Which of the following conditions is the MOST common?

A. *Postpartum blues*

B. *Postpartum depression*

C. *Postpartum infanticide*

D. *Postpartum panic attacks*

E. *Postpartum psychosis*

Q1 The answer is: (A) A.

As is the case with other medications, four types of risk are typically cited with respect to potential use of antidepressants during pregnancy: (1) risk of pregnancy-loss or miscarriage, (2) risk of organ malformation or teratogenesis, (3) risk of neonatal toxicity or withdrawal syndromes during the acute neonatal period, and (4) risk of long-term neurobehavioral sequelae.

To provide guidance to physicians seeking information on the reproductive safety of various prescription medications, the US Food and Drug Administration has established a system that classifies medications into five risk categories (A, B, C, D, and X) based on data derived from human and animal studies. Medications in category A are designated as safe for use during pregnancy, whereas category X drugs are contraindicated and are known to have risks to the fetus that outweigh any benefit to the patient. Most psychotropic medications are classified as category C agents, for which human studies are lacking and for which "risk cannot be ruled out." No psychotropic drugs are classified as safe for use during pregnancy (category A).

Unfortunately, this system of classification is often ambiguous and may lead some to make unwarranted conclusions. For example, certain tricyclic antidepressants (TCAs) have been labeled as category D agents, indicating "positive evidence of risk," although the pooled available data do not support this assertion and, in fact, suggest that these drugs are safe for use during pregnancy. Therefore, the physician must rely on other sources of information when counseling patients about the potential use of psychotropic medications during pregnancy. Randomized, placebo-controlled studies that examine the effects of medication use on pregnant populations are unethical for obvious reasons. Therefore much of the data related to the profile of reproductive safety for a medication are derived from retrospective studies and case reports. More recently, studies that have evaluated the reproductive safety of antidepressants have used a more rigorous prospective design. Data supporting reproductive safety of fluoxetine and citalopram are particularly robust.

Q2 The answer is: (E) Paroxetine.

In situations in which pharmacologic treatment during pregnancy is indicated, the clinician should attempt to select the safest medication regimen, using, if possible, medications with the safest reproductive profile. Fluoxetine, with the most extensive literature supporting its reproductive safety, is a first-line choice. The TCAs and bupropion have been relatively well characterized in this setting and should also be considered as first-line agents. Among the TCAs, desipramine and nortriptyline are preferred because they are less anticholinergic and the least likely to induce orthostatic hypotension during pregnancy. The amount of literature on the reproductive safety of the newer selective serotonin reuptake inhibitors, including citalopram, is growing, and these agents may be useful in certain settings.

Paroxetine, however, should be avoided when possible given the increased risk of cardiac malformations with first-trimester exposure to this medication. The US Food and Drug Administration changed the paroxetine pregnancy category label from C to D in late 2005, given unpublished reports from a Swedish registry and a US claims database that associated first-trimester exposure to paroxetine with a greater risk of atrial and ventricular septal defects.

In patients with depression who have not responded to either fluoxetine or a TCA, these newer agents may be considered, acknowledging that information on their reproductive safety is limited. When prescribing medications during pregnancy, every attempt should be made to simplify the medication regimen. For instance, one may select a more sedating TCA for a woman with depression and insomnia, instead of using a selective serotonin reuptake inhibitor in combination with trazodone or a benzodiazepine.

Q3 The answer is: (A) True.

Patients with severe depression who are acutely suicidal or psychotic who require hospitalization can be safely and effectively treated with electroconvulsive therapy (ECT). In a review of the 300 case reports of ECT during pregnancy published over the past 50 years, four premature labors and no premature ruptures of membranes have been reported. Given its relative safety, ECT may also be considered an alternative to conventional pharmacotherapy for women who wish to avoid extended exposure to psychotropic medications during pregnancy, or for women who fail to respond to standard antidepressants.

Q4 The answer is: (E) Lithium.

Concerns regarding fetal exposure to lithium have typically been based on early reports of higher rates of cardiovascular malformations (e.g., Ebstein anomaly) following prenatal exposure to this drug. More recent data suggest the risk of cardiovascular malformations following prenatal exposure to lithium are smaller than previous estimates (1 per 2000 vs. 1 per 1000). Prenatal screening with a high-resolution ultrasound and fetal echocardiography is recommended at or about 16 to 18 weeks of gestation to screen for cardiac anomalies. Nonetheless, for the woman with bipolar disorder who is faced with a decision regarding use of lithium during pregnancy, it is appropriate to counsel such a patient about the very small risk of organ dysgenesis associated with prenatal exposure to this medicine. Preliminary data suggest that there are no gross developmental deficits with lithium exposure when looking at neurobehavioral outcomes in children exposed to lithium *in utero*. Although lithium appeared to have a statistically significant impact on certain outcomes (e.g., gestational age, birth weight, Apgar scores, and Bayley scores), the effect was relatively small and appeared to have little clinical relevance.

Q5 The answer is: (E) Valproic acid.

Compared with lithium and lamotrigine, prenatal exposure to some anticonvulsants is associated with a far greater risk for organ malformation. An association between prenatal exposure to mood stabilizers (including valproic acid and carbamazepine) and neural tube defects (3% to 8%) and spina bifida (1%) also has been observed. Fetal exposure to anticonvulsants has been associated not only with relatively high rates of neural tube defects, such as spina bifida, but also with multiple anomalies (including midface hypoplasia [also known as the "anticonvulsant face"], congenital heart disease, cleft lip and/or palate, growth retardation, and microcephaly). Factors that may increase the risk for teratogenesis include high maternal serum anticonvulsant levels and exposure to more than one anticonvulsant. This finding of dose-dependent risk for teratogenesis is at variance with that of other psychotropic medications (e.g., antidepressants). Thus, when using anticonvulsants during pregnancy, the lowest effective dose should be used, and anticonvulsant levels should be monitored closely, and the dosage adjusted appropriately.

Information about the reproductive safety of newer anticonvulsants (including gabapentin, oxcarbazepine, and topiramate) sometimes used to treat patients with bipolar disorder remains sparse. Other efforts are underway to accumulate data from prospective registries regarding teratogenic risks across a broad range of anticonvulsants. The North American Antiepileptic Drug Pregnancy Registry was recently established to collect such information rapidly and efficiently (www.aedpregnancyregistry.org).

Prenatal screening following anticonvulsant exposure for congenital malformations (including cardiac anomalies) with fetal ultrasound at 18 to 22 weeks of gestation is recommended. The possibility of fetal neural tube defects should be evaluated with maternal serum alpha-fetoprotein and ultrasonography. In addition, 4 mg/day of folic acid before conception and during the first trimester for women receiving anticonvulsants is recommended. Supplemental folic acid's ability to attenuate the risk of neural tube defects in the setting of anticonvulsant exposure has not been examined.

Lamotrigine is another mood stabilizer that is an option for pregnant women with bipolar disorder. Although previous reports have not shown an elevated risk of malformations associated with lamotrigine exposure, data from the North American Antiepileptic Drug Pregnancy Registry indicate increased risk of oral cleft in infants exposed to lamotrigine during the first trimester; the prevalence was approximately 9 per 1000 births.

Q6 The answer is: (B) False.

The data indicate that all psychotropic medications (including antidepressants, antipsychotic agents, lithium carbonate, and benzodiazepines) are secreted into breast milk. However, concentrations of these agents in breast milk vary considerably. The amount of medication to which an infant is exposed depends on several factors: the maternal dosage of medication, frequency of dosing, and rate of maternal drug metabolism. Typically, peak concentrations in the breast milk are attained approximately 6 to 8 hours after the medication is ingested. Thus, the frequency of feedings and the timing of the feedings can influence the amount of drug to which the nursing infant is exposed. By restricting breastfeeding to times during which breast milk drug concentrations would be at their lowest (either shortly before or immediately after dosing medication), exposure may be reduced; however, this approach may not be practical for newborns, who typically feed every 2 to 3 hours.

The nursing infant's chances of experiencing toxicity are dependent not only on the amount of medication ingested but also on how well the ingested medication is metabolized. The liver metabolizes most psychotropics. During the first few weeks of a full-term infant's life, there is a lower capacity for hepatic drug metabolism, which is about one-third to one-fifth of the adult capacity. Over the next few months, the capacity for hepatic metabolism increases significantly, and by about 2 to 3 months of age it surpasses that of adults. In premature infants or in infants with signs of compromised hepatic metabolism (e.g., hyperbilirubinemia), breastfeeding typically is deferred because these infants are less able to metabolize drugs and are thus more likely to experience toxicity.

Over the past 5 years, data have accumulated regarding the use of various psychotropics during breastfeeding. Much data has accumulated on the use of antidepressants in women who are nursing. The available data on the TCAs, fluoxetine, paroxetine, and sertraline during breastfeeding have been encouraging and suggest that the amounts of drug to which the nursing infant is exposed is low, and that significant complications related to neonatal exposure to psychotropic medications in breast milk appear to be rare. Typically, very low or nondetectable levels of drug have been detected in the infant serum, and one recent report indicates that exposure during nursing does not result in clinically significant blockade of serotonin (5-hydroxytryptamine) reuptake in infants. Although less information is available on other antidepressants, serious adverse events related to exposure to these medications have not been reported.

For women with bipolar disorder, breastfeeding may pose more significant challenges. First, on-demand breastfeeding may significantly disrupt the mother's sleep, and thus may increase her vulnerability to relapse during the acute postpartum period.

Second, there have been reports of toxicity in nursing infants related to exposure to various mood stabilizers, including lithium and carbamazepine, in breast milk. Lithium is excreted at high levels in the mother's milk, and infant serum levels are relatively high, about one-third to one-half of the mother's serum levels, thereby increasing the risk of neonatal toxicity. Reported signs of toxicity include cyanosis, hypotonia, and hypothermia. More recent data, however, indicate that the infant serum level of lithium is relatively low, about one-fourth of maternal levels, and that the risk of serious adverse events in the nursing infant is relatively low. Although breastfeeding typically is avoided in women taking lithium, the lowest possible effective dosage should be used, and both maternal and infant serum lithium levels should be followed in mothers who breastfeed. In collaboration with the pediatrician, the child should be monitored closely for signs of lithium toxicity, and lithium levels, thyroid-stimulating hormone, blood urea nitrogen, and creatinine should be monitored every 6 to 8 weeks while the child is nursing.

Q7 The answer is: (D) 50%.
The postpartum period has typically been considered a time of risk for the development of affective disorder. Although several studies suggest rates of depression during the postpartum period equal to those in nonpuerperal controls, other research has identified subgroups of women at risk for postpartum worsening of mood. At highest risk are women with a history of postpartum psychosis; up to 70% of women who have had one episode of puerperal psychosis will experience another episode following a subsequent pregnancy. Similarly, women with histories of postpartum depression are at significant risk, with rates of postpartum recurrence as high as 50%. Women with bipolar disorder also appear to be particularly vulnerable during the postpartum period, with rates of postpartum relapse ranging from 30% to 50%. The extent to which a history of major depression influences risk for postpartum illness is less clear. However, in all women (with or without histories of major depression) the emergence of depressive symptoms during pregnancy significantly increases the likelihood of postpartum depression.

Q8 The answer is: (A) Postpartum blues.
During the postpartum period, up to 85% of women experience some degree of mood disturbance. For most women the symptoms are mild; however, 10% to 15% of women experience clinically significant symptoms. Postpartum depressive disorders typically are divided into three categories: (1) postpartum blues, (2) nonpsychotic major depression, and (3) puerperal psychosis. Because these three diagnostic subtypes overlap significantly, it is not clear if they actually represent three distinct disorders. It may be more useful to conceptualize these subtypes as existing along a continuum, in which postpartum blues is the mildest and postpartum psychosis is the most severe form of puerperal psychiatric illness.

Postpartum blues does not indicate psychopathology, but it is common and occurs in approximately 50% to 85% of women following delivery. Symptoms of reactivity of mood, tearfulness, and irritability are, by definition, time limited and typically remit by the 10th postpartum day. As postpartum blues is associated with no significant impairment of function and is time limited, no specific treatment is indicated. Symptoms that persist beyond 2 weeks require further evaluation and may suggest an evolving depressive disorder. In women with a history of recurrent mood disorder, the blues may herald the onset of postpartum major depression.

Several studies describe a prevalence of postpartum major depression of between 10% and 15%. The signs and symptoms of postpartum depression usually appear over the first 2 to 3 months following delivery, and generally are indistinguishable from characteristics of major depression that occur at other times in a woman's life. The symptoms of postpartum depression include depressed mood, irritability, and loss of interest in usual activities. Insomnia, fatigue, and loss of appetite are frequently described. Postpartum depressive symptoms also coexist with anxiety and obsessional symptoms, and women may have generalized anxiety, panic disorder, or hypochondriasis. Although it may sometimes be difficult to diagnose depression in the acute puerperium given the normal occurrence of symptoms suggestive of depression (e.g., sleep and appetite disturbance, low libido), it is an error to dismiss neurovegetative symptoms, such as severe decreased energy, profound anhedonia, and guilty ruminations as normal features of the puerperium. In its most severe form, postpartum depression may result in profound dysfunction. Risk factors for postpartum depression include prenatal depression, prenatal anxiety, and a history of depression.

Postpartum psychosis is a psychiatric emergency. The clinical picture is most frequently consistent with mania or a mixed state and may include symptoms of restlessness, agitation, sleep disturbance, paranoia, delusions, disorganized thinking, impulsivity, and behaviors that place mother and infant at risk. The typical onset is within the first 2 weeks after delivery, and symptoms may appear as early as the first 48 to 72 hours postpartum. Although investigators have debated whether postpartum psychosis is a discrete diagnostic entity or a manifestation of bipolar disorder, treatment should follow the same algorithm to treat acute manic psychosis (including hospitalization and potential use of mood stabilizers, antipsychotic medications, benzodiazepines, or ECT).

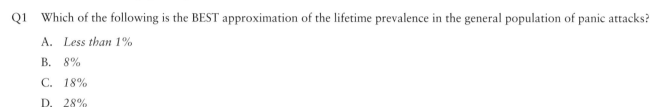

Chapter 32
Anxiety Disorders
Multiple-Choice Questions

Select the appropriate answer.

Q1   Which of the following is the BEST approximation of the lifetime prevalence in the general population of panic attacks?

    A. *Less than 1%*

    B. *8%*

    C. *18%*

    D. *28%*

    E. *More than 40%*

Q2   According to the recent National Comorbidity Survey–Replication (NCS-R), what is the BEST approximation of the lifetime prevalence rate for panic disorder?

    A. *0.7%*

    B. *4.7%*

    C. *12.7%*

    D. *20.7%*

    E. *32.7%*

Q3   True or False. Increased rates of suicide and suicide attempts have been associated with panic disorder.

    A. *True*

    B. *False*

Q4   Which of the following statements is LEAST likely to be accurate?

    A. *Childhood physical and sexual abuse do not appear to increase the risk for the later development of panic disorder*

    B. *Panic disorder has a heritability of approximately 40%*

    C. *The pathogenesis and maintenance of panic disorder is likely the result of a complex interaction of biological, psychological, and environmental factors*

    D. *The risk of panic disorder is increased eight-fold in first-degree relatives of patients with the disorder*

    E. *Twin studies have demonstrated that monozygotic twins have a significantly greater concordance rate for panic disorder than do dizygotic twins*

Q5   Which of the following BEST characterizes the condition marked by a persistent fear of situations that involve performance, evaluation, or potential scrutiny by others?

    A. *Generalized anxiety disorder (GAD)*

    B. *Obsessive-compulsive disorder*

    C. *Panic disorder (PD)*

    D. *Posttraumatic stress disorder*

    E. *Social anxiety disorder (SAD)*

Q6 True or False. Panic disorder is MORE prevalent than is social anxiety disorder.

    A. *True*

    B. *False*

Q7 Which of the following conditions is BEST characterized by excessive anxiety and worry occurring more days than not for at least 6 months about several events or activities (such as work or school performance)?

    A. *Generalized anxiety disorder (GAD)*

    B. *Obsessive-compulsive disorder*

    C. *Panic disorder (PD)*

    D. *Posttraumatic stress disorder*

    E. *Social anxiety disorder (SAD)*

Chapter 32

Answers

Q1 The answer is: (D) 28%.
The characteristic feature of panic disorder (PD) is the presence of recurrent panic attacks, or paroxysms of extreme anxiety, which are sudden, intense bursts of anxiety or fear accompanied by an array of physical symptoms (e.g., rapid heart rate, dizziness, shortness of breath, sweating, or nausea). Panic attacks themselves are relatively common in the general population, with lifetime prevalence rates reported at approximately 28% in a recent large-scale community sample. The diagnosis of PD, however, requires the presence of recurrent panic attacks (at least some of which have been unexpected), along with at least 1 month of persistent worry about the possibility of future attacks, worry about the implications or consequences of panic attacks, development of situational avoidance, or other behavioral changes that occur because of the attacks (e.g., repeated emergency department or physician visits owing to fears of an undiagnosed medical condition).

Q2 The answer is: (B) 4.7%.
Results from the recent National Comorbidity Survey–Replication (NCS-R) reported lifetime and 12-month prevalence rates of PD at 4.7% and 2.7%, respectively. Notably, those rates are somewhat higher than findings from the original NCS and the Epidemiological Catchment Area study. It is unclear whether these discrepancies represent an increasing prevalence over the past several decades or are due to differences in diagnostic methods and criteria. Given the salient and distressing physical symptoms experienced by people with PD, it is not surprising that prevalence rates of this condition are even higher in primary medical settings, with reports ranging from 3% to 8%.

Q3 The answer is: (A) True.
The presence of comorbidity in PD bodes poorly for a variety of psychological, functional, and treatment outcomes. For instance, increased rates of suicide and suicide attempts have been associated with PD, with some research suggesting that inflated rates of lifetime suicide attempts are the result of co-occurring psychiatric conditions (such as depression or alcohol abuse); however, recent evidence suggests that the presence of PD is associated with increased rates of suicide attempts, even when comorbidity and a history of childhood abuse is accounted for. Similarly, the lifetime risk of suicide attempts in patients with PD and major depressive disorder is more than double that of the two disorders independently.

Q4 The answer is: (A) Childhood physical and sexual abuse do not appear to increase the risk for the later development of panic disorder.
Consistent with etiologic models of other anxiety-related conditions, the pathogenesis and maintenance of PD is likely the result of a complex interaction of biological, psychological, and environmental factors. In support of a genetic transmission of PD, twin studies have demonstrated that monozygotic twins have a significantly greater concordance rate for PD than do dizygotic twins. Further, the risk of PD is increased eight-fold in first-degree relatives of patients with the disorder. A recent review of twin and family studies suggests that PD has a heritability of approximately 40%, with additional significant contributions from unique environmental effects (greater than 50%), and only a relatively small (less than 10%) contribution from common (familial) environmental factors.

Stressful life events also appear to be important in the etiology of PD. Some research has found that approximately 80% of patients with PD report major life stressors within the 12 months preceding the onset of the disorder, suggesting that stressful life events may contribute to the timing of the onset of the disorder. Childhood physical and sexual abuse also appear to increase the risk for the later development of PD. Moreover, symptom severity has been correlated with negative life events (including interpersonal conflicts, physical or health-related problems, and work-related difficulties), whereas the presence of chronic life stressors has been shown to worsen the course of PD.

Q5 The answer is: (E) Social anxiety disorder (SAD).
The fundamental characteristic of social anxiety disorder (SAD) is a marked and persistent fear of situations that involve performance, evaluation, or potential scrutiny by others. People with SAD fear that they will act in ways or show anxiety symptoms that will be embarrassing or humiliating, or that may result in negative evaluation by others. Consequently, the feared social interaction or performance situations are avoided, or else endured with intense distress and anxiety.

Q6 The answer is: (B) False.
Results from the recent NCS-R reported lifetime and 12-month prevalence rates of PD at 4.7% and 2.7%, respectively.

SAD is even more common, with lifetime prevalence rates in Western countries ranging between 7% and 13%. Variations in prevalence rates depend on diagnostic criteria (e.g., *Diagnostic and Statistical Manual of Mental Disorders*(DSM)-III, DSM-III-R, or DSM-IV), diagnostic threshold (e.g., required level of distress or impairment necessary to meet diagnostic criteria), and method of assessment (e.g., self-report surveys or interviews). Results from the recent NCS-R indicate that SAD occurs at a lifetime prevalence of approximately 12.1% in the general population, making it the fourth most prevalent psychiatric disorder behind major depressive disorder, alcohol dependence, and specific phobia.

Q7 The answer is: (A) Generalized anxiety disorder (GAD).
Generalized anxiety disorder (GAD) is characterized by persistent, excessive, and difficult-to-control worry and tension about a variety of events and activities in one's daily life. Common worries concern financial matters, work/school, relationships, minor matters (e.g., punctuality or small household repairs), one's own health or the health/safety of loved ones, and community or world affairs. The worry must be associated with at least three out of six of the following psychological and somatic symptoms: (1) feeling keyed up, restless, or on edge; (2) fatigability; (3) irritability; (4) muscle tension; (5) impaired concentration; and (6) disrupted sleep.

Although autonomic hyperactivity (e.g., shortness of breath, rapid heart rate, or dizziness) was included in earlier versions of the DSM, and continues to be used in the *International Classification of Diseases, Tenth Edition*, numerous studies suggest that people with GAD do not differ from anxious and nonanxious controls on self-report and physiological indices of autonomic activity. In contrast, muscle tension consistently differentiates people with GAD from anxious and nonanxious controls, suggesting that this may represent a particularly important diagnostic feature of GAD. According to the DSM, the worry and associated feelings of anxiety and tension must be present for more days than not for at least a 6-month period to the point in which the person experiences significant distress or marked impairment in social, occupational, or day-to-day function.

Obsessive-Compulsive Disorder and Obsessive-Compulsive and Related Disorders

Multiple-Choice Questions

Select the appropriate answer.

Q1   What is the approximate percent of the world's population that suffers from obsessive-compulsive disorder (OCD) at some point in their lives?

A. *Less than 1%*

B. *2% to 3%*

C. *7% to 8%*

D. *12% to 13%*

E. *19% to 20%*

Q2   Which of the following is LEAST often considered to be an obsessive-compulsive-related disorder (OCRD)?

A. *Body dysmorphic disorder*

B. *Illness anxiety disorder*

C. *Perseveration*

D. *Tourette disorder*

E. *Trichotillomania (TTM)*

Q3   True or False. Numerous lines of evidence support the genetic basis for obsessive-compulsive disorder and obsessive-compulsive-related disorder.

A. *True*

B. *False*

Q4   Which of the following brain structures is LEAST likely to be implicated in the pathophysiology of obsessive-compulsive disorder?

A. *Amygdala*

B. *Anterior cingulate cortex*

C. *Caudate*

D. *Cerebellum*

E. *Orbitofrontal cortex*

Q5   Which of the following tests is MOST often used to record the severity and lifetime presence of specific symptoms of obsessive-compulsive disorder?

A. *BDI*

B. *BPRS*

C. *HANDS*

D. *Y-BOCS*

E. *Y-MRS*

Chapter 33

Answers

Q1 The answer is: (B) 2% to 3%.

Approximately 2% to 3% of the world's population suffers from obsessive-compulsive disorder (OCD) at some point in their lives, and higher rates will suffer from obsessive-compulsive-related disorders (OCRDs). Most individuals with OCD spend an average of 17 years before they receive an appropriate diagnosis and treatment for this illness.

The disorder has been listed as one of the 10 most disabling illnesses by the World Health Organization, whereas the National Comorbidity Survey Replication indicated that OCD is the anxiety disorder with the highest percentage (50.6%) of serious cases.

Q2 The answer is: (C) Perseveration.

Perseveration, often involving repetition (e.g., of a word, a phrase, hand gestures, or numbers on a clock), is not made worse by the prevention of the action, as is the case with symptoms of OCD; it often results from frontal lobe dysfunction.

Putative OCRDs include somatoform disorders (e.g., body dysmorphic disorder and hypochondriasis), tic disorders (e.g., Tourette disorder), and impulse-control disorders (e.g., trichotillomania [TTM] and pathological skin picking).

Q3 The answer is: (A) True.

Numerous lines of evidence support the genetic basis for OCD and OCRDs. Twin and family aggregation studies of OCD report higher-than-expected rates of OCD in relatives. This was confirmed in a meta-analysis of five OCD family studies that included 1209 first-degree relatives, which calculated a significantly increased risk of OCD among relatives of probands (8.2%) versus controls (2.0%) (odds ratio[OR] = 4.0). However, in studies ascertained through children or adolescents, familial risk appears to be even higher (9.5% to 17%) than that for those with later-onset OCD.

No large systematic twin studies have focused exclusively on OCD. A recent review of OCD twin studies dating back to 1929 concluded that obsessive-compulsive symptoms are heritable, with genetic influences ranging from 45% to 65% in children, and from 27% to 47% in adults.

Molecular genetic studies have begun to provide evidence that specific genes play a role in the manifestation of OCD. It is highly likely that OCD is an oligogenic disorder with several genes that are important for the expression of the syndrome. Currently, none of the four linkage studies for OCD or OCD symptoms reported genome-wide significance. The following regions have been suggestive for susceptibility loci: 1_q, 6_q, 9_p, 19_q, 7_p, and 15_q.

OCD candidate genes have been studied based on their function and their position in the genome. Serotonin-related genes considered in OCD include those coding for the serotonin transporter (5-HT_T) and receptors 5-HT_{2A}, 5-HT_{2B}, 5-HT_{2C}, and 5-HT_{1B}, as well as the serotonin enzyme, tryptophan hydroxylase. Dopamine-related genes studied in OCD include dopamine transporter genes, D_2, D_3, and D_4 receptors, catechol-O-methyltransferase and monoamine oxidase $_A$ enzymes. Glutamate-related genes associated with OCD include *GRIK*, *GRIN*$_{2B}$, and *SLC-*$_{1A1}$. Other genes that are associated with OCD include the white matter genes, *OLIG*$_2$ and *MOG*.

With respect to family studies of OCRDs, among the relatives of OCD probands significantly higher-than-expected rates were found of body dysmorphic disorder (OR = 5.4), somatoform disorders (OR = 3.9), grooming disorders (OR = 1.8), and all spectrum disorders combined (OR = 2.7). Relatives of OCD probands have elevated rates of Tourette disorder and chronic tics (4.6%) versus relatives of controls (1%), regardless of a diagnosis of Tourette disorder in the probands. This is especially true in families with earlier-onset OCD. Moreover, relatives of Tourette disorder probands have elevated rates of OCD as compared with controls. It has also been suggested that TTM has an underlying genetic basis. In the only twin study exploring the genetic basis for TTM, a significantly greater concordance rate was present among monozygotic (31.9%) than dizygotic (0%) twins for "clinically significant hairpulling."

Q4 The answer is: (D) Cerebellum.

Neuroimaging findings indicate that OCD involves subtle structural and functional abnormalities of the orbitofrontal cortex, the anterior cingulate cortex, the caudate, the amygdala, and the thalamus. The nodes of the implicated frontal cortico-basal ganglia-thalamo-cortical circuit are interconnected via two principal white matter tracts—the cingulum bundle and the anterior limb of the internal capsule.

The basal ganglia are likely associated with abnormal compulsions of OCD. Damage to this region in both humans and animal models results in behaviors that resemble compulsions. Prefrontal and orbito-frontal regions are responsible for filtering information received by the brain, and for suppressing unnecessary responses to external stimuli; these may be more associated with the obsessive symptoms of OCD. There is also evidence of brain white matter involvement in OCD. Patients with OCD have significantly more gray matter, less white matter, and abnormalities of white matter than do normal controls, which suggests a possible developmental etiologic process.

Q5 The answer is: (D) Y-BOCS.

The Yale-Brown Obsessive Compulsive Scale (Y-BOCS) and checklist should be used to record the severity and lifetime presence of specific symptoms. There is also a child version of this scale, the Children's Yale-Brown ObsessiveCompulsive Scale (CY-BOCS). Alternatively, the Obsessive-Compulsive Inventory or the Obsessive-Compulsive Checklist may be used. Regarding the history of present illness, the duration and severity of symptoms and their precipitating, exacerbating, and ameliorating factors should be elucidated. Functional consequences of these symptoms in home, work, and social environments and the level of insight, resistance, and control over symptoms should also be assessed. Family insight and accommodation of symptoms (which permits their perpetuation) are other important factors to be determined. In the assessment of past psychiatric history, the duration of time at the maximum dosage of every past medication trial should be recorded. The length and success of past behavior or cognitive therapies and other psychotherapies also needs to be established.

The Beck Depression Inventory (BDI) is a 21-item scale on which patients must rate their symptoms on a scale from 0 to 3; the total score is tallied. The BDI tends to focus more on cognitive symptoms of depression, and it excludes atypical symptoms (such as weight gain and hypersomnia).

The Brief Psychiatric Rating Scale (BPRS) is an 18-item scale that evaluates a range of positive and negative symptoms, as well as other categories (such as depressive mood, mannerisms, posturing, hostility, and tension). Each item is rated on a 7-point scale following a clinical interview. It has been used to assess psychotic symptoms in patients with both primary psychotic disorders and secondary psychoses, such as depression with psychotic features, but not OCD.

The Harvard Department of Psychiatry National Depression Screening Day Scale (HANDS) is a self-administered scale that includes 10 questions about depression symptoms and is scored based on the experience of symptoms from 0 or "none of the time" to 3 or "all of the time;" it does not screen for OCD.

The Young Mania Rating Scale (Y-MRS) is a clinician-rated scale of 11 items used to detect symptoms of mania, not OCD.

Trauma and Posttraumatic Stress Disorder

Multiple-Choice Questions

Select the appropriate answer.

Q1   What is the BEST approximation for the occurrence of a symptom cluster of acute stress disorder (ASD) in individuals exposed to trauma?

A.   *Less than 10%*

B.   *10% to 30%*

C.   *30% to 50%*

D.   *50% to 70%*

E.   *More than 70%*

Q2   True or False. Women have a higher lifetime prevalence of posttraumatic stress disorder (PTSD) than do men.

A.   *True*

B.   *False*

Q3   True or False. The development of posttraumatic stress disorder after a traumatic experience is the exception rather than the rule.

A.   *True*

B.   *False*

Q4   True or False. Psychiatric comorbidity is the rule rather than the exception in posttraumatic stress disorder.

A.   *True*

B.   *False*

Q5   True or False. The estimated genetic heritability of posttraumatic stress disorder is approximately 30% to 40% after controlling for traumatic exposure.

A.   *True*

B.   *False*

Q6   True or False. Most of the recovery that takes place following the development of posttraumatic stress disorder occurs more than 1 year following the trauma.

A.   *True*

B.   *False*

Chapter 34

Answers

Q1 The answer is: (B) 10% to 30%.

The *Diagnostic and Statistical Manual of Mental Disorders* (DSM)-IV introduced a new diagnostic category, acute stress disorder (ASD), to recognize brief stress reactions to traumatic events that are manifest in the first month following a trauma. In addition to a shorter duration (2 days to 4 weeks), ASD comprises a less restrictive set of posttraumatic stress disorder (PTSD) symptoms in each of the three cluster types; however, with the addition of dissociative symptoms (one must meet three out of five symptoms).

Empirical studies have suggested that the ASD symptom cluster occurs in 10% to 30% of individuals exposed to trauma.

Prospective studies suggest that 72% to 83% of those diagnosed with ASD go on to develop PTSD 6 months after trauma, and 63% to 80% have PTSD 2 years after the trauma.

Preliminary research has suggested that the employment of specific treatment approaches (e.g., exposure therapy, cognitive therapy, stress management) for ASD leads to lower rates of later PTSD (approximately 15% to 25% 6 months after trauma) relative to patients with ASD who are either untreated or who receive general supportive counseling (approximately 60% to 70% have PTSD at 6 months). Despite evidence regarding the prevalence and use of the diagnosis of ASD, unresolved issues remain, not only with regard to its emphasis on dissociative symptoms, but also as to whether ASD and PTSD may in fact represent the same disorder, the latter merely differentiated by the arbitrary month-long duration criterion. In other words, ASD may simply exemplify "acute PTSD" as defined in the earlier DSM-III.

Q2 The answer is: (A) True.

Although the lifetime prevalence of PTSD in the general community is 8% to 9%, women show a higher lifetime prevalence (10% to 14%) than do men (5% to 6%).

Exposure to potentially traumatizing events in the general population is the rule rather than the exception. In the National Comorbidity Survey (NCS), the lifetime prevalence of exposure to any traumatic event (based on DSM-III-R criteria) was 60% for men and 50% for women. The lifetime prevalence of exposure to any trauma increases to nearly 90% when the broader DSM-IV exposure criteria are employed. More than half of individuals with trauma exposure report exposure to more than one event. The median number of distinct traumatic events among individuals exposed to any trauma is nearly five.

Events involving assault (e.g., rape, military combat, kidnap/torture, physical assault, and molestation) are experienced by roughly 40% of the population, whereas other direct experiences of trauma (e.g., motor vehicle accidents, natural disasters, witnessing others being killed or injured, or being diagnosed with a life-threatening illness) have an estimated lifetime prevalence rate of 60%. The nature and type of trauma experienced by men and women differ considerably. Men more frequently report exposure to physical attacks, to combat, to being threatened with a weapon, to being held captive/kidnapped, and to witnessing others injured or killed. Men are twice as likely as women to be exposed to assaults, with nearly 35% being mugged or threatened with a weapon. Women more often report being raped, sexually molested, neglected as children, or physically abused. More than 40% of women have experienced interpersonal violence (including sexual violence and intimate partner violence).

Exposure to all classes of trauma in both men and women peaks during late adolescence/early adulthood (ages 16 to 20 years). This is reflected in the median age of onset (23 years) for PTSD. Exposure to assaultive violence declines precipitously after this period, whereas all other classes of trauma exposure decline only modestly with advancing age, or not at all in the case of sudden unexpected death of a close friend or relative (an event that peaks in middle age). In general, the decline in all types of trauma following early adulthood appears to be steeper for women, suggesting that in women the risk of PTSD is especially pronounced during adolescence and early adulthood. The demographic variables of race, education, and income level do not appear to affect the risk of exposure to most types of trauma; the clear exception is assaultive violence, which has a two-fold increase in exposure prevalence for non-whites versus whites, for those with less education versus those with a college education, and for those with low incomes versus high incomes.

Q3 The answer is: (A) True.

Despite the high prevalence of traumatic exposure, the development of PTSD is the exception rather than the rule. The overall conditional probability of PTSD after a traumatic event is 9.2%. However, the risk of PTSD varies substantially with the type of trauma experienced. Assaultive violence in general demonstrates the highest probability (over 20%) of leading to PTSD, whereas learning about traumatic events of others carries the lowest probability (2%). Specific traumatic events that carry the highest conditional probability for PTSD include rape (50% or greater), torture/kidnap (50%), combat (nearly 40%), and childhood physical abuse or sexual molestation (25% to 50%). Women exposed to trauma are in general more than twice as likely (13% to 20%) to develop PTSD as are men (6% to 8%). This general two-fold increase in risk of PTSD in women is maintained after controlling for the distribution of trauma types. However, women's increased vulnerability to PTSD does not appear to be equally generalizable to all types of trauma. Specifically, the increased risk of a woman developing PTSD occurs predominantly after an assault, in which women demonstrate a conditional PTSD with a probability of 35% (vs. 6% in men). A significant portion of this sex difference appears attributable to the greater likelihood that women, relative to men, will meet the avoidance/numbing symptoms required for the diagnosis.

Q4 The answer is: (A) True.

Psychiatric comorbidity is the rule rather than the exception in PTSD. The NCS has estimated the percentage of a lifetime history of other psychiatric disorders in individuals diagnosed with PTSD at nearly 90% in men and 80% in women. In fact, nearly 60% of men and 45% of women with PTSD report more than three comorbid psychiatric conditions. Major depressive disorder (MDD) is among the most common of comorbid conditions for both men and women (affecting nearly 50%). Alcohol abuse (in the majority) and conduct disorder (over 40%) are also highly comorbid in men. Additionally, there is a three- to seven-fold increased risk for both men and women with PTSD to be diagnosed with other anxiety disorders, including generalized anxiety disorder, panic disorder, and specific phobias. High levels of psychiatric comorbidity in PTSD may result from the substantial symptom overlap between PTSD and disorders such as MDD (with a loss of interest, social withdrawal, insomnia, and poor concentration) and other anxiety disorders (manifest by hyperarousal and avoidance).

NCS results suggest that more often than not, PTSD is primary with respect to comorbid affective disorders and substance abuse disorders, but secondary with respect to comorbid anxiety disorders (and for men, comorbid conduct disorder). Most studies have failed to find an increased risk of MDD or drug abuse for trauma-exposed individuals who are not diagnosed with PTSD. The same has been found for alcohol abuse or dependence in men, but not women. This suggests that MDD and substance abuse (with the exception of alcohol abuse in women) are not likely to be psychiatric conditions that independently occur outside of PTSD in response to trauma; rather they appear more likely either to be the result of PTSD (i.e., an emotional response to impairment with "self-medication" through substance abuse) or to share antecedent genetic or environmental factors (i.e., with a shared liability for both PTSD and depression/substance abuse).

Q5 The answer is: (A) True.

An understanding of relevant risk factors for the development of PTSD is complicated by the fact that independent risks may exist for an increased exposure to traumatic events, and to an increased susceptibility for the development of PTSD once exposed to traumatic events. Research into the genetics of PTSD illustrates this complexity. Combat and civilian twin studies have repeatedly estimated the genetic heritability of exposure to trauma as between 35% and 50%. Furthermore, exposure to different types of trauma may be differentially mediated by genetic factors. The likelihood of exposure to traumatic events involving assaultive violence appears to be highly influenced by genetics (with a heritability greater than 50%), whereas event exposure involving nonassaultive trauma appears to be largely nongenetic. It has been proposed that one pathway underlying genetic predisposition to traumatic exposure may be mediated through heritable personality traits (e.g., neuroticism, antisocial behavior, extroversion, and sensation-seeking) that increase the risk of experiencing a traumatic event. It has been reported, for example, that the likelihood of experiencing a violent assault is predicted by antisocial personality traits, as well as the more non-pathological personality style of "being open to new ideas and experiences," with genetic factors accounting for upward of 10% of the relationship between personality and trauma exposure. Once exposed to a traumatic event, the conditional risk of PTSD also appears to be substantially influenced by genetics. Both combat and civilian trauma twin studies estimate the genetic heritability of PTSD to be approximately 30% to 40% after controlling for trauma exposure. Genetic heritability appears to be comparable among the three symptom clusters (i.e., re-experiencing, avoidance/numbing, and arousal). It remains unclear as to whether genetic factors for risk of PTSD are different for men and women or for different trauma types. Some preliminary gene studies have identified specific dopamine- or serotonin-transporter-linked polymorphic regions that may be linked to PTSD susceptibility. However, these findings have yet to be fully replicated.

Q6 The answer is: (B) False.
Recovery from PTSD appears to be most pronounced within the first year following trauma exposure. Large-scale epidemiologic studies suggest a remission rate of approximately 25% at 6 months and 40% at 1 year. The rate of recovery following the first year slows, with the median time to remission estimated at between 2 and 3 years. The NCS has estimated that the median time to remission for treated samples is approximately 36 months, whereas the median time to remission in untreated individuals increases to 64 months. Regardless of treatment, more than 30% of individuals diagnosed with PTSD appear never to remit. If PTSD remission has not occurred within 6 to 7 years after the trauma, the chance for significant recovery thereafter appears to be quite small. An estimated 10% to 15% of all Vietnam combat veterans, and nearly 30% of those with high or very high combat exposure, were found to have PTSD 12 years following the cessation of combat. Twenty-eight percent of adult survivors of the Buffalo Creek flood failed to show remission from PTSD after 14 years. In a longitudinal prospective study of Israeli veterans from the 1982 Lebanon War, 20% of individuals who experienced combat stress reactions maintained a diagnosis of chronic PTSD for 20 years following the war. Many of the risk factors for the development of PTSD also appear to be relevant to increased risk for a chronic course (e.g., comorbidity, multiple trauma exposures, negative social support, and trauma severity). In addition, the presence and intensity of avoidance and numbing symptoms may specifically predispose toward a chronic, rather than a remitting, course of illness in PTSD.

Dissociative Disorders

Multiple-Choice Questions

Select the appropriate answer.

Q1   Which of the following disorders was previously called multiple personality disorder?

   A.   *Depersonalization disorder*

   B.   *Dissociative amnesia*

   C.   *Dissociative fugue*

   D.   *Dissociative identity disorder*

   E.   *Dissociative disorder not otherwise specified*

Q2   Which of the following conditions was formerly called psychogenic amnesia?

   A.   *Depersonalization disorder*

   B.   *Dissociative amnesia*

   C.   *Dissociative fugue*

   D.   *Dissociative identity disorder*

   E.   *Dissociative disorder not otherwise specified*

Q3   In which of the following conditions is the sufferer MOST likely to engage in sudden unexpected travel away from one's place of daily activities, with an inability to recall some or all of one's past?

   A.   *Depersonalization disorder*

   B.   *Dissociative amnesia*

   C.   *Dissociative fugue*

   D.   *Dissociative identity disorder*

   E.   *Dissociative disorder not otherwise specified*

Q4   In which of the following conditions is the sufferer MOST likely to feel like an automaton or like he or she is living in a movie?

   A.   *Depersonalization disorder*

   B.   *Dissociative amnesia*

   C.   *Dissociative fugue*

   D.   *Dissociative identity disorder*

   E.   *Dissociative disorder not otherwise specified*

Q5   In which of the following conditions are approximate answers (i.e., those in which the correct set of the response is given, but the answer is inaccurate) MOST often given to simple questions?

A.   *Depersonalization disorder*

B.   *Dissociative amnesia*

C.   *Dissociative fugue*

D.   *Dissociative identity disorder*

E.   *Ganser syndrome*

Chapter 35

Answers

Q1 The answer is: (D) Dissociative identity disorder.

Among the dissociative disorders, dissociative identity disorder, previously called multiple personality disorder, has received the most attention over the last 2 decades, and has endured considerable controversy. Aspects of this controversy involve the ongoing debate regarding the interplay of society and psychiatric nosology, as well as the relationship of dissociative phenomena to consciousness; pathology involves "the presence of two or more distinct identities or personality states (each with its own relatively enduring pattern of perceiving, relating to, and thinking about the environment and the self)." In addition, "at least two of these identities" must periodically "take control of the person's behavior." Finally, there must be a demonstrated "inability to recall important personal information that is too extensive to be explained by ordinary forgetfulness."

An essential aspect of dissociative identity disorder is the amnestic quality for alternate personalities displayed by the primary personality. However, in many instances, different personality states have varying levels of awareness of other personalities (often called "alters") and often a dominant personality state exists that is cognizant of all the various personalities. The term "coconsciousness" has been used to describe the simultaneous experience of multiple entities at one time. Thus, one personality may be aware of another's feelings regarding an ongoing experience.

Q2 The answer is: (B) Dissociative amnesia.

Dissociative amnesia (previously termed psychogenic amnesia) involves "an inability to recall important personal information, usually of a traumatic nature, that is too extensive to be explained by normal forgetfulness." Dissociative amnesia may be global, involving a total loss of important personal information, or it may be more localized, in which patients cannot recall specific episodes of behavior or traumatic experiences. These experiences may include self-mutilation, criminal or sexual behaviors, traumatic events, or even marital or financial crises.

The incidence in men and women appears to be equal, and large segments of the general population may suffer brief amnestic periods following a significant large-scale disaster.

Q3 The answer is: (C) Dissociative fugue.

Dissociative fugue is probably the rarest of the dissociative disorders and is characterized by "the sudden unexpected travel away from one's place of daily activities, with inability to recall some or all of one's past." Often, patients suffering from dissociative fugue will assume entirely new identities during their fugue episode. Like dissociative amnesia, fugue is typically triggered by a traumatic event, and thus appears to be more common during wartime or after natural disasters. Patients suffering from dissociative fugue may appear normal, although they often become confused and distressed when asked questions about their personal history.

Dissociative fugue occurs primarily in adults, usually between the second and fourth decades of life. Although men appear to be affected as often as women, during war, the incidence of men suffering from dissociative fugue increases. Although fugues may last several years, most episodes last from a few days to a few months. Alternative diagnoses include brain pathology leading to fugue states, drug-induced fugues secondary to alcoholic or drug-related blackouts, and factitious disorders or malingering. In addition, some cultural syndromes (e.g., Amok and Latah) may mimic fugue states.

Q4 The answer is: (A) Depersonalization disorder.

Depersonalization disorder is characterized by "persistent or recurrent episodes after.. ... of detachment or estrangement from one's self." Often, patients with symptoms of depersonalization will "feel like an automaton or like he or she is living in a movie."

However, reality testing remains intact in those who suffer from depersonalization disorder, representing an important distinction from what would otherwise be seen as primarily a psychotic process.

Studies have suggested that as many as 50% of people will at some point endorse transient symptoms of depersonalization, and in most cases these symptoms cause little disruption and are not considered pathological. However, frequent depersonalization can be quite disruptive, interfering with daily function and preventing the integration of new experiences. Also, although transient depersonalization is roughly equal among men and women, depersonalization disorder is about twice as common in women as it is in men. Depersonalization disorder usually begins by late adolescence or early adulthood, with most episodes lasting from hours to weeks at a time. Symptoms of depersonalization have also been described in those with severe depression or psychosis, among patients taking illicit substances, and as a result of specific brain damage, migraines, or seizures.

Q5 The answer is: (E) Ganser syndrome.
Ganser syndrome (sometimes called "prison psychosis") is classified as a dissociative disorder not otherwise specified. It is characterized by the provision of approximate answers, that is, offering half-correct answers to simple inquiries, such as answering "Five" to the question, "What is two plus two?" The correct set of the response is given, but the answer is inaccurate. Ganser syndrome is often reported in incarcerated populations.

Sexual Disorders and Sexual Dysfunction

Multiple-Choice Questions

Select the appropriate answer.

Q1 Which of the following statements is LEAST accurate?

A. *A biopsychosocial model for understanding the female sexual response complements increased efforts at discovering unique pharmacologic therapies to treat female sexual disorders*

B. *Increasing recognition that sexual disorders have an organic, rather than a purely psychological, basis has transformed treatment strategies*

C. *It is important to screen routinely for sexual problems; a sexual history typically facilitates diagnosis*

D. *Phosphodiesterase (PDE)-1 inhibitors have revolutionized the treatment of male erectile disorders*

E. *Sexual disorders are common in both men and women and are associated with significant distress*

Q2 Which of the following is/are characterized by recurrent, intense sexual urges that involve unusual objects or activities?

A. *Dyspareunia*

B. *Gender identity disorders*

C. *Paraphilias*

D. *Parasomnias*

E. *Sexual dysfunction*

Q3 Which of the following is NOT one of the four distinct phases of the human sexual response (as delineated by Masters and Johnson) that are experienced in a linear progression?

A. *Desire*

B. *Excitement (arousal)*

C. *Orgasm (rhythmic muscular contractions)*

D. *Plateau (maximal arousal before orgasm)*

E. *Resolution (return to baseline)*

Q4 Which of the following conditions is the LEAST common?

A. *Female orgasmic disorder*

B. *Male orgasmic disorder*

C. *Premature ejaculation*

D. *Secondary (acquired) erectile dysfunction (ED)*

E. *Vaginismus*

Q5   Which of the following agents is LEAST likely to induce sexual dysfunction?

A.   *Fluoxetine*

B.   *Methyldopa*

C.   *Sildenafil*

D.   *Thiazide diuretics*

E.   *Thioridazine*

Q6   Which of the following terms BEST defines "sexual arousal by touching and rubbing against a non-consenting person."

A.   *Exhibitionism*

B.   *Fetishism*

C.   *Frotteurism*

D.   *Pedophilia*

E.   *Voyeurism*

Chapter 36

Answers

Q1 The answer is (D) Phosphodiesterase (PDE)-1 inhibitors have revolutionized the treatment of male erectile disorders.

The mainstay of treatment for erectile dysfunction (ED) is the use of oral PDE-5 inhibitors (e.g., sildenafil, vardenafil, and tadalafil), which can help men with a wide range of conditions; they are easy to use and have few adverse effects. The PDE-5 inhibitors are effective in the treatment of antidepressant-induced ED and retarded ejaculation. Of note, the PDE-5 inhibitors are metabolized by P450 3A4 and 2C9 isoenzyme systems. Patients who take potent inhibitors (including grapefruit juice, cimetidine, ketoconazole, erythromycin, and ritonavir) of these P450 isoenzyme systems should have a lower starting dose of a PDE-5 inhibitor. Statins may also help improve the efficacy of PDE-5 inhibitors.

Q2 The answer is: (C) Paraphilias.

Paraphilias are characterized by recurrent, intense sexual urges that involve unusual objects or activities.

Dyspareunia is a disorder defined as persistent genital pain associated with sexual intercourse.

Gender identity disorders involve persistent cross-gender identification and discomfort with one's assigned sex.

Parasomnias are sleep disorders characterized by activities that are carried out during sleep (e.g., talking, walking, or urinating) that would be considered normal if performed during wakefulness.

Sexual dysfunction is characterized by disturbances in sexual desire and/or psychophysiological changes in the sexual response cycle.

Q3 The answer is: (A) Desire.

Masters and Johnson developed the first model of the human sexual response, consisting of a linear progression through four distinct phases: (1) excitement (arousal); (2) plateau (maximal arousal before orgasm); (3) orgasm (rhythmic muscular contractions); and (4) resolution (return to baseline). Following resolution, a refractory period exists in men. Desire was not one of the stages described.

Kaplan modified the Masters and Johnson model by introducing a desire stage; this model emphasized the importance of neuropsychological input in the human sexual response. The Kaplan model consisted of three stages: (1) desire; (2) excitement/arousal (including an increase in peripheral blood flow); and (3) orgasm (muscular contraction).

Q4 The answer is: (B) Male orgasmic disorder.

Female orgasmic disorder is defined as a recurrent delay in, or absence of, orgasm following a normal sexual excitement phase. Some women who can have orgasm with direct clitoral stimulation find it impossible to reach orgasm during intercourse. This is a normal variant of sensitivity that requires the pairing of direct clitoral contact with intercourse. Female orgasmic disorder has a lifetime prevalence of 35%. Approximately 5% to 8% of afflicted individuals are totally anorgasmic. Moreover, 30% to 40% of afflicted individuals are unable to achieve orgasm without clitoral stimulation during intercourse.

Male orgasmic disorder ("retarded ejaculation") is defined as a persistent delay or absence of orgasm following normal sexual excitement. It is infrequent, with a lifetime prevalence of 2%; it occurs in men who are usually under age 35 years, and who are sexually inexperienced. Retarded ejaculation is usually restricted to failure to reach orgasm in the vagina during intercourse. Orgasm can usually occur with masturbation and/or from a partner's manual or oral stimulation.

Premature ejaculation is defined as recurrent ejaculation with minimal sexual stimulation before, on, or shortly after penetration and before the person wishes it (most often less than 2 minutes after penetration or on fewer than 10 thrusts). The lifetime prevalence of premature ejaculation is 15%. Premature ejaculation affects 30% of men. Prolonged periods of no sexual activity make premature ejaculation worse. If the problem is chronic and untreated, secondary impotence often occurs.

Male erectile disorder, or ED ("impotence"), is defined as the inability of a male to maintain an erection sufficient to engage in intercourse; it is considered a problem if it occurs in more than 25% of attempts.

Roughly 20 to 30 million American men suffer from ED; this symptom accounts for more than 500,000 ambulatory care visits to health care professionals annually.

Primary (lifelong) ED occurs in 1% of men under age 35 years. Secondary (acquired) ED occurs in 40% of men over age 60 years; this figure increases to 73% in men who are age 80 years.

Vaginismus is defined as recurrent involuntary spasm of the musculature of the outer third of the vagina, interfering with sexual intercourse. The frequency of this disorder is unknown, but it probably accounts for less than 10% of female sexual disorders. The diagnosis is often made on routine gynecologic examination when contraction of the vaginal outlet occurs as either the examining finger or the speculum is introduced. There is a high incidence of associated pelvic pathology. Lifelong vaginismus has an abrupt onset, at the first attempt at penetration, and has a chronic course. Acquired vaginismus may occur suddenly, following a sexual trauma or a medical condition.

Q5 The answer is: (C) Sildenafil.
Sildenafil and other oral PDE-5 inhibitors are effective in the treatment of antidepressant-induced ED and retarded ejaculation. The other agents listed are known to cause or exacerbate sexual dysfunction.

Q6 The answer is: (C) Frotteurism.
Exhibitionism is exposure of genitals to unsuspecting strangers in public.

Fetishism is sexual arousal using non-living objects (e.g., female lingerie).

Frotteurism is sexual arousal by touching and rubbing against a non-consenting person.

Pedophilia is sexual activity with a prepubescent child; the person must be at least age 16 years and be 5 years older than the victim.

Voyeurism is sexual arousal by watching an unsuspecting person who is naked, disrobing, or engaging in sexual activity.

Eating Disorders: Evaluation and Management

Multiple-Choice Questions

Select the appropriate answer.

Q1   Which of the following disorders is MOST common in the United States?

  A.   *Anorexia nervosa (AN)*

  B.   *Binge-eating disorder (BED)*

  C.   *Bulimia nervosa (BN)*

  D.   *Schizophrenia*

  E.   *Somatization disorder*

Q2   Which of the following conditions is BEST characterized by a refusal to maintain, or attain, a minimally healthful body weight?

  A.   *Anorexia nervosa (AN)*

  B.   *Binge-eating disorder (BED)*

  C.   *Bulimia nervosa (BN)*

  D.   *Schizophrenia*

  E.   *Somatization disorder*

Q3   Which of the following conditions is MOST closely associated with the development of low bone mineral density?

  A.   *Anorexia nervosa (AN)*

  B.   *Binge-eating disorder (BED)*

  C.   *Bulimia nervosa (BN)*

  D.   *Schizophrenia*

  E.   *Somatization disorder*

Q4   True or False. Laxatives do NOT remove ingested calories.

  A.   *True*

  B.   *False*

Q5   Which of the following is the MOST accurate equation for the calculation of body mass index (BMI)?

  A.   *Weight (in kg)/height (in meters)^2*

  B.   *Weight (in kg)/height (in meters)*

  C.   *Weight (in lb)/height (in feet)^2*

  D.   *Weight (in lb)/height (in inches)*

  E.   *Weight (in lb)/height (in inches)^2*

Chapter 37

Answers

Q1 The answer is: (B) Binge-eating disorder (BED).

Binge-eating disorder (BED) appears to be the most common eating disorder, with a lifetime prevalence ranging between 2.9% and 3.5% in females.

The lifetime prevalence of anorexia nervosa (AN) has been estimated from several large international twin cohorts (ranging from 0.5% to 2.2% for females). An estimate of the lifetime prevalence of AN combined with eating disorder not otherwise specified resembling AN is over 3%. Bulimia nervosa (BN) is more common than is AN, with a reported lifetime prevalence in adult women ranging from 1.1% to 2.9%. An estimate of the lifetime prevalence of BN-like syndromes is considerably higher (8%).

The prevalence of eating disorders appears to vary by sex, ethnicity, and the type of population studied. Eating disorders are substantially more common among females than males. Binge-eating is relatively more common among males (about 40% of cases), but still is more common in females. Eating disorders occur in culturally, ethnically, and socioeconomically diverse populations.

The incidence of eating disorders ascertained by case registries probably underestimates the true incidence for several reasons. Data from the National Comorbidity Survey Replication indicated that fewer than half of individuals with an eating disorder access any kind of health care service for their illness. Many of those affected are known to avoid or to postpone clinical care for the condition. In addition, both BN and BED may occur without clinical signs, making them difficult, if not impossible, to recognize in a clinical setting without patient disclosure of symptoms, which may not be forthcoming. Furthermore, whereas AN may manifest with a variety of clinical signs, including emaciation, many patients effectively conceal their symptoms; up to 50% of cases of eating disorders may be missed in clinical settings.

Schizophrenia has a prevalence of 0.2% to 2.0%, and somatization has a prevalence of 0.2% to 2.0% among women and 0.2% in men.

Q2 The answer is: (A) Anorexia nervosa (AN).

AN is characterized and distinguished by a refusal to maintain, or attain, a minimally healthful body weight. In addition to a low body weight, AN is characterized in Western populations by a fear of becoming fat, and by a disturbance in body experience that can range from a denial of serious medical consequences to a distorted perception of one's size and its importance. For postmenarchal females, amenorrhea of at least 3 months'duration is a diagnostic criterion.

BN is characterized by recurrent episodes of binge-eating and behaviors aimed at the prevention of weight gain or purging calories. These behaviors, termed "inappropriate compensatory behaviors,"include induced vomiting; laxative, enema, and diuretic misuse; stimulant abuse; diabetic underdosing of insulin; fasting; and excessive exercise. To meet criteria for the syndrome, patients need to engage in both bingeing and inappropriate compensatory behaviors at least twice weekly for at least 3 months. Two subtypes, "purging type" and "non-purging type," are distinguished. Individuals who prevent weight gain (by exercise or by fasting) fall into the latter subtype. In addition, individuals with BN are excessively concerned with body shape and weight.

BED is characterized by recurrent episodes of binge-eating. Unlike in individuals with BN, there are no recurrent behaviors to purge calories, or to prevent weight gain from the binge episodes. Binge episodes are accompanied by at least three of five correlates (these include eating rapidly, until uncomfortably full, when not hungry, alone to avoid embarrassment) and are associated with distress. Individuals must experience these episodes (on average) once each week for at least 3 months to meet provisional *Diagnostic and Statistical Manual of Mental Disorders* criteria for BED.

Q3 The answer is: (A) Anorexia nervosa (AN).

Although cardiac complications may be the most dangerous for patients with AN, osteoporosis is among the most permanent. Loss of bone mass can be rapid and remain low despite disease recovery; it represents a lifelong risk of increased fractures. The association of low bone mineral density is established in adolescent girls, as well as boys. Of importance, effects on bone mass can be seen with brief disease duration, with significant reductions in bone mass being reported in girls who have been ill for less than 1 year. Skeletal impact can be severe.

Factors that contribute to low bone mineral density in AN include hormonal and nutritional abnormalities, and risks associated with excess exercise, smoking, and alcohol use. Endocrine factors include hypogonadism, low levels of insulin-like growth factor-I, and hypercortisolemia. In AN, normal puberty is disrupted with prolonged estrogen deficiency and lack of growth hormone effects. Maximal bone mass is achieved during adolescence and early adult life. Therefore, suppression of bone formation by undernutrition during adolescence leaves affected girls particularly vulnerable to inadequate peak bone mass formation.

BN, BED, schizophrenia, and somatization disorder are not closely linked with profound weight loss and osteoporosis.

Q4 The answer is: (A) True.
Laxatives do *not* remove ingested calories. Their futility as a weight loss vehicle notwithstanding, they are the most commonly abused agents by eating-disordered patients, second only to vomiting as a form of purging. Patients who try to stop their abuse of laxatives may experience both rebound edema and refractory constipation. Protocols are available for abrupt cessation of laxatives and temporary measures to restore normal bowel function. Others find gradual tapering of laxatives better tolerated, especially in outpatients.

Q5 The answer is: (A) Weight (in kg)/Height (in meters)^2.
A healthful body weight is assessed in relation to age, height, and sometimes sex and frame. Although the clinical context guides whether a weight is consistent with AN, a commonly recognized guideline is a weight that falls below 85% of that expected for height or a body mass index (BMI) less than 17.5 kg/m^2 in adults. Although commenting on "ideal weight" in adults is relatively straightforward, there are no standardized tables or formulas available for children and adolescents. This is largely related to the fact that growth patterns are highly variable and can change monthly. Both the American Academy of Pediatrics and the American Psychiatric Association have set forth practice guidelines that encourage providers to determine an individual adolescent's goal weight range using past growth charts, menstrual history, midparental height, and even bone age as guides. The Centers for Disease Control and Prevention recommends use of growth charts, which plot BMI for age (2 to 20 years) and sex. Children who fall below the fifth percentile in BMI for age are considered underweight, and those who fall between 5% and 85% are deemed "average weight." Clearly, there is considerable variation in the "normal" range. Therefore following the expected trajectory for a child based on the pediatrician's past records is often most helpful.

The expected body weight for adult women is calculated by the following equation: (100 lb + 5 lb/inch above 5 feet) ± 10%.

Chapter 38

Grief, Bereavement, and Adjustment Disorders

Multiple-Choice Questions

Select the appropriate answer.

Q1 Which of the following terms BEST defines "the physical and emotional pain precipitated by a significant loss"?

   A. *Adjustment disorder with depressive features*

   B. *Denial*

   C. *Grief*

   D. *Major depression*

   E. *Psychotic depression*

Q2 Which of the following terms BEST describes a condition in which there is a sense of disbelief regarding the death, anger, and bitterness over the death, recurrent pangs of painful emotions, and a preoccupation with thoughts of the lost loved one (that often include distressing intrusive thoughts related to the death)?

   A. *Acute grief*

   B. *Anticipatory grief*

   C. *Complicated grief*

   D. *Delayed grief*

   E. *Unresolved grief*

Q3 Which of the following is perhaps the BEST treatment of grief?

   A. *Listening to the mourner's experience and providing support*

   B. *Prescribing an atypical antipsychotic*

   C. *Prescribing a sedative-hypnotic*

   D. *Prescribing a selective serotonin reuptake inhibitor*

   E. *Providing advice to the mourner (e.g., that the mourners should be stoic and keep his or her emotional displays to a minimum)*

Q4 Which of the following statements is LEAST accurate?

   A. *As the mourning process proceeds, the grieving person may experience himself or herself in new ways that may lead to the development of a new identity (e.g., an orphan, an only child, a widow, or a single parent)*

   B. *Emotional and cognitive responses to the death of a loved one may include anger, guilt, regret, anxiety, intrusive images, and feelings of being overwhelmed, relieved, or lonely*

   C. *Mourners mourn in the same way across cultures*

   D. *The death of a loved one can profoundly shift the dynamics of a survivor's relationships with family, friends, and coworkers*

   E. *The mourner's connection with the deceased may be maintained through symbolic representations, adoption of traits of the deceased, cultural rituals, or various means of continued contact (e.g., dreams or attempts at communication)*

Q5   Which of the following is NOT a primary psychotherapeutic task of working with a bereaved person?

A.   *Establishing a relationship with the grieving individual on his or her own terms*

B.   *Exploring the loss as fully as possible*

C.   *Identifying strengths and supports*

D.   *Insisting that the grieving person speak about the deceased*

E.   *Providing support*

Chapter 38
Answers

Q1 The answer is: (C) Grief.

Grief may be defined as the physical and emotional pain precipitated by a significant loss. The loss may be of a person or pet, but it can also be of a meaningful place, job, or an object. A closely related term to grief is bereavement, which literally means to be robbed by death.

Death and loss are part of the human condition; therefore, everyone is at risk for the experience of grief. However, the diagnosis of pathological grief is often complicated by the fact that normal grief often varies in its duration and intensity, is shaped by sociocultural influences, and does not necessarily proceed smoothly from one phase to another.

In a bereaved psychiatric patient, prevention of relapse (of the patient's mental disorder) may be achieved by providing support and by optimizing psychotropic medications.

Q2 The answer is: (C) Complicated grief.

Complicated grief includes a sense of disbelief regarding the death, anger, and bitterness over the death, recurrent pangs of painful emotions, and a preoccupation with thoughts of the lost love one (that often includes distressing intrusive thoughts related to the death). Clinical complications may include social/occupational/familial dysfunction, and/or health-compromising behaviors (e.g., non-compliance with prescribed medical treatment), anxiety, and physical morbidity.

Acute grief is the first stage of the process of bereavement. Symptoms may begin immediately following the loss or may be delayed.

Anticipatory grief involves a grief reaction that occurs in anticipation of an impending loss; its symptoms include anger, guilt, anxiety, irritability, sadness, feelings of loss, and decreased ability to perform usual tasks.

Delayed grief involves the absence of the expression of grief at the time of loss.

Unresolved grief involves a persistence of grief symptoms that can reach extremes of intensity, duration, or tenacity.

Q3 The answer is: (A) Listening to the mourner's experience and providing support.

Perhaps the most common treatment of grief involves the simple listening to the mourner's experience, and the provision of support. Family members, community members, and primary care providers provide the most support to mourners.

Two categories of mourners come to the attention of a psychiatrist: those individuals already in treatment for a previously diagnosed psychiatric condition, and those whose concern about pathological grief is the initiating complaint.

Psychiatric patients with any kind of pathological grief may benefit from a review of their psychoactive medications.

Besides providing support during the time of grief, an additional goal of treatment is the prevention of a relapse of the patient's mental disorder (e.g., a temporary increase in sleep medications may be helpful if insomnia threatens to overwhelm a patient's ability to cope).

Q4 The answer is: (C) Mourners mourn in the same way across cultures.

Not everyone mourns in the same way. Mourners may employ some of the strategies (e.g., involvement with others, distraction, avoidance, rationalization, the direct expression of feelings, disbelief or denial, use of faith or religious guidance, or indulgence in "forbidden" activities).

Mourners have the right to mourn because of the love held for the deceased. Not everyone expects the same type of treatment.

As the mourning process proceeds, the grieving person may experience himself or herself in new ways that may lead to the development of a new identity (e.g., an orphan, an only child, a widow, or a single parent).

Emotional and cognitive responses to the death of loved ones may include anger, guilt, regret, anxiety, intrusive images of feelings of being overwhelmed, relieved, or lonely.

The death of a loved one can profoundly shift the dynamics of the survivor's relationships with family, friends, and coworkers.

The mourner's connection with the deceased may be maintained through symbolic representations, adoption of traits of the deceased, cultural rituals, or various means of continued contact (e.g., dreams or attempts at communication).

Q5 The answer is: (D) Insisting that the grieving person speak about the deceased.

Appropriate intervention of acute grief often involves creating a balance between legitimizing a loss, expressing sorrow, and involving oneself in the ceremonies that surround grief. As not everyone grieves in the same way or at the same time, forcing a person to deal with loss in a proscribed manner makes little sense.

Instead, it is reasonable to relate to the grieving individual (on his or her own terms), explore the loss as fully as possible, identify strengths and supports, and provide support.

Chapter 39

Personality and Personality Disorders

Multiple-Choice Questions

Select the appropriate answer.

Q1   Which of the following MOST closely approximates the percentage of the general population with a personality disorder?

A.   *Less than 5%*

B.   *10% to 15%*

C.   *20% to 25%*

D.   *30% to 35%*

E.   *More than 50%*

Q2   Which of the following is generally considered to be the "father of personality psychology"?

A.   *Gordon Allport*

B.   *Aaron Beck*

C.   *Sigmund Freud*

D.   *Jerome Kagan*

E.   *Alexander Thomas*

Q3   Which of the following is NOT considered to be one of the five most common names given to categories in the Five-Factor Model of personality traits?

A.   *Agreeableness*

B.   *Aggressiveness*

C.   *Conscientiousness*

D.   *Extroversion*

E.   *Neuroticism*

Q4   Which of the following categories of personality disorders would BEST be applied to a patient with a borderline personality disorder?

A.   *Cluster A*

B.   *Cluster B*

C.   *Cluster C*

D.   *Cluster D*

E.   *Cluster E*

Q5 Which of the following is MOST closely associated with a personality disorder in which a person has little desire for relationships and has few emotional ties?

A. *Antisocial personality disorder*

B. *Borderline personality disorder*

C. *Paranoid personality disorder*

D. *Schizoid personality disorder*

E. *Schizotypal personality disorder*

Q6 Which of the following is MOST closely associated with a personality disorder in which a person embraces unusual beliefs to a degree that exceeds cultural and subcultural norms?

A. *Antisocial personality disorder*

B. *Borderline personality disorder*

C. *Paranoid personality disorder*

D. *Schizoid personality disorder*

E. *Schizotypal personality disorder*

Q7 Which of the following is MOST closely associated with a personality disorder in which a person engages in socially irresponsible behaviors, and has a pervasive disregard for the rights of others?

A. *Antisocial personality disorder*

B. *Borderline personality disorder*

C. *Paranoid personality disorder*

D. *Schizoid personality disorder*

E. *Schizotypal personality disorder*

Q8 Which of the following is MOST closely associated with a personality disorder in which a person has an impaired capacity to form stable relationships, has affective instability, impulsivity, identity disturbance, and recurrent suicidal thinking?

A. *Antisocial personality disorder*

B. *Borderline personality disorder*

C. *Paranoid personality disorder*

D. *Schizoid personality disorder*

E. *Schizotypal personality disorder*

Q9 Which of the following is MOST closely associated with a personality disorder in which a person has an overwhelming and pathological self-absorption?

A. *Antisocial personality disorder*

B. *Borderline personality disorder*

C. *Narcissistic personality disorder*

D. *Paranoid personality disorder*

E. *Schizoid personality disorder*

Q10 Which of the following is MOST closely associated with a personality disorder in which a person has an excessive discomfort or fear in intimate and social relationships that results in self-protection from social interactions?

A. *Antisocial personality disorder*

B. *Avoidant personality disorder*

C. *Borderline personality disorder*

D. *Narcissistic personality disorder*

E. *Schizoid personality disorder*

Chapter 39

Answers

Q1 The answer is: (B) 10% to 15%.

Personality disorders are common conditions that affect 10% to15% of the general population.

Furthermore, 25% to 50% of individuals who seek outpatient mental health care have either a primary or a comorbid personality disorder.

The percentage of psychiatric inpatients with a personality disorder is estimated to be approximately 80%.

Personality disorders as a group are among the most frequent disorders treated by psychiatrists.

Q2 The answer is: (A) Gordon Allport.

Gordon Allport, the father of personality psychology, defined personality as "the dynamic organization within the individual of those psychophysical systems that determine his characteristic behavior and thought."

Aaron Beck pioneered cognitive therapy, whereas Sigmund Freud is called the "father of psychoanalysis."

Jerome Kagan and colleagues from Harvard University (expanding on the work of Dr. Alexander Thomas and Dr. Stella Chess at New York University) have studied temperament (e.g., inhibited and uninhibited) in infants.

Q3 The answer is: (B) Aggressiveness.

The Five-Factor Model does not argue that all personality traits are represented within the broad domains; however, it provides a reasonably comprehensive coverage of the most important traits that people use to describe themselves and others. The most common names given to these categories are agreeableness, conscientiousness, extroversion, neuroticism, and openness.

Aggressiveness is not one of the common features.

Agreeableness is primarily an interpersonal trait. Individuals who are high in agreeableness are cooperative, easygoing, and tend to have smooth relationships, often at the expense of self-assertion. Individuals who score low on this trait, however, are disagreeable, oppositional, express their anger easily, and tend to have relationships that are frequently disrupted by conflict.

Extroversion is associated with positive emotional experiences and an optimistic outlook on life. Individuals who are high in extroversion tend to be outgoing, to like social interactions, to be responsive to intermittent positive reinforcement, and to display high behavioral persistence. High levels of extroversion are thought to be protective against psychiatric illness, and should an illness develop, to respond more consistently to various treatment modalities. The opposite end of the extroversion spectrum is known as introversion. Individuals with this trait are often solitary, socially withdrawn, less influenced by certain types of positive reinforcement, and have a slower personal pace. Both neuroticism and extroversion have a high degree of heritability.

Conscientiousness is associated with self-control and a focused and organized approach to life. Individuals high in conscientiousness are achievement-oriented goal-setters who can delay immediate gratification to obtain their long-term desired outcome. They are considered responsible, reliable, and dependable. Individuals low in conscientiousness tend to be careless, disorganized, impulsive, and irresponsible. They easily give in to the prospect of immediate or very near-term gratification.

Neuroticism reflects the degree of negative emotion and pessimism a person generally experiences. Individuals who are high in neuroticism tend to be "worriers," and they expect and fear the worst from every experience. Neuroticism is a robust predictor for the development of a psychiatric illness at some point during the life cycle, and it is often associated with low self-esteem, depression, and anxiety. Individuals low in neuroticism are emotionally stable and they deny being bothered by anxiety, irritability, or anger.

Openness describes an individual's interest in engaging in, or willingness to engage in, new and various intellectual and cultural experiences. It is a reflection of curiosity and imagination; it should not to be confused with extroversion. Individuals who are high in openness enjoy a wide range of intellectual and cultural experiences (such as art, theater, poetry, and philosophy). Individuals who are low on this trait, however, may be no less intelligent, but have less interest in esoteric intellectual pursuits. Rather, they concentrate on learning and on experiences that are more practical and applicable to their life.

Q4 The answer is: (B) Cluster B.

The *Diagnostic and Statistical Manual of Mental Disorders* recognizes 10 major personality disorders, which are organized into three clusters (based on shared diagnostic features): (1) cluster A personality disorders, which share the common features of being odd and eccentric (paranoid, schizoid, and schizotypal personality disorders); (2) cluster B personality disorders, which share the common features of being dramatic, emotional, and erratic (antisocial, borderline, histrionic, and narcissistic personality disorders); and (3) cluster C personality disorders, which share the common features of being anxious and fearful (avoidant, dependent, and obsessive-compulsive personality disorders). As a rule, patients often display traits of more than one personality disorder, and if they meet diagnostic criteria for another one, it should be diagnosed along with the primary one.

Q5 The answer is: (D) Schizoid personality disorder.

Individuals with a schizoid personality disorder are loners who are emotionally detached and indifferent to the world around them. They have little desire for relationships and have few emotional ties, even with family members. They express little or no discomfort over their detachment. With respect to employment, they prefer noncompetitive and isolative jobs with non-human themes (such as mathematics, philosophy, or astronomy). They may greatly enjoy solitary pursuits, such as computer games and puzzles. On interview, their thinking is clear and their reality testing is intact. The best caricature of the person with a schizoid personality would be the single, unfashionable, laboratory-oriented, absent-minded professor.

Q6 The answer is: (E) Schizotypal personality disorder.

The essential features of the schizotypal personality disorder are cognitive, perceptual, and behavioral eccentricities, and a pervasive discomfort with close relationships. Patients with this personality disorder frequently embrace unusual beliefs (such as telepathy, clairvoyance, and magical thinking) to a degree that exceeds cultural and subcultural norms. Socially, they are inept and uncomfortable. The style of their clothing may be inappropriate and strange, further reflecting their eccentric nature. Their speech is often vague, digressive, or inappropriately abstract, and they may talk to themselves in public. The content of that speech may also reflect ideas of reference, bodily illusions, and paranoia, but there is usually an absence of formal thought disorders, and reality testing is intact. Under periods of stress, however, these patients may decompensate into brief psychotic states.

Q7 The answer is: (A) Antisocial personality disorder.

The key features of antisocial personality disorder are repetitive unlawful acts, socially irresponsible behaviors, and a pervasive disregard for the rights of others. Antisocial behaviors develop early in adolescence, before age 15 years. These individuals are so unconcerned with the feelings and rights of others that they are morally bankrupt and lack a sense of remorse. Such people seem completely unable to project themselves into the feelings of others and they are bereft of empathy. Superficially, they can be charming and engaging, yet beneath the facade, individuals live in a world filled with illegal activity, deceit, promiscuity, substance abuse, and assaultive behaviors. Because patients with this disorder are so indifferent to how their actions affect others, antisocial personality disorder is the personality disorder most resistant to treatment.

Q8 The answer is: (B) Borderline personality disorder.

Borderline personality disorder has attracted the most research and clinical interest of all the personality disorders. Central to this disorder is an impaired capacity to form stable interpersonal relationships. Other salient features include affective instability (with rapidly shifting mood swings), impulsivity, identity disturbance (described as chronic boredom or emptiness), recurrent manipulative suicidal and parasuicidal behaviors (e.g., self-mutilation), and idealization/devaluation ("splitting"). When faced with real or perceived separation, these patients often react with intense fear and anger. Under stress, the borderline patient may also experience brief reactive psychotic states (also known as "micropsychotic episodes"). Also, they are more likely to have various dissociative phenomena in stressful and in affectively intense situations.

Q9 The answer is: (C) Narcissistic personality disorder.

The hallmark of narcissistic personality disorder is an overwhelming and pathological self-absorption. These individuals possess a grandiose sense of self-importance or uniqueness; they are preoccupied with fantasies of success and feel that the people with whom they associate need also be special and unique. They are blindly ambitious, often breaking conventional rules and exploiting others to meet their self-serving ends. They lack empathy for others (although less so than the antisocial patient) and can react with disappointment and rage when another's needs interfere with their desires. Beneath the facade of self-sufficiency and arrogance lies a fragile individual who is so hypersensitive to issues of self-esteem that if he or she is criticized in even the slightest manner, the reaction is intense emotion and rage.

Q10 The answer is: (B) Avoidant personality disorder.

The core feature of avoidant personality disorder is an excessive discomfort or fear in intimate and social relationships that results in the pathological avoidance of social interactions (as a means of self-protection). For example, to guard against what they fear might be potentially embarrassing or humiliating situations, these individuals exaggerate the risks of ordinary, but unplanned, tasks so as not to deviate from a safe and predictable daily routine. Although genuinely desiring relationships, they are unwilling to enter into them because of real or perceived signs of humiliation, rejection, or negative feedback. If, however, they manage to negotiate a relationship, it is only with the assurance of uncritical acceptance. Because of this pervasive awkwardness and shyness, they suffer from very low self-esteem. Because their chronic avoidant behavior reduces anticipatory anxiety through negative reinforcement (i.e., the removal of a noxious situation), this behavior pattern is powerfully entrenched and difficult to modify.

TREATMENT APPROACHES

Psychiatric Neuroscience: Incorporating Pathophysiology into Clinical Case Formulation

Multiple-Choice Questions

Select the appropriate answer.

Q1 Which of the following was awarded a Nobel Prize in 2000 for work characterizing information processing in the brain at the molecular level?

  A. *Julius Axelrod*

  B. *Ulf von Euler*

  C. *Eric Kandel*

  D. *Bernard Katz*

  E. *Emil Kraeplin*

Q2 Which of the following was the FIRST to describe plaques in the brains of patients with dementia?

  A. *Alois Alzheimer*

  B. *Paul Broca*

  C. *Ulf von Euler*

  D. *Phineas Gage*

  E. *Emil Kraeplin*

Q3 Which of the following brain territories is the MOST likely to be considered as the major relay station for incoming sensory information and other critical circuitry?

  A. *Amygdala*

  B. *Cerebellum*

  C. *Hippocampus*

  D. *Nucleus accumbens*

  E. *Thalamus*

Q4 Which of the following won a Nobel Prize in 1906 for demonstrating that neurons act as physically discrete functional units within the brain, communicating with each other through specialized junctions?

  A. *Julius Axelrod*

  B. *Santiago Ramon y Cajal*

  C. *Ulf von Euler*

  D. *Eric Kandel*

  E. *Bernard Katz*

Q5   Which of the following is the MAJOR excitatory neurotransmitter in the brain?

A.   *Acetylcholine*

B.   *Dopamine*

C.   *Endorphin*

D.   *Gamma-aminobutyric acid*

E.   *Glutamate*

Q6   Which of the following is MOST likely to be thought of as capable of imparting either rapid or gradual change in the function of the postsynaptic neuron?

A.   *Acetylcholine receptors*

B.   *Dopamine receptors*

C.   *Endorphin receptors*

D.   *Gamma-aminobutyric acid receptors*

E.   *Glutamate receptors*

Q7   Which of the following substances is MOST closely linked with the nigrostriatal system, the mesolimbic system, the mesocortical system, and the tuberoinfundibular system?

A.   *Acetylcholine*

B.   *Dopamine*

C.   *Endorphin*

D.   *Gamma-aminobutyric acid*

E.   *Glutamate*

Q8   In which of the following structures is serotonin primarily synthesized?

A.   *Amygdala*

B.   *Basal ganglia*

C.   *Hippocampus*

D.   *Raphe nuclei*

E.   *Thalamus*

Q1 The answer is: (C) Eric Kandel.
The work of Julius Axelrod, Ulf von Euler, and Bernard Katz on neurotransmitters and their mechanisms of release, reuptake, and metabolism was recognized with a Nobel Prize in 1970. Later, converging work characterizing information processing in the brain at a molecular level earned Arvid Carlsson, Paul Greengard, and Eric Kandel the 2000 Nobel Prize at the end of the decade of the brain.

Q2 The answer is: (A) Alois Alzheimer.
Neuropathology was clearly in fashion in the late 1800s and early 1900s, when Alois Alzheimer first described plaques in the brain of his patient with dementia, and identified frontal cortex abnormalities in schizophrenia.

Q3 The answer is: (E) Thalamus.
The thalamus is a major relay station for incoming sensory information and other critical circuitry, including connections between association cortices (via the mediodorsal nucleus) and outputs regulating motor activity. The mediodorsal nucleus, a critical relay station between association cortices, is a region of the thalamus found to be smaller in some neuropathological studies of patients with schizophrenia. The basal ganglia orchestrate multiple functions; the dorsal striatum plays an important role in motor control, whereas the ventral striatum (in particular, the nucleus accumbens) plays key roles in emotion and learning via connections with the hippocampus, amygdala, and prefrontal cortex. The hypothalamus plays a critical role in neuroendocrine regulation of the internal milieu. Via its effects on pituitary hormone release and connections to other regions of the brain, the hypothalamus exerts homeostatic effects on numerous psychiatrically relevant factors including mood, motivation, sexual drive, hunger, temperature, and sleep. Finally, a number of discrete nuclei in the brainstem synthesize key modulatory neurotransmitters, exerting major effects on brain function via their widespread projections to striatal and corticolimbic regions of the brain. These neuromodulatory nuclei include the dopaminergic ventral tegmental area (VTA) in the midbrain, serotonergic raphe nuclei in the brainstem, noradrenergic locus ceruleus neurons in the pons, and cholinergic neurons of the basal forebrain and brainstem.

Although the cerebellum has traditionally been known for its role in motor coordination and learning, it has more recently been implicated in cognitive and affective processes as well.

Q4 The answer is: (B) Santiago Ramon y Cajal.
The Spanish neuroanatomist Santiago Ramon y Cajal prolifically and painstakingly documented the cellular diversity of the nervous system. Based on his observations, Ramon y Cajal proposed that neurons act as physically discrete functional units within the brain, communicating with each other through specialized junctions. This theory became known as the "neuron doctrine"; Ramon y Cajal's enormous contributions were recognized with a Nobel Prize in 1906.

Q5 The answer is: (E) Glutamate.
The major excitatory neurotransmitter in the brain is glutamate (commonly used by projection neurons), whereas the major inhibitory neurotransmitter in the brain is gamma-aminobutyric acid, which is commonly used by local interneurons.

Q6 The answer is: (E) Glutamate receptors.
Glutamate receptors are varied in structure and function, capable of imparting either rapid or gradual change in the function of the postsynaptic neuron. The ionotropic family of glutamate receptors, which includes N-methyl-D-aspartate, alpha-amino-3-hydroxy-5-methyl-isoxazolepropionic acid, and kainate receptors, act rapidly by opening channels for Na+ and (to a variable degree) calcium ion influx. This influx causes postsynaptic depolarization, which, if present in sufficient force, causes the neuron to fire. The metabotropic glutamate receptors effect gradual change in neuronal function. These seven membrane-

spanning G protein-coupled receptors are linked to cytoplasmic enzymes via G proteins embedded within the cell membrane. Once activated, these enzymes can induce second-messenger cascades that can influence intracellular processes, including gene transcription.

Q7 The answer is: (B) Dopamine.

Although glutamate and gamma-aminobutyric acid are found throughout the brain, other neurotransmitter systems are localized to specific neural pathways. The monoamines (e.g., norepinephrine, serotonin, dopamine), as well as acetylcholine, are synthesized in several discrete brainstem nuclei, yet project widely, affecting a majority of brain systems. Dopamine, a catecholamine neurotransmitter, affects many brain regions that are consistently implicated in psychiatric disorders.

There are four major dopamine projections, each with great relevance to neuropsychiatric phenomena. The name of each projection indicates the location of the dopaminergic cell bodies, and the region targeted by their axons; for example, the nigrostriatal system consists of dopamine cell bodies in the substantia nigra, with axons projecting to the striatum. Degeneration of the nigrostriatal pathway leads to extrapyramidal motor symptoms (such as tremor, bradykinesia, and rigidity) as seen in Parkinson disease. An analogous mechanism underlies extrapyramidal symptoms associated with antipsychotic medications, which block dopamine receptors in the striatum.

Dopamine neurons in the mesolimbic pathway project from the VTA, also in the midbrain, to limbic and paralimbic structures including the nucleus accumbens, amygdala, hippocampus, septum, anterior cingulate cortex, and orbitofrontal cortex. Given the importance of these downstream structures to emotion, sensory perception, and memory, it has been speculated that altered activity in the mesolimbic pathway may underlie the perceptual disturbances common to positive symptoms of schizophrenia, hallucinogen use, and even temporal lobe seizures. The mesolimbic pathway is also implicated in the addictive actions of drugs of abuse, which share the common feature of enhancing dopamine release in the nucleus accumbens. In addition, loss of midbrain nigrostriatal dopaminergic neurons in Parkinson disease may spread to VTA neurons, and this may underlie the depressive symptoms commonly seen in Parkinson disease.

Mesocortical dopamine neurons also have their cell bodies in the VTA, but project to the neocortex, primarily the prefrontal cortex. Release of dopamine in the prefrontal cortex is believed to affect the efficiency of information processing, attention, and wakefulness. Altered availability of prefrontal dopamine may underlie cognitive impairment in schizophrenia, attention deficit hyperactivity disorder, Parkinson disease, and other neuropsychiatric conditions.

The tuberoinfundibular dopamine system projects from the arcuate nucleus of the hypothalamus to the stalk of the pituitary gland. When released in the pituitary, dopamine inhibits the secretion of prolactin. Individuals who take dopamine-blocking medications (including some antipsychotics) are therefore at risk for hyperprolactinemia, which can in turn cause menstrual cycle abnormalities, galactorrhea, gynecomastia, and sexual dysfunction.

Q8 The answer is: (D) Raphe nuclei.

The serotonin system is involved in many processes in psychiatry including, most prominently, mood, sleep, and psychosis. Serotonin (5-hydroxytryptamine, a monoamine and indolamine) is synthesized from the amino acid tryptophan by tryptophan hydroxylase. Serotonin is synthesized in midline neurons of the brainstem known as the raphe nuclei. Serotonergic neurons project diffusely to numerous targets (including cerebral cortex, thalamus, basal ganglia, midbrain dopaminergic nuclei, hippocampus, and amygdala).

Like the catecholamines, serotonin is transported into vesicles by the vesicular monoamine transporter. Serotonin is subsequently released into the synaptic cleft, and after receptor binding, is inactivated either by presynaptic reuptake via the serotonin transporter (SERT) or degradation via monoamine oxidase. The SERT is a critical molecule in neuropsychopharmacology. Drugs that block the SERT prolong serotonin's action; these agents include the selective serotonin reuptake inhibitors commonly used in treating depression and anxiety disorders. Like the norepinephrine transporter and dopamine transporter, SERT is also a common target of drugs of abuse. For example, both cocaine and amphetamine prolong the action of serotonin by inhibiting SERT. Similarly, the club drug ecstasy (3,4-methyl enedioxy methamphetamine) is a fast-acting SERT inhibitor; ecstasy may also be neurotoxic to serotonergic neurons in the dorsal raphe.

Chapter 41

The Pharmacotherapy of Anxiety Disorders

Multiple-Choice Questions

Select the appropriate answer.

Q1 True or False. The typical starting dose of a selective serotonin reuptake inhibitor (SSRI) or a serotonin–norepinephrine reuptake inhibitor (SNRI)for an anxiety disorder is equivalent to that for the treatment of major depression.

    A. *True*

    B. *False*

Q2 True or False. The tricyclic antidepressants (TCAs) imipramine and clomipramine have demonstrated efficacy for the treatment of panic disorder.

    A. *True*

    B. *False*

Q3 True or False. Monoamine oxidase inhibitors (MAOIs) have been systematically studied in panic disorder and found to be highly efficacious for this condition.

    A. *True*

    B. *False*

Q4 Which of the following agents is LEAST likely to be associated with a significant withdrawal syndrome after prolonged use followed by an abrupt taper?

    A. *Alprazolam*

    B. *Clonazepam*

    C. *Lorazepam*

    D. *Oxazepam*

    E. *Temazepam*

Q5 Which of the following classes of agents is MOST likely to reduce somatic symptoms of arousal associated with panic and anxiety, but is more useful as augmentation for incomplete response rather than as initial monotherapy?

    A. *Benzodiazepines*

    B. *Beta-blockers*

    C. *Monoamine oxidase inhibitors (MAOIs)*

    D. *Serotonin–norepinephrine reuptake inhibitors(SNRIs)*

    E. *Selective serotonin reuptake inhibitors (SSRIs)*

Chapter 41

Answers

Q1 The answer is: (B) False.
Because selective serotonin reuptake inhibitors (SSRIs) and serotonin–norepinephrine reuptake inhibitors (SNRIs) have the potential to cause initial restlessness, insomnia, and increased anxiety, and because panic patients are sensitive to somatic sensations, the starting dose of these should be low for patients with anxiety disorders, typically half (or less) of the usual starting dose (e.g., fluoxetine 5 to 10 mg/day, sertraline 25 mg/day, paroxetine 10 mg/day [or 12.5 mg/day of the controlled-release formulation], controlled-release venlafaxine 37.5 mg/day) for the treatment of major depression to minimize the early anxiogenic effect. Doses can usually be raised gradually based on clinical response and side effects, starting after about 1week of acclimation to typical therapeutic doses, although more gradual upward titration is sometimes necessary in particularly sensitive individuals. Although the nature of the dose-response relationship for the SSRIs in panic is still being assessed, doses for this indication are in the typical antidepressant range, and sometimes higher, that is, fluoxetine 20 to 40 mg/day, paroxetine 20 to 60 mg/day (25 to 72.5 mg/day of the controlled-release formulation), sertraline 100 to 200 mg/day, citalopram 20 to 60 mg/day, escitalopram 10 to 20 mg/day, fluvoxamine 150 to 250 mg/day, and controlled-release venlafaxine 75 to 225 mg/day (although some patients may respond at lower doses).

Q2 The answer is: (A) True.
Imipramine (Tofranil) was the first pharmacologic agent shown to be efficacious in panic disorder. Until it was supplanted by the SSRIs, SNRIs, and benzodiazepines, the tricyclic antidepressants (TCAs) were typically the first-line, "gold standard" pharmacologic agents for panic disorder. Numerous, randomized controlled trials demonstrate the efficacy of imipramine and clomipramine for panic disorder, with supportive evidence for other TCAs. There is some evidence that clomipramine may have superior antipanic properties when compared with the other TCAs, possibly related to its greater potency for serotonergic uptake. The efficacy of the TCAs is comparable to that of the newer agents for panic disorder, but they are now used less frequently because of their greater side effect burden, including associated anticholinergic effects, orthostasis, weight gain, cardiac conduction delays, and greater lethality in overdose. The side effect profile of the TCAs are associated with a high drop-out rate (30% to 70%) in most studies. The SSRIs/SNRIs appear to have a broader spectrum of efficacy than the TCAs (which are less efficacious for conditions such as social phobia and obsessive-compulsive disorder) with the exception of clomipramine, which may present with comorbid panic disorder.

Similar to recommendations for the use of the SSRIs and SNRIs, treatment with the TCAs should be initiated with lower doses (e.g., 10 mg/day for imipramine) to minimize the "activation syndrome" (involving restlessness, jitteriness, palpitations, and increased anxiety) noted on initiation of treatment. Typical antidepressant doses (e.g., 100 to 300 mg/day for imipramine) may ultimately be used to control the symptoms of panic disorder. In cases of poor response or intolerability to treatment with standard doses, use of TCA plasma levels, especially for imipramine, nortriptyline (Pamelor), and desipramine (Norpramin), may be informative.

Q3 The answer is: (B) False.
Despite their reputation for efficacy, the monoamine oxidase inhibitors (MAOIs) have not been systematically studied in panic disorder as defined by the current nomenclature; there is, however, at least one study predating the use of current diagnostic criteria that likely included panic-disordered patients and reported results consistent with efficacy for the MAOI phenelzine. Although clinical lore suggests that MAOIs may be particularly effective for patients with panic disorder refractory to other agents, there are actually no data to address this issue.

Because of the need for careful dietary monitoring (including proscriptions against tyramine-containing foods and ingestion of sympathomimetic and other agents) to reduce the risks of hypertensive reactions and serotonin syndrome, the MAOIs are typically used after failure with safer and better-tolerated agents. Use of MAOIs is further associated with a side effect profile that includes insomnia, weight gain, orthostatic hypotension, and sexual disturbance.

Q4 The answer is: (B) Clonazepam.

Benzodiazepines remain widely used for panic and other anxiety disorders, likely due to their effectiveness, tolerability, rapid onset of action, and ability to be used on an "as-needed" basis for situational anxiety.

Despite their generally favorable tolerability, benzodiazepine administration is associated with side effects that include sedation, ataxia, and memory impairment (particularly problematic in the elderly and those with prior cognitive impairment). However, even after a relatively brief period of regular dosing, rapid discontinuation of benzodiazepines may result in significant withdrawal symptoms; for instance, over two-thirds of patients with panic disorder who discontinued alprazolam experienced a discontinuation syndrome (involving increased anxiety and agitation). Discontinuation of longer-acting agents (such as clonazepam) may result in fewer and less intense withdrawal symptoms after an abrupt taper. Patients with a high level of sensitivity to somatic sensations may find withdrawal-related symptoms particularly distressing, and a slow taper as well as the addition of cognitive-behavioral therapy during discontinuation may be helpful to reduce distress associated with benzodiazepine discontinuation.

A gradual taper is recommended for all patients treated with daily benzodiazepines for more than a few weeks to reduce the likelihood of withdrawal symptoms including, in rare cases, seizures.

Q5 The answer is: (B) Beta-blockers.

Beta-blockers reduce the somatic symptoms of arousal associated with panic and anxiety but may be more useful as augmentation for incomplete response rather than as initial monotherapy. Recently, pindolol, a beta-blocker with partial antagonist effects at the 5-HT1$_A$ receptor, was effective in a small double-blind randomized controlled trial of patients with panic disorder remaining symptomatic despite initial treatment.

Antipsychotic Drugs

Multiple-Choice Questions

Select the appropriate answer.

Q1 In which of the following decades was the newly synthesized agent chlorpromazine first studied and approved for use by the US Food and Drug Administration?

   A. *1930s*

   B. *1940s*

   C. *1950s*

   D. *1960s*

   E. *1970s*

Q2 Which of the following MOST closely matches the percentage of subjects in the "Clinical Antipsychotic Trials of Intervention Effectiveness" (CATIE) study who completed the 18-month trial still taking their originally assigned antipsychotic?

   A. *Less than 10%*

   B. *25%*

   C. *40%*

   D. *60%*

   E. *75%*

Q3 Which of the following agents has the GREATEST propensity for inducing tardive dyskinesia (TD)?

   A. *Aripiprazole*

   B. *Clozapine*

   C. *Haloperidol*

   D. *Olanzapine*

   E. *Ziprasidone*

Q4 Which of the following statements is MOST likely to be accurate?

   A. *Neuroleptic-induced dystonias usually occur between the second and fourth week of initiating neuroleptic treatment, or after a dose increase, and often affect the neck, tongue, or back*

   B. *Older patients started on high-potency conventional antipsychotic medication are especially at risk for developing acute dystonic reactions several weeks after exposure to antipsychotic medication*

   C. *Prophylaxis with anticholinergic agents (such as benztropine 1 to 2 mg twice daily) substantially reduces the likelihood of dystonic reactions in high-risk patients*

   D. *The incidence of dystonia decreases by approximately 8% per year of age until it is almost negligible after age 20 years*

   E. *The occurrence of dystonia early in treatment rarely jeopardizes future compliance with antipsychotic medication*

Q5   Which of the following agents is MOST closely associated with little or no weight gain?

A.   *Clozapine*

B.   *Olanzapine*

C.   *Quetiapine*

D.   *Risperidone*

E.   *Ziprasidone*

Q6   To which of the following drug classes does clozapine belong?

A.   *Benzisoxazoles*

B.   *Butyrophenones*

C.   *Dibenzodiazepines*

D.   *Phenothiazines*

E.   *Thienobenzodiazepines*

Q7   Which of the following first-generation antipsychotic agents has the LOWEST potency?

A.   *Haloperidol*

B.   *Perphenazine*

C.   *Thioridazine*

D.   *Thiothixene*

E.   *Trifluoperazine*

Chapter 42

Answers

Q1 The answer is: (C) 1950s.

In 1952, Henri Laborit, a French naval surgeon, was experimenting with combinations of preoperative medications to reduce the autonomic stress of surgical procedures. He tried a newly synthesized antihistamine, chlorpromazine, and was impressed by its calming effect. He noted that patients seemed indifferent about their impending surgery, yet they were not overly sedated. Convinced that the medication had potential for psychiatric patients, Laborit urged colleagues to test his hypothesis. Eventually a surgical colleague told his brother-in-law, the psychiatrist Pierre Deniker, about Laborit's discovery.

Deniker and Jean Delay, who was the chairman of his department, experimented with chlorpromazine and found remarkable tranquilizing effects in their most agitated and psychotic patients. They noted in 1955 that chlorpromazine and the dopamine-depleting agent, reserpine, shared antipsychotic efficacy and neurologic side effects that resembled Parkinson disease. They coined the term "neuroleptic" to describe these effects.

Smith-Kline purchased chlorpromazine from the French pharmaceutical company, Rhone-Poulenc, and in 1954 chlorpromazine received approval from the US Food and Drug Administration for the treatment of psychosis. Almost immediately, the care of psychotic patients was transformed.

Q2 The answer is: (B) 25%.

In 1999, the National Institutes of Mental Health, recognizing that almost all information regarding the new antipsychotics had come from industry-supported efficacy trials of uncertain generalizability, awarded a competitive contract to Dr. Jeffrey Lieberman to conduct a large, multicenter trial to assess the effectiveness and tolerability of these agents under more representative treatment conditions. Results of the "Clinical Antipsychotic Trials of Intervention Effectiveness" (CATIE) study were first published in 2005. The study was conducted at 57 diverse sites across the United States and included 1493 representative patients with schizophrenia who were randomly assigned to risperidone, olanzapine, quetiapine, ziprasidone, or the conventional comparator, perphenazine, for an 18-month double-blind trial. Dosing was flexible; the range of doses for each drug was selected based on patterns of clinical use (in consultation with the manufacturers). Ziprasidone became available and was added after the study was roughly 40% completed; aripiprazole was not available and was not included. Patients with tardive dyskinesia (TD) at study entry were not randomized to perphenazine, and their data were excluded from analyses comparing the atypical agents with perphenazine. Patients who failed treatment with their first assigned agent could be randomized again in subsequent phases; one re-randomization pathway featured open-label clozapine for treatment-resistant patients and one pathway featured ziprasidone for treatment-intolerant patients. The secondary randomization pathway did not include perphenazine.

One striking finding of the CATIE study was that only 26% of subjects completed the 18-month trial still taking their originally assigned antipsychotic.

Q3 The answer is: (C) Haloperidol.

Of the agents listed, only haloperidol is considered a conventional antipsychotic, and as such conveys a greater risk of TD than do atypical antipsychotics. The risk for developing TD with conventional agents is about 5% per year of exposure, with a lifetime risk possibly as high as 50% to 60%. Risperidone and olanzapine have been associated with substantially lower rates of TD compared with conventional agents, and it is expected that the atypical agents as a class will share this advantage; however, because the incidence of TD is low, it will require very large trials of long duration to establish a difference—the CATIE study failed to detect a difference in TD rates between perphenazine and atypical agents.

Q4 The answer is: (C) Prophylaxis with anticholinergic agents (such as benztropine 1 to 2 mg twice daily) substantially reduces the likelihood of dystonic reactions in high-risk patients.

Dystonias are sustained spasms that can affect any muscle group. Neuroleptic-induced dystonias usually occur within the first 4 days of initiating neuroleptic treatment, or after a dose increase, and often affect the neck, tongue, or back. Dystonia may also manifest as lateral deviation of the eyes (opisthotonus) or stridor (laryngeal spasm). Younger patients started on high-potency conventional antipsychotic medication are especially at risk for developing acute dystonic reactions during the first week of exposure to antipsychotic medication. The incidence of dystonia decreases by about 4% per year of age until it is almost negligible after age 40 years. Dystonia is a frightening and uncomfortable experience. The occurrence of dystonia early in treatment seriously jeopardizes future compliance with antipsychotic medication, so it is important to anticipate and treat this side effect aggressively. The best method of prevention comes from use of an atypical antipsychotic. When high-potency neuroleptics are started, prophylaxis with anticholinergic agents (such as benztropine 1 to 2 mg twice daily) substantially reduces the likelihood of dystonic reactions in high-risk patients.

Q5 The answer is: (E) Ziprasidone.
Several of the atypical agents, particularly clozapine and olanzapine, can cause considerable weight gain, which is highly variable and currently not predictable. Risperidone and quetiapine are associated with intermediate weight gain, and ziprasidone and aripiprazole appear to produce little or no weight gain.

Q6 The answer is: (C) Dibenzodiazepines.
Clozapine is a tricyclic dibenzodiazepine derivative. Risperidone is a benzisoxazole derivative. Olanzapine is a thienobenzodiazepine derivative, chemically related to clozapine. Haloperidol is a butyrophenone. Chlorpromazine is a phenothiazine.

Q7 The answer is: (C) Thioridazine.
Low-potency agents and their milligram equivalents follow: they include chlorpromazine (100 mg), thioridazine (85 mg), and mesoridazine (50 mg); mid-potency agents include loxapine (15 mg), molindone (10 mg), and perphenazine (10 mg); and high-potency agents include trifluoperazine (5 mg), thiothixene (5 mg), fluphenazine (2 mg), haloperidol (2 mg), and pimozide (1 mg).

Antidepressants

Multiple-Choice Questions

Select the appropriate answer.

Q1 Which of the following agents was noted in the 1950s to possess antidepressant efficacy in patients suffering from tuberculosis?

A. *Chlorpromazine*

B. *Diphenhydramine*

C. *Iproniazid*

D. *Nortriptyline*

E. *Phenelzine*

Q2 Which of the following syndromes is characterized by alterations in cognition (e.g., disorientation and confusion), behavior (e.g., agitation and restlessness), autonomic nervous system function (e.g., fever, shivering, diaphoresis, and diarrhea), and neuromuscular activity (e.g., ataxia, hyperreflexia, and myoclonus)?

A. *Catatonia*

B. *Delirium*

C. *Neuroleptic malignant syndrome*

D. *Serotonin syndrome*

E. *Wernicke encephalopathy*

Q3 Which of the following is the time that MOST experts favor for a continuation of antidepressant therapy following the achievement of remission after an episode of major depression?

A. *2 weeks*

B. *4 weeks*

C. *8 weeks*

D. *16 weeks*

E. *26 weeks*

Q4 Which of the following selective serotonin reuptake inhibitors (SSRIs) is NOT US Food and Drug Administration–approved for the treatment of depression?

A. *Citalopram*

B. *Fluvoxamine*

C. *Fluoxetine*

D. *Paroxetine*

E. *Sertraline*

Q5   Which of the following drugs is BEST classified as a norepinephrine dopamine reuptake inhibitor?

A. *Atomoxetine*

B. *Bupropion*

C. *Duloxetine*

D. *Trazodone*

E. *Venlafaxine*

Q6   Which of the following is classified as a secondary amine tricyclic antidepressant (TCA)?

A. *Amitriptyline*

B. *Clomipramine*

C. *Desipramine*

D. *Doxepin*

E. *Imipramine*

Q7   Which of the following agents is LEAST likely to cause anticholinergic symptoms?

A. *Amitriptyline*

B. *Doxepin*

C. *Paroxetine*

D. *Phenelzine*

E. *Thioridazine*

Chapter 43

Answers

Q1 The answer is: (C) Iproniazid.

The precursors of two of the major contemporary antidepressant families, the monoamine oxidase inhibitors (MAOIs) and the tricyclic antidepressants (TCAs), were discovered by serendipity in the 1950s.

Specifically, the administration of iproniazid, an antimycobacterial agent, was first noted to possess antidepressant effects in patients with depression suffering from tuberculosis. Shortly thereafter, iproniazid was found to inhibit monoamine oxidase (MAO), and was involved in the catabolism of serotonin, norepinephrine, and dopamine.

In parallel, imipramine was initially developed as an antihistamine, but Kuhn and colleagues in 1958 discovered that of some 500 imipramine-treated patients with various psychiatric disorders, only those with endogenous depression with mental and motor retardation showed a remarkable improvement during 1 to 6 weeks of daily imipramine therapy. The same compound was also found to inhibit the reuptake of serotonin and norepinephrine. Thus it was the discovery of the antidepressant effects of iproniazid and imipramine that led to the development of the MAOIs and TCAs, but also such discovery was instrumental in the formulation of the monoamine theory of depression. In turn, guided by this theory, the subsequent development of compounds selective for the reuptake of either serotonin or norepinephrine or both was designed, rather than accidental. As a result, over the last few decades, chemical alterations of these first antidepressants have resulted in the creation of a wide variety of monoamine-based antidepressants, with a variety of mechanisms of action.

Q2 The answer is: (D) Serotonin syndrome.

MAOIs act by inhibiting MAO, an enzyme found on the outer membrane of mitochondria, in which it catabolizes a number of monoamines including dopamine, norepinephrine, and serotonin. After reuptake, norepinephrine, serotonin, and dopamine are either reloaded into vesicles for subsequent release or broken down by the enzyme MAO.

MAO is present in two forms (MAO_A and MAO_B), which differ in their substrate preferences, inhibitor specificities, tissue expression, and cell distribution. MAO_A preferentially oxidizes serotonin and is irreversibly inactivated by low concentrations of the acetylenic inhibitor clorgyline. MAO_B preferentially oxidizes phenylethylamine and benzylamine and is irreversibly inactivated by low concentrations of pargyline and deprenyl. Dopamine, tyramine, and tryptamine are substrates for both forms of MAO. In the gastrointestinal tract and the liver, MAO catabolizes a number of dietary pressor amines (such as dopamine, tyramine, tryptamine, and phenylethylamine).

For this reason, consumption of certain foods (that contain high levels of dietary amines) while on an MAOI may precipitate a hypertensive crisis, characterized by hypertension, hyperpyrexia, tachycardia, tremulousness, and cardiac arrhythmias. The same reaction may also occur during coadministration of dopaminergic agents and MAOIs, whereas the coadministration of MAOIs with other antidepressants that potentiate serotonin could result in serotonin syndrome due to toxic central nervous system serotonin levels. The serotonin syndrome is characterized by alterations in cognition (e.g., disorientation and confusion), behavior (e.g., agitation and restlessness), autonomic nervous system function (e.g., fever, shivering, diaphoresis, and diarrhea), and neuromuscular activity (e.g., ataxia, hyperreflexia, and myoclonus). Considering that MAO enzymatic activity requires approximately 14 days to be restored, such food or medications should be avoided for 2 weeks after the discontinuation of an irreversible MAOI ("MAOI wash-out period"). Serotonergic and dopaminergic antidepressants are typically discontinued 2 weeks before the initiation of an MAOI, except for fluoxetine, which needs to be discontinued 5 weeks in advance, owing to its longer half-life.

Q3 The answer is: (E) 26 weeks.

Originally, based on studies with TCAs, patients with unipolar depressive disorders were observed to be at high risk for relapse when treatment was discontinued within the first 16 weeks of therapy. Therefore, in treatment-responders, most experts favor a continuation of antidepressant therapy for a minimum of

6 months following the achievement of remission. The value of continuation therapy for several months to prevent relapse into the original episode has also been established for virtually all of the newer agents.

Risk of recurrence after this 6- to 8-month continuation period (that is, the development of a new episode after recovery from the index episode) is particularly elevated in patients with a chronic course before recovery, residual symptoms, and multiple prior episodes (three or more). For these individuals, the optimal duration of maintenance treatment is unknown, but it is measured in years. Based on research to date, prophylactic efficacy of an antidepressant has been observed for as long as 5 years with clear benefit.

In contrast to the initial expectation that maintenance therapy would be effective at dosages lower than that required for acute treatment, the current consensus is that full-dose therapy is required for effective prophylaxis. Approximately 20% to 30% of patients who are treated with each of the classes of antidepressants will experience a return of depressive symptoms despite continued treatment. In such patients, a dose increase of the antidepressant is typically the first-line approach.

Q4 The answer is: (B) Fluvoxamine.

The overall efficacy of the selective serotonin reuptake inhibitors (SSRIs) in the treatment of depression is equivalent to the other antidepressants, whereas all six of the SSRIs appear to be equally effective in the treatment of depression. Because of their favorable side effect profile, the SSRIs are used as first-line treatment in most cases, with more than 90% of clinicians indicating that SSRIs were their first line of treatment. Despite the tolerability and the widespread efficacy of the SSRIs, there is mounting evidence to suggest that patients with depression with certain characteristics (including comorbid anxiety disorders and a greater number of somatic symptoms [such as pain, headaches, and fatigue]) respond less well to SSRIs than those without such characteristics.

Only one of the SSRIs, fluvoxamine, is not approved for the treatment of depression in the United States, as it is approved only for the treatment of obsessive-compulsive disorder.

Because of their relatively low sideeffect burden, the starting dose of SSRIs is often the minimally effective daily dose: 10 mg for escitalopram (Lexapro); 20 mg for fluoxetine (Prozac), paroxetine (Paxil), and citalopram (Celexa); 50 mg for sertraline (Zoloft); and 100 mg for fluvoxamine (Luvox). Starting at lower doses, and increasing the dose shortly thereafter (i.e., after 1 to 2 weeks) may further improve tolerability. Maximum therapeutic doses for SSRIs are typically one-fold to two-fold greater than the starting dose.

Q5 The answer is: (B) Bupropion.

The norepinephrine dopamine reuptake inhibitor bupropion appears to be as effective as the SSRIs in the treatment of depressive as well as anxiety symptoms in depression. Bupropion is a phenethylamine compound that is effective for the treatment of major depressive disorder. Bupropion is structurally related to amphetamine and the sympathomimetic diethylpropion, and it primarily blocks the reuptake of dopamine and norepinephrine and has minimal or no affinity for postsynaptic receptors. Although some researchers have argued that bupropion's effect on norepinephrine is primarily through an increase in presynaptic release, there is still convincing evidence for binding of both norepinephrine and dopamine transporters.

Venlafaxine, duloxetine, and milnacipran share the property of being relatively potent reuptake inhibitors of serotonin and norepinephrine and are therefore considered selective norepinephrine reuptake inhibitors. Of these, only venlafaxine and duloxetine are approved for the treatment of depression in the United States.

Reboxetine acts by selectively inhibiting the norepinephrine transporter, thereby increasing synaptic norepinephrine levels. Atomoxetine also selectively inhibits the reuptake of norepinephrine. These agents are called norepinephrine reuptake inhibitors.

Trazodone and nefazodone are classified as serotonin receptor antagonists/agonists, whereas mirtazapine and mianserin are alpha2-adrenergic receptor antagonists.

Q6 The answer is: (C) Desipramine.

The TCAs may be subdivided into tertiary amines and secondary amines (their demethylated secondary amine derivatives). In addition, maprotiline (Ludiomil), which is classified as a tetracyclic antidepressant, is commonly grouped with the TCAs due to similarities in dosing, mechanism of action, and side effects.

Tertiary amine TCAs include amitriptyline (Elavil, Adepril), imipramine (Tofranil, Antidepril), trimipramine (Surmontil, Herphonal), clomipramine (Anafranil, Clopress), and doxepin (Sinequan, Deptran).

Secondary amine TCAs are nortriptyline (Pamelor, Aventyl), desipramine (Norpramin, Metylyl), protriptyline (Vivactil, Concordin), and amoxapine (Ascendin, Defanyl).

Q7 The answer is: (D) Phenelzine

Anticholinergic-like side effects occur in patients treated with MAOIs, although they are not due to muscarinic antagonism. These side effects are less severe than those seen with TCAs, although patients on phenelzine may experience dry mouth. Elderly patients may develop constipation or urinary retention. Alternatively, nausea and diarrhea have been reported by some patients. Sweating, flushing, or chills also may occur with their use.

Chapter 44

Pharmacologic Approaches to Treatment-Resistant Depression

Multiple-Choice Questions

Select the appropriate answer.

Q1   Which of the following BEST approximates the lifetime prevalence of major depressive disorder (MDD)?

A.   *3% to 7%*

B.   *7% to 11%*

C.   *13% to 17%*

D.   *17% to 21%*

E.   *21% to 25%*

Q2   According to data from randomized controlled trials, approximately what percentage of patients will achieve full remission (absence or near absence of symptoms) with adequate pharmacotherapy?

A.   *10% to 20%*

B.   *30% to 40%*

C.   *50% to 60%*

D.   *70% to 80%*

E.   *90% to 100%*

Q3   True or False. Adequate antidepressant therapy is typically considered to consist of one or more trials with antidepressant medications with established efficacy in major depressive disorder (MDD), with doses considered to be effective (e.g., superior to placebo in controlled clinical trials) for long enough to produce a robust therapeutic effect (e.g., 12 weeks).

A.   *True*

B.   *False*

Q4   True or False. Patients with depression and high ratings of anxiety symptoms are LESS likely to respond to antidepressant treatment than are those without prominent anxiety.

A.   *True*

B.   *False*

Q5   Which of the following strategies is probably the MOST common approach to the pharmacologic management of treatment-resistant depression (TRD)?

A.   *Augmentation with buspirone*

B.   *Augmentation of the psychotropic with lithium*

C.   *Augmentation of the psychotropic with thyroid hormone*

D.   *Raising the dose of the antidepressant being used*

E.   *Switching to another antidepressant*

Q1 The answer is: (D) 17% to 21%.
Major depressive disorder (MDD) has a lifetime prevalence of 17% to 21%, with about twice as many women affected as men. In any 12-month period, the prevalence of MDD is approximately 6.7%, with over 80% of those with MDD having moderate to severe depression. Unfortunately, most patients do not receive timely treatment, even though the disorder disrupts function at work, home, and school.

Q2 The answer is: (B) 30% to 40%.
The National Comorbidity Replication study showed that approximately 38% of those who experience an episode of major depression receive at least minimally adequate care in mental health specialty or general medical settings, while the majority of patients receive inadequate treatment. For those patients who receive adequate pharmacotherapy, it is estimated from randomized controlled trials of antidepressants that only approximately 30% to 40% will achieve full remission (absence or near absence of symptoms); the rest fail to reach remission. Approximately 10% to 15% fail to respond (with at least a 50% improvement). Non-response is associated with disability and higher medical costs, and partial response or response without remission is associated with higher relapse and recurrence rates.

Q3 The answer is: (A) True.
Adequate antidepressant therapy is typically considered to consist of one or more trials with antidepressant medications with established efficacy in MDD, with doses considered to be effective (e.g., superior to placebo in controlled clinical trials) for a sufficient period to produce a robust therapeutic effect (e.g., 12 weeks).

Q4 The answer is: (A) True.
A commonly studied contributing factor to treatment-resistant depression (TRD) is psychiatric comorbidity. Substance abuse, and even moderate consumption of alcohol, has also been associated with worse response to antidepressant treatment. Other forms of psychiatric comorbidity (such as MDD with comorbid anxiety disorders [anxious depression]) have also been associated with a poorer response to antidepressant treatment. This is consistent with the observation that anxious depression (defined as depression with high ratings of anxiety symptoms) is less likely to respond to antidepressant treatment. One may argue that the negative effect of anxiety disorder's comorbidity is mostly related to specific forms of anxiety disorders (such as panic disorder or obsessive-compulsive disorder). In fact, depressed patients with lifetime panic disorder showed a poor recovery in response to psychotherapy or pharmacotherapy in a large primary care study, and a lifetime burden of panic-agoraphobic spectrum symptoms predicts a poorer response to interpersonal psychotherapy.

Q5 The answer is: (D) Raising the dose of the antidepressant being used.
From a pharmacologic standpoint, raising the dose of the antidepressant is a common approach to TRD. The dose of an antidepressant is usually raised within the recommended therapeutic dose range. In a survey of 412 psychiatrists from across the United States, respondents indicated their preferred strategies when a patient failed to respond to 8 weeks or more of an adequate dose of a selective serotonin reuptake inhibitor (SSRI). Interestingly, in the case of partial response, raising the dose was the first choice for 82% of the respondents, whereas raising the dose was endorsed by only 27% of the respondents in the case of non-response, with the remainder of the respondents selecting either switching a medication or an augmentation strategy.

Among the most widely studied augmentation agents is lithium (at greater than 600 mg/day) when added to tricyclic antidepressants (TCAs), monoamine oxidase inhibitors, and SSRIs. Disadvantages of lithium augmentation include relatively low response rates.

Thyroid hormone (25 to 50 mcg/day) augmentation is another option that has received attention. L-triiodothyronine (T3) has been thought to be superior to thyroxine (T4). The disadvantages of thyroid augmentation are that all published controlled studies involved TCAs, and only uncontrolled studies involved SSRIs.

Buspirone, a 5-HT1$_A$ partial agonist (commonly prescribed at 10 to 30 mg bid), used early on in open augmentation trials of antidepressants, should augment SSRIs by blunting the negative feedback of increased synaptic serotonin effects on the presynaptic 5-HT1$_A$ receptor. Disadvantages are that the data are equivocal. The only two placebo-controlled studies showed that buspirone was no better than placebo.

Pindolol, a beta-blocker and a 5-HT1$_A$ antagonist (often prescribed at 2.5 mg tid), was initially thought to have great potential because of its ability to block the negative feedback of serotonin on presynaptic 5-HT1$_A$ receptors (like buspirone). Disadvantages from published studies include that the dose used may be too low (according to positron emission tomography studies), and that no response was found in a group of 10 patients with TRD, and no difference from placebo was found in two TRD studies.

Dopaminergic agonists have been particularly interesting because they bring in a mechanism of action missing from antidepressants. Pergolide (0.25 to 2 mg/day), amantadine (100 to 200 mg bid), pramipexole (0.125 to 1 mg tid), and ropinirole (0.5 to 1.75 mg tid) have been found to be helpful in uncontrolled studies in patients with MDD. Disadvantages include the side effect of nausea (with the older compounds) and a lack of controlled studies. Advantages include that pramipexole, ropinirole, and amantadine have also been used to treat SSRI-induced sexual dysfunction.

Traditional psychostimulants that affect dopamine as potential augmenting agents include methylphenidate (at 10 to 40 mg/day) and dextroamphetamine (at 5 to 20 mg/day). These have augmented TCAs, monoamine oxidase inhibitors, and SSRIs. Disadvantages of stimulants are that the only two controlled trials in TRD were negative. Clinicians may also avoid using them because of their abuse potential in patients with a history of substance abuse, which is frequently comorbid with MDD.

Atypical antipsychotics are being used with increased frequency by clinicians for non-psychotic MDD. Evidence suggests that risperidone (0.5 to 2 mg/day), olanzapine (5 to 20 mg/day), ziprasidone (40 to 80 mg bid), quetiapine (25 to 300 mg/day), and aripiprazole (15 to 30 mg bid) are helpful. A recent meta-analysis of published and unpublished trials of atypical antipsychotic augmentation of antidepressants in TRD suggests that atypical antipsychotics may all have the potential to augment antidepressant effects. Disadvantages include intolerability (especially the risk of a metabolic syndrome) and cost issues. In addition, long-term side effects of the atypical antipsychotics for non-psychotic MDD are not known. Advantages of this approach are that they may help manage anxiety and agitation.

One of the more innovative sets of augmentations involves one-carbon metabolism. Folate and related compounds participate in the transfer of methyl groups involved in neurotransmitter synthesis and DNA regulation. Alpert and colleagues found that open augmentation with methylfolate (15 to 30 mg/day) resulted in a statistically significant improvement in depression scores. The same group found that open addition of S-adenosylmethionine (SAMe, 800 to 1600 mg/day) also had promise, and they are currently conducting two double-blind, placebo-controlled studies in TRD: one of L-methylfolate and one of SAMe. The disadvantages are that there are no controlled studies yet, and that SAMe use is not covered by insurance (because it is an over-the-counter medication). The advantages are that these are naturally occurring substances that are often very acceptable for most patients.

Several anticonvulsants have been studied as augmentation agents. These include lamotrigine (100 to 300 mg/day), gabapentin (300 to 1800 mg/day), topiramate (100 to 300 mg/day), carbamazepine (200 to 400 mg/day), and valproic acid (500 to 1000 mg/day). Disadvantages of this approach include potential tolerability issues with some of the anticonvulsants (e.g., sedation or weight gain), and the specific risk of Stevens-Johnson syndrome with lamotrigine that necessitates a slow dose escalation. Potential advantages of anticonvulsants are that they may help mitigate anxiety symptoms.

Benzodiazepines not only treat anxiety but also help with core depressive symptoms when added to an antidepressant.

Augmentation with glutamatergic drugs also offers a promising strategy.

Electroconvulsive Therapy

Multiple-Choice Questions

Select the appropriate answer.

Q1   True or False. Remission rates associated with use of electroconvulsive therapy (ECT) exceed those associated with use of antidepressants for depression.

A.   *True*

B.   *False*

Q2   Which of the following is the MOST common indication for ECT?

A.   *Depression*

B.   *Mania*

C.   *Neuroleptic malignant syndrome*

D.   *Parkinson disease*

E.   *Psychotic illness*

Q3   True or False. Congestive heart failure in a person with depression is an absolute contraindication for use of ECT.

A.   *True*

B.   *False*

Q4   True or False. A space-occupying brain lesion in a person with depression is an absolute contraindication for use of ECT.

A.   *True*

B.   *False*

Q5   Which of the following classes of medications should be DISCONTINUED before ECT?

A.   *Benzodiazepines*

B.   *Monoamine oxidase inhibitors*

C.   *Neuroleptics*

D.   *Selective serotonin reuptake inhibitors*

E.   *Tricyclic antidepressants*

Chapter 45

Answers

Q1 The answer is: (A) True.

Electroconvulsive therapy (ECT) remains an indispensable treatment because of the large number of patients with depression who are unresponsive to drugs or who are intolerant to their side effects. In the largest clinical trial of antidepressant medication, only 50% of patients with depression achieved a full remission, whereas an equal percentage were non-responders or achieved only partial remission. However, remission rates of 70% to 90% have been reported in clinical trials of ECT. ECT is currently the most promising prospect for addressing the unmet worldwide need for effective treatment of individuals suffering from depression.

Q2 The answer is: (A) Depression.

Major depression is the most common indication for ECT. The symptoms that predict a good response to ECT are those of major depression. Young, healthy patients can safely receive four or more different drug regimens before moving to ECT, whereas older patients with depression may be unable to tolerate more than one drug trial without developing serious medical complications.

Psychotic illness is the second most common indication for ECT. Although it is not a routine treatment for schizophrenia, ECT, in combination with a neuroleptic, may result in sustained improvement in up to 80% of drug-resistant patients with chronic schizophrenia. Young patients with psychosis conforming to the schizophreniform profile (i.e., with acute onset, positive psychotic symptoms, affective intactness, and medication resistance) are more responsive to ECT than are those with chronic schizophrenia, and they may have a full and enduring remission of their illness with treatment.

Mania also responds well to ECT, but drug treatment remains the first-line therapy. Nevertheless, in controlled trials, ECT is as effective as lithium (or more so), and in drug-refractory mania, more than 50% of cases have remitted with ECT. ECT is highly effective in the treatment of medication-resistant mixed affective states and refractory bipolar disorder in adolescents.

Patients who are severely malnourished, dehydrated, and exhausted (such as patients with protracted depressive illness) are medically at risk and should be treated promptly after careful rehydration. Patients with complicating medical illness (e.g., cardiac arrhythmia or coronary artery disease) are often more safely treated with ECT than with an antidepressant. Patients with delusional depression may be resistant to antidepressant therapy but respond to ECT 80% to 90% of the time. Patients with catatonia respond promptly to ECT. ECT is effective in up to 75% of patients with catatonia, regardless of the underlying cause, and is the treatment of choice as a primary treatment for most patients with catatonia. ECT has been reported to be effective in neuroleptic malignant syndrome, but intensive supportive medical treatment, discontinuation of neuroleptic therapy, use of dantrolene, and use of bromocriptine are still the essential steps of management.

Q3 The answer is: (B) False.

The cardiac conditions that most often worsen under this autonomic stimulus that accompanies ECT are ischemic heart disease, hypertension, congestive heart failure, and cardiac arrhythmia. These conditions, if properly managed, have proved to be surprisingly tolerant to ECT. The idea that general anesthesia is contraindicated within 6 months of a myocardial infarction has acquired a certain sanctity, which is surprising considering the ambiguity of the original data. A more rational approach involves careful assessment of the cardiac reserve, a reserve that is needed as cardiac work increases during ECT. Vascular aneurysms should be repaired before ECT if possible, but in practice, they have proved surprisingly durable during treatment. Critical aortic stenosis should be surgically corrected before ECT to avoid ventricular overload during the seizure. Patients with cardiac pacemakers generally tolerate ECT uneventfully, although proper pacer function should be ascertained before treatment. Implantable cardioverter defibrillators should be converted from demand mode to fixed mode by placing a magnet over the device before ECT. Patients with compensated congestive heart failure generally tolerate ECT well, although a transient decompensation into pulmonary edema for 5 to 10 minutes may occur in patients with a baseline ejection fraction below 20%. It is unclear whether the underlying cause is a neurogenic stimulus to the lung parenchyma or a reduction in cardiac output because of increased heart rate and blood pressure.

Q4 The answer is: (B) False.
The brain is physiologically stressed during ECT. Cerebral oxygen consumption approximately doubles, and cerebral blood flow increases several-fold. Increases in intracranial pressure and the permeability of the blood–brain barrier also develop. These acute changes may increase the risk of ECT in patients with a variety of neurologic conditions.

Space-occupying brain lesions were previously considered an absolute contraindication to ECT, and earlier case reports described clinical deterioration when ECT was given to patients with brain tumors. Reports indicate, however, that with careful management, patients with meningioma or chronic subdural hematoma may be safely treated. Recent cerebral infarction probably represents the most common intracranial risk factor. Case reports of ECT after recent cerebral infarction indicate that the complication rate is low, and consequently ECT is often the treatment of choice for poststroke depression. The interval between infarction and time of ECT should be determined by the urgency of treatment for depression.

ECT has been safe and efficacious in patients with hydrocephalus, arteriovenous malformations, cerebral hemorrhage, multiple sclerosis, systemic lupus erythematosus, Huntington disease, and intellectual disability. Patients with depression and Parkinson disease note improvement of both disorders with ECT, and Parkinson disease alone may constitute an indication for ECT. Patients with depression with preexisting dementia are likely to develop especially severe cognitive deficits secondary to ECT, but most return to their baseline after treatment, and many improve.

Q5 The answer is: (A) Benzodiazepines.
Benzodiazepines are antagonistic to the ictal process and should be discontinued. Even short-acting benzodiazepines may have a long half-life in a sick, elderly person and make effective treatment less likely.

Antidepressant medications do not necessarily have to be discontinued before ECT, considering that there is little evidence of a harmful interaction. Indeed, there is preliminary evidence that neuroleptics, tricyclic antidepressants, selective serotonin reuptake inhibitors, and mirtazapine are not only safe to prescribe during a course of ECT but also may enhance the therapeutic effectiveness of the treatment. Monoamine oxidase inhibitors may be safely given during a course of ECT, if sympathomimetic drugs are not administered. Early case reports described excessive cognitive disturbance and prolonged apnea in a small percent of patients receiving lithium during ECT, but more recent data indicate that this is a rare complication, and that concurrent administration of lithium is usually safe.

For sedation, patients receiving ECT usually do well with a sedating atypical antipsychotic (such as quetiapine [Seroquel]) or a non-benzodiazepine hypnotic, such as hydroxyzine (Vistaril).

Anticonvulsants prescribed as mood stabilizers are usually discontinued before ECT, but in a recent series of patients with bipolar disorder, the concurrent administration of lamotrigine did not interfere with treatment and facilitated transition to maintenance pharmacotherapy. In the patient with a pre-existing seizure disorder, the anticonvulsant regimen should be continued for patient safety. The elevated seizure threshold can almost always be overridden with an ECT stimulus, and patients managed in this manner usually have the same clinical response as patients not taking anticonvulsants.

Chapter 46

Neurotherapeutics

Multiple-Choice Questions

Select the appropriate answer.

Q1 Which of the following treatments has received US Food and Drug Administration approval for treatment-resistant depression and treatment-resistant epilepsy?

A. *Anterior capsulotomy*

B. *Anterior cingulotomy*

C. *Limbic leucotomy*

D. *Subcaudate tractotomy*

E. *Vagus nerve stimulation (VNS)*

Q2 Which of the following ablative neurosurgical procedures was often used indiscriminately in the middle of the 20th century?

A. *Anterior capsulotomy*

B. *Anterior cingulotomy*

C. *Frontal lobotomy*

D. *Limbic leucotomy*

E. *Subcaudate tractotomy*

Q3 Which of the following involves use of a magnetic field introduced on the scalp surface to non-invasively generate focal electrical stimulation of the cortical surface?

A. *Electroconvulsive therapy*

B. *Functional magnetic resonance imaging*

C. *Repetitive transcranial magnetic stimulation (rTMS)*

D. *Single-photon emission computed tomography*

E. *Vagus nerve stimulation (VNS)*

Q4 Which of the following conditions was MOST likely the first target for the therapeutic uses of deep brain stimulation (DBS)?

A. *Alzheimer disease*

B. *Huntington disease*

C. *Obsessive-compulsive disorder (OCD)*

D. *Parkinson disease*

E. *Treatment-resistant depression*

Chapter 46

Answers

Q1 The answer is: (E) Vagus nerve stimulation (VNS).

Vagus nerve stimulation (VNS) was approved for use in treatment-resistant epilepsy in 1994 in Europe and in 1997 in the United States. VNS has been approved for treatment-resistant depression (TRD) and bipolar disorder in Europe and Canada since 2001. Finally, in July 2005, the US Food and Drug Administration approved VNS for TRD. Implantation of the VNS device involves surgical placement of electrodes around the left vagus nerve via an incision in the neck (only the left vagus nerve is used for VNS because the right vagus nerve has parasympathetic branches to the heart). A second incision is used to place an internal pulse generator (IPG) subcutaneously in the left subclavicular region, and the wire between the electrodes on the vagus nerve and the IPG is connected by means of subcutaneous tunneling between the two incision sites. After a 2-week postoperative recovery period, the IPG can be turned on, and electrical stimulation of the left vagus nerve can be initiated.

Q2 The answer is: (C) Frontal lobotomy.

Concerns regarding ablative neurosurgery for psychiatric indications arose following the indiscriminate use of crude procedures, such as frontal lobotomy, in the middle of the 20th century. These procedures were associated with severe adverse events including frontal lobe symptoms (e.g., apathy). In the latter half of the 20th century, neurosurgeons began to use much smaller lesions in well-targeted and specific brain regions. As a result, the incidence of adverse events dropped precipitously. Currently used procedures include anterior cingulotomy, subcaudate tractotomy, limbic leucotomy (which is a combination of an anterior cingulotomy and a subcaudate tractotomy), and anterior capsulotomy. All of these procedures use craniotomy techniques.

Q3 The answer is: (C) Repetitive transcranial magnetic stimulation (rTMS).

Although VNS stimulates the brain indirectly via the vagus nerve, therapeutic interventions that directly stimulate the brain have also been studied for the treatment of psychiatric illness. Repetitive transcranial magnetic stimulation (rTMS), the most studied of such interventions, uses a strong magnetic field introduced on the scalp surface to non-invasively generate focal electrical stimulation of the cortical surface. In contrast to the generalized seizure associated with electroconvulsive therapy, the focal stimulation resulting from rTMS does not produce a seizure. Therefore rTMS can be administered in an office setting without the use of anesthesia. Also, the focal stimulation resulting from rTMS does not cause cognitive side effects that may occur following treatment with electroconvulsive therapy. Although rTMS is not currently approved for the treatment of major depressive disorder in the United States, it is approved for the treatment of major depressive disorder in Canada and Israel.

Q4 The answer is: (D) Parkinson disease.

Deep brain stimulation (DBS) involves the placement of electrodes in, as the name indicates, deep brain regions so that electrical stimulation can be delivered in a targeted manner. Therefore by its very nature, DBS is more invasive than is VNS or cortical stimulation (e.g., via rTMS). However, it also allows for access to a wider range of target brain structures. As is the case with VNS and surgical cortical stimulation techniques, after placement, the DBS electrodes are attached to subcutaneous IPGs on the chest wall that provide power for the electrical stimulation and allow for transcutaneous adjustment of stimulation parameters.

The first therapeutic use of DBS was for Parkinson disease. Just as ablative limbic system surgery has been used to treat refractory psychiatric illness, ablative striatal procedures (such as pallidotomy) have been used for patients with treatment-refractory Parkinson disease. Investigators began to explore DBS as an alternative to ablative procedures for Parkinson disease. DBS of the subthalamic nucleus has been used since 1987 for Parkinson disease. Since then, over 35,000 patients with Parkinson disease have had DBS electrodes implanted in different brain regions associated with the pathophysiology of the illness; the majority of patients have benefited from the procedure.

Clinical trials of DBS for TRD and for refractory obsessive-compulsive disorder (OCD) are underway. All of the clinical trials of DBS for refractory OCD have used bilateral anterior limbs of the internal capsule as the electrode target. All of the published results suggest that DBS at this location appears to be efficacious for patients with treatment-refractory OCD. For OCD, the target region of the anterior limb of the internal capsule was chosen based on the success of ablative anterior capsulotomy at this site. Although initial results are encouraging, DBS remains an experimental procedure; it is not yet approved for general clinical use for psychiatric disorders.

Lithium and Its Role in Psychiatry

Multiple-Choice Questions

Select the appropriate answer.

Q1 In which year was lithium first approved by the US Food and Drug Administration for the treatment of mania?

A. *1949*

B. *1956*

C. *1963*

D. *1970*

E. *1982*

Q2 True or False. Hyponatremia will lead to an increase in one's lithium level.

A. *True*

B. *False*

Q3 Which of the following lithium levels are generally considered to be solidly in the therapeutic range for treatment of mood disorders?

A. *0.1 to 0.3 mEq/L*

B. *0.4 to 0.6 mEq/L*

C. *0.6 to 0.8 mEq/L*

D. *1.0 to 1.2 mEq/L*

E. *1.3 to 1.5 mEq/L*

Q4 Which of the following is/are the LEAST common side effect(s) of lithium treatment?

A. *Cognitive complaints*

B. *Gastrointestinal disturbance*

C. *Sinus arrhythmia*

D. *Tremor*

E. *Weight gain*

Q5 Which of the following has been associated with lithium use during the first trimester of pregnancy?

A. *Ebstein anomaly*

B. *Edelstein anomaly*

C. *DaCosta syndrome*

D. *Goldberg anomaly*

E. *Goldstein anomaly*

Chapter 47

Answers

Q1 The answer is: (D) 1970.

The history of lithium's use in psychiatry is instructive, both in understanding its present role and in tracing the development of psychopharmacology in general. The first modern description of the application of lithium to treat mania occurred in 1949 by an Australian named John Cade, who observed that lithium had calming effects on animals and then treated a series of 10 agitated manic patients. In fact, however, descriptions of lithium treatment date back to at least the US Civil War. An 1883 textbook by Union Army Surgeon General William Hammond recommended the use of lithium bromide to treat manic or agitated patients, although he later downplayed the importance of lithium. In the early 1900s, a Danish physician, Lange, published a case series reporting the treatment of manic patients with lithium carbonate. There is little evidence that lithium was studied further, however, until Garrod proposed that lithium urate could be used to treat gout, opening the door to its broader therapeutic application.

Unfortunately, despite some early study by Mogen Schou and others, lithium's wider adoption in the United States was hindered by concerns about lithium toxicity. Lithium chloride had been used as a sodium substitute in the 1940s until several deaths were reported from lithium toxicity among hyponatremic patients.

Lithium was initially perceived as too dangerous for clinical application, and it was only in 1970 that lithium was approved by the US Food and Drug Administration for the treatment of mania.

Q2 The answer is: (A) True.

In the kidney, lithium is primarily reabsorbed in the proximal renal tubules, with some subsequent absorption in the loop of Henle. Importantly, in contrast to sodium, no significant absorption occurs in the distal tubules. Therefore thiazide diuretics, which act distally, will tend to increase lithium levels by up to 50%, whereas those that act more proximally generally have less effect on lithium levels.

More broadly, hydration status can affect lithium levels: individuals who become salt-avid (e.g., because of hypovolemia or hyponatremia, perhaps in the context of vomiting, diarrhea, or long-distance running) will cause their lithium levels to increase.

Q3 The answer is: (C) 0.6 to 0.8 mEq/L.

Lithium carbonate is available in 300 mg capsules or tablets, as well as 300 mg and 450 mg slow-release forms. A liquid, lithium citrate, is also available in 300 mg/5 mL form. For most patients, the immediate-release lithium carbonate is initiated first, with a switch to another form only to maximize tolerability if necessary.

The narrow therapeutic window for lithium treatment complicates lithium dosing. Indeed, in its early application lithium levels of 0.8 to 1.2 mEq/L were advised, whereas more recently levels of 0.6 to 0.8 mEq/L—and perhaps even lower in some cases—have been advocated. The optimal dose is driven, not merely by considerations of efficacy, but by tolerability as well: that is, the "best" dose for prevention of recurrence may be too high for some patients to tolerate.

Typically, the clinician will begin 600 mg once daily at bedtime, and then increase it to 900 mg at bedtime. After 5 days, a lithium level is checked, and the dose is increased or decreased as required to attain a level in the 0.6 to 0.8 mEq/L range.

Q4 The answer is: (C) Sinus arrhythmia.

Although rare, lithium can cause a depression of firing at the sinoatrial node, contributing to sinus arrhythmias. Lithium may also cause benign electrocardiogram abnormalities, most typically an appearance resembling hypokalemia, including widening of the QRS complex and an increased PR interval.

Weight gain is common among lithium-treated patients, and although the mechanism is not known, it is not merely a result of lithium-induced edema. Some studies suggest that up to half of lithium-treated patients will experience a 5% to 10% increase in weight.

Cognitive complaints are common among lithium-treated patients, sometimes characterized as feeling "foggy" or "cloudy." Adjunctive thyroid hormone is sometimes used in an attempt to ameliorate these symptoms; however, there are no well-established means of treating such complaints, other than decreasing the lithium dose.

Gastrointestinal side effects are common among lithium-treated patients, and may include upper (nausea, vomiting, and dyspepsia) and lower (diarrhea and cramping) gastrointestinal symptoms. Because slow-release formulations are absorbed lower in the gut, they are more often associated with the latter symptoms, whereas immediate-release formulations are more often associated with the former symptoms. In many cases, dividing dosages or dosing with food can minimize or eliminate these symptoms.

Tremor is common with lithium treatment, even at therapeutic levels and particularly following each dose when peak levels are achieved. This tremor, which resembles a benign physiological tremor, may be exacerbated by caffeine and by anxiety. It is typically managed by changing the timing of the lithium dose (to ensure peak levels during sleep) and when necessary by adding a beta-adrenergic blocker. This may be used on either an as-needed or a standing basis, depending on patient preference.

Q5 The answer is: (A) Ebstein anomaly.

Lithium use during the first trimester of pregnancy has been associated with a potentially life-threatening cardiac abnormality, known as Ebstein anomaly, a spectrum of changes that typically includes insufficiency of the tricuspid valve and hypoplasia of the right ventricle. The risk appears to be about 10-fold greater among children of lithium-treated patients compared with those in the general population, although the absolute risk is still quite low (on the order of 1 in 2000). This risk must also be balanced against the substantial dangers to the fetus in a mother with uncontrolled bipolar disorder during pregnancy.

The Use of Antiepileptic Drugs in Psychiatry

Multiple-Choice Questions

Select the appropriate answer.

Q1 Which of the following anticonvulsants is MOST often considered as a first-line agent for the maintenance treatment of bipolar disorder?

    A. *Carbamazepine*

    B. *Gabapentin*

    C. *Lamotrigine*

    D. *Lithium carbonate*

    E. *Valproic acid*

Q2 Which of the following agents is MOST likely to cause a serious rash requiring hospitalization?

    A. *Carbamazepine*

    B. *Gabapentin*

    C. *Lamotrigine*

    D. *Lithium carbonate*

    E. *Valproic acid*

Q3 Which of the following was the first anticonvulsant studied as a treatment for mania?

    A. *Carbamazepine*

    B. *Gabapentin*

    C. *Lamotrigine*

    D. *Lithium carbonate*

    E. *Valproic acid*

Q4 Which of the following statements is LEAST likely to be accurate?

    A. *More than 90% of plasma valproic acid is protein-bound*

    B. *The therapeutic plasma levels of valproic acid generally used for the treatment of mania are the same as those used for anticonvulsant therapy (50 to 100 mcg/mL), and the total daily dosage required to achieve these levels typically ranges from 500 mg to greater than 1500 mg*

    C. *Valproic acid is metabolized by the hepatic cytochrome P450 2D6 (CYP2D6)system and, like carbamazepine, autoinduces its own metabolism*

    D. *Valproic acid has been associated with potentially fatal hepatic failure, usually occurring within the first 6 months of treatment; it most frequently occurs in children under age 2 years, and in persons with preexisting liver disease*

    E. *Valproic acid may produce teratogenic effects, including spina bifida (1%) and other neural tube defects*

Q5   True or False. Based on its use as an anticonvulsant, dosages of carbamazepine typically range from 400 mg to 1200 mg/day, and therapeutic plasma levels range from 4 to 12 mcg/mL.

    A. *True*

    B. *False*

Q6   Which of the following statements is LEAST likely to be accurate?

    A. *Carbamazepine is an anticonvulsant structurally related to the tricyclic antidepressants*

    B. *Carbamazepine is metabolized by the hepatic cytochrome P450 2D6 (CYP2D6) system*

    C. *Carbamazepine is rapidly absorbed (peak plasma levels within 4 to 6 hours) after oral administration*

    D. *The half-life of carbamazepine ranges from 13 to 17 hours*

    E. *Twenty percent of plasma carbamazepine is protein-bound*

Q7   True or False. Carbamazepine induces the cytochrome P450 (CYP) enzymes, causing an increase in the rate of its own metabolism over time (as well as that of other drugs metabolized by the cytochrome P450 [CYP] system).

    A. *True*

    B. *False*

Chapter 48

Answers

Q1 The answer is: (E) Valproic acid.

The acute antimanic efficacy of valproic acid has been established by several controlled studies. The largest trial of valproate for the maintenance treatment of bipolar disorder ($n = 372$) failed to find a difference between valproate, lithium, and placebo for the primary outcome measure (time to any mood episode). Unfortunately, no other adequately powered maintenance studies of valproate exist. Valproate is not approved by the US Food and Drug Administration for the maintenance treatment of bipolar disorder. Despite this lack of evidence, it has been recommended as a first-line prophylactic treatment of bipolar disorder in multiple treatment guidelines.

The use of gabapentin as a treatment for bipolar disorder became popular in the late 1990s, propelled in part by the drug's favorable qualities: no need for blood monitoring, few interactions with other drugs, simple metabolism, and the perception of good tolerability (at least compared with the established treatments, including lithium and valproate, for bipolar disorder). Even as studies demonstrated its ineffectiveness for mania (gabapentin was significantly worse than placebo as an adjunctive treatment for mania), its use persisted.

Lamotrigine is an anticonvulsant that inhibits voltage-gated sodium channels and reduces glutamate levels. Given the prominence of depression and depressive relapses in bipolar disorder, lamotrigine offers a significant advance in the long-term management of bipolar depression. Lamotrigine is approved for the maintenance treatment of bipolar disorder, and is efficacious when compared to placebo in maintenance studies.

Lithium, a first-line treatment for bipolar disorder, is not considered an anticonvulsant.

Carbamazepine (in extended-release form) was recently found to be effective for acute mania in a large, placebo-controlled trial. No large-scale trials have compared it with other antimanic drugs, so its relative efficacy is unknown. There are no data establishing carbamazepine as an effective maintenance treatment in bipolar disorder, although some have suggested that carbamazepine may be more effective in rapid cycling, dysphoric mania, mixed states, and "ultrarapid cycling."

Q2 The answer is: (C) Lamotrigine.

Although allergic reactions can occur after administration of essentially all medications, rash arises in up to 8% of lamotrigine-treated adults, and serious rash that requires hospitalization is seen in up to 0.5% of lamotrigine-treated individuals. Because of the possibility of Stevens-Johnson syndrome, toxic epidermal necrolysis, or angioedema, all rashes should be regarded as potentially serious and be monitored closely; to minimize serious rashes, the dose should be increased at the rate suggested in the package insert.

Q3 The answer is: (A) Carbamazepine.

Carbamazepine was the first anticonvulsant studied as a treatment for mania. More than 19 studies (most of which were small case series or open trials) evaluated carbamazepine for the treatment of mania, and until recently it was used in bipolar disorder despite little scientific support for its use. Recently, however, carbamazepine (in extended-release form) was found to be effective for acute mania in a large, placebo-controlled trial. No large-scale trials have compared it with other antimanic drugs, so its relative efficacy is unknown.

Q4 The answer is: (C) Valproic acid is metabolized by the hepatic cytochrome P450 2D6 (CYP2D6) system and, like carbamazepine, autoinduces its own metabolism.

Valproic acid is metabolized by the hepatic CYP2D6 system but, unlike carbamazepine, does not autoinduce its own metabolism.

More than 90% of plasma valproic acid is protein-bound.

The therapeutic plasma levels of valproic acid generally used for the treatment of mania are the same as those used for anticonvulsant therapy (50 to 100 mcg/mL), and the total daily dosage required to achieve these levels typically ranges from 500 mg to greater than 1500 mg.

Valproic acid has been associated with potentially fatal hepatic failure, usually occurring within the first 6 months of treatment; it most frequently occurs in children under age 2 years, and in persons with preexisting liver disease.

Valproic acid may produce teratogenic effects, including spina bifida (1%) and other neural tube defects.

Q5 The answer is: (A) True.
Based on its use as an anticonvulsant, dosages of carbamazepine typically range from 400 mg to 1200 mg/day, and therapeutic plasma levels range from 4 to 12 mcg/mL.

Q6 The answer is: (E) Twenty percent of plasma carbamazepine is protein-bound.
Eighty percent, not 20%, of plasma carbamazepine is protein-bound.

Carbamazepine is an anticonvulsant structurally related to the tricyclic antidepressants. Carbamazepine is metabolized by the hepatic CYP2D6 system. Carbamazepine is rapidly absorbed (peak plasma levels within 4 to 6 hours) after oral administration. The half-life of carbamazepine ranges from 13 to 17 hours.

Q7 The answer is: (A) True.
Carbamazepine induces the cytochrome P450 (CYP) enzymes, causing an increase in the rate of its own metabolism over time (as well as that of other drugs metabolized by the CYP system). Because of this, the dose of the drug should be monitored by serum levels every 2 to 3 months and raised if necessary. Concomitant administration of carbamazepine with oral contraceptives, warfarin, theophylline, doxycycline, haloperidol, tricyclic antidepressants, lamotrigine, or valproic acid leads to decreased plasma levels of these other drugs. Concomitant administration of drugs that inhibit the CYP system will increase plasma levels of carbamazepine; these drugs include fluoxetine, cimetidine, erythromycin, isoniazid, calcium-channel blockers, and propoxyphene. Concomitant administration of phenobarbital, phenytoin, and primidone causes a decrease in carbamazepine levels through induction of the CYP enzymes.

Chapter 49

Pharmacotherapy of Attention-Deficit/Hyperactivity Disorder Across the Life Span

Multiple-Choice Questions

Select the appropriate answer.

Q1 Which of the following disorders is LEAST likely to be comorbid with attention-deficit/hyperactivity disorder (ADHD)?

A. Conduct disorder

B. Major depression

C. Obsessive-compulsive disorder

D. Oppositional defiant disorder

E. Schizophrenia

Q2 Stimulants are thought to be effective in ADHD because of their ability to increase intrasynaptic concentrations of norepinephrine and what other neurotransmitter?

A. Acetylcholine

B. Cholecystokinin

C. Dopamine (DA)

D. Glutamate

E. Serotonin

Q3 Which of the following agents for the treatment of ADHD was removed from the market in 2005?

A. Atomoxetine

B. Clonidine

C. Dextroamphetamine

D. Methylphenidate (MPH)

E. Pemoline

Q4 True or False. Stimulants may have a mild negative impact on growth velocity in youths with ADHD.

A. True

B. False

Q5 True or False. Stimulant treatment results in nearly a twofold reduction in the risk for substance abuse among youths treated with a stimulant for ADHD, as compared with youths receiving no pharmacotherapy for their ADHD.

A. True

B. False

Q1 The answer is: (E) Schizophrenia.

Attention-deficit/hyperactivity disorder (ADHD) is a common psychiatric condition shown to occur in 3% to 10% of school-age children worldwide, and in up to 4% of adults. The classic triad of impaired attention, impulsivity, and excessive motor activity characterizes ADHD, although many patients may manifest only inattentive symptoms. ADHD usually persists, to a significant degree, from childhood through adolescence and into adulthood. Most children, adolescents, and adults with ADHD suffer significant functional impairment(s) in multiple domains, as well as comorbid psychiatric and/or learning disorders.

Several types of studies inform us about ADHD and comorbid psychiatric disorders, including cross-sectional clinical and epidemiologic studies of ADHD in children and adults; family genetic studies (which study the distribution of psychiatric disorders in adoptive and biological families of ADHD children and adults); prospective longitudinal follow-up studies (that observe the development of ADHD in patients from childhood through adolescence and into adulthood); and studies of referred ADHD adults. These studies demonstrate that ADHD is frequently comorbid with oppositional defiant disorder, conduct disorder, multiple anxiety disorders (panic disorder, obsessive-compulsive disorder, tic disorders), mood disorders (e.g., depression, dysthymia, and bipolar disorder), learning disorders (e.g., auditory processing problems and dyslexia), and substance use disorders (SUDs). These studies demonstrate that ADHD is not a feature of, or a precursor to, these comorbid conditions, and that these comorbid disorders are not the result of methodological artifacts. Moreover, some of these comorbid disorders segregate independently of ADHD (e.g., conduct disorder, bipolar disorder, and anxiety disorders), whereas others cosegregate within families (e.g., depression).

Q2 The answer is: (C) Dopamine (DA).

Stimulants increase intrasynaptic concentrations of dopamine (DA) and norepinephrine. Methylphenidate (MPH) primarily binds to the DA transporter protein, blocking the reuptake of DA, and increasing intrasynaptic DA from reserpine-insensitive DA pools. Although amphetamines diminish presynaptic reuptake of DA by binding to DA transporter protein, these compounds also travel into the DA neuron, cause release of DA from vesicles into the cytoplasm, prevent repackaging of DA from the cytoplasm into the vesicles, and promote release of DA from reserpine-sensitive vesicles in the presynaptic neuron. In addition, stimulants (amphetamine more than MPH) increase levels of norepinephrine and serotonin (5-HT) in the interneuronal space, although compared with their effects on DA, these effects are relatively minor. Although group studies comparing MPH and amphetamines generally demonstrate similar efficacy, their pharmacodynamic differences may explain why a particular patient may respond to, or tolerate, one stimulant preferentially over another. It is necessary to appreciate that although the efficacy of amphetamine and MPH are similar, their potency differs, such that 5 mg of amphetamine is approximately equivalent to 10 mg of MPH.

Q3 The answer is: (E) Pemoline.

Pemoline (Cylert) is a central nervous system stimulant that is structurally different from both MPH and amphetamine, and that seems to enhance central dopaminergic transmission. Although a variety of studies have demonstrated pemoline's efficacy, the overall risk of liver toxicity appears to be 10 to 25 times the background risk; therefore the US Food and Drug Administration concluded that the risks of this medication outweighed the benefits and pemoline was removed from the market in the United States on October 24, 2005 (www.fda.gov/cder/drug/InfoSheets/HCP/pemolineHCP.htm). Although pemoline will remain available from pharmacies and wholesalers until supplies are exhausted, clinicians are advised to transition patients to alternative treatments.

Q4 The answer is: (A) True.

The impact of stimulant treatment on growth remains a concern, and the data are conflicting. For instance, ADHD youths treated with a stimulant medication continuously over a 24-month period experienced a deceleration of about 1 cm per year. Despite this slowing, except for those subjects in the lowest percentile for height, these children remained within the normal curves. Recently Biederman and colleagues reported on growth deficit in girls with ADHD. Although statistically significant differences were observed between girls with ADHD and controls, these deficits were modest, only evident in early adolescence, unrelated to weight deficits or stimulant treatment, and not significant after correcting for age and parental height. The finding of small height differences in preadolescent girls is consistent with Spencer and associates' earlier work in boys, and results from additional long-term studies. Although stimulants may have a mild negative impact on growth velocity, perhaps more related to ADHD than its treatment, height and weight should be monitored but will not pose significant clinical problems for most patients.

Q5 The answer is: (A) True.
Many adolescents and young adults with ADHD have either a past or current alcohol and/or drug use disorder. Comorbidity within ADHD increases the risk of SUD. Patients with ADHD frequently misuse a variety of substances (including alcohol, marijuana, cocaine, stimulants, opiates, and nicotine). In fact, children with ADHD start smoking cigarettes (with nicotine) an average of 2 years earlier than their non-ADHD peers and have increased rates of smoking as adults, more difficulty quitting smoking, and heightened symptoms of nicotine withdrawal. Furthermore, patients with ADHD appear to develop substance dependence more rapidly, and their dependence lasts longer compared with controls. Considering that the rates of substance abuse in patients with ADHD are increased, concerns persist that stimulant treatment contributes to subsequent substance abuse. Wilens and colleagues performed a pooled analysis of six studies that examined the relationship between stimulant treatment and substance abuse. Their meta-analysis revealed that stimulant treatment resulted in a 1.9-fold reduction in risk for later substance abuse among youths treated with a stimulant for ADHD, as compared with those youths receiving no pharmacotherapy for their ADHD. The protective effect was greater through adolescence and less into adulthood. Longitudinal follow-up also suggested that stimulant pharmacotherapy of ADHD does not increase risk of developing an SUD. A recent population-based study observed reduced risk of SUD in boys with ADHD (20.3% vs. 27.4%; odds ratio, 0.5; 95% confidence interval, 0.3 to 0.9) treated with stimulants over the course of 17-year follow-up.

Chapter 50

Drug–Drug Interactions in Psychopharmacology

Multiple-Choice Questions

Select the appropriate answer.

Q1 True or False. Pharmacodynamic interactions are those that involve a change in the plasma level and/or tissue distribution of one drug by coadministration of another drug.

A. *True*

B. *False*

Q2 Which of the following agents is highly protein-bound?

A. *Diazepam*

B. *Gabapentin*

C. *Lithium*

D. *Memantine*

E. *Venlafaxine*

Q3 Which of the following agents skips phase 1 metabolism and undergoes only phase 2 reactions?

A. *Alprazolam*

B. *Chlordiazepoxide*

C. *Clorazepate*

D. *Diazepam*

E. *Lorazepam*

Q4 True or False. Only prescribed substances can act as an inhibitor of metabolic enzymes.

A. *True*

B. *False*

Q5 True or False. Inducers tend to have a noticeable effect on plasma levels of substrates more rapidly than do inhibitors.

A. *True*

B. *False*

Q6 True or False. The proportion of frankly poor metabolizers with respect to P450 2D6 appears to be higher among whites (approximately 5% to 10%) than among Asian and African Americans (approximately 1% to 3%).

A. *True*

B. *False*

Q7 Which of the following antipsychotic agents is classified as a diphenylbutylpiperidine?

A. *Aripiprazole*

B. *Olanzapine*

C. *Pimozide*

D. *Quetiapine*

E. *Thiothixene*

Q8 True or False. Lower-potency antipsychotics are generally MORE sedating than are high-potency antipsychotics.

A. *True*

B. *False*

Q9 Which of the following agents when prescribed to a lithium-treated patient will MOST likely lower the serum lithium level?

A. *Captopril*

B. *Hydrochlorothiazide*

C. *Ibuprofen*

D. *Losartan*

E. *Theophylline*

Q10 True or False. Valproate does NOT induce hepatic microsomes.

A. *True*

B. *False*

Q11 Which of the following is the LEAST protein-bound?

A. *Citalopram*

B. *Escitalopram*

C. *Fluvoxamine*

D. *Fluoxetine*

E. *Venlafaxine*

Q12 Which of the following classes of medications possess class 1A antiarrhythmic activity and can lead to depression of cardiac conduction that can result in heart block or ventricular arrhythmias when combined with quinidine-like agents?

A. *Benzodiazepines*

B. *Monoamine oxidase inhibitors*

C. *Selective serotonin reuptake inhibitors*

D. *Serotonin norepinephrine reuptake inhibitors*

E. *Tricyclic antidepressants (TCAs)*

Q13 Prompt intervention with which of the following agents may be lifesaving when a hypertensive crisis occurs in conjunction with use of a monoamine oxidase inhibitor?

A. *Flumazenil*

B. *Naloxone*

C. *Phentolamine*

D. *Phenylpropanolamine*

E. *Physostigmine*

Q1 The answer is: (B) False.

Pharmacokinetic, not pharmacodynamic, interactions are those that involve a change in the plasma level and/or tissue distribution of one drug by virtue of coadministration of another drug. These interactions occur due to effects at one or more of the four pharmacokinetic processes by which drugs are acted on by the body: absorption, distribution, metabolism, and excretion. An example of a pharmacokinetic drug–drug interaction is the inhibition of the metabolism of lamotrigine by valproic acid, thereby raising lamotrigine levels and increasing the risk of hypersensitivity reactions (such as Stevens-Johnson syndrome).

Pharmacodynamic interactions are those that involve a known pharmacologic effect at biologically active (receptor) sites. These interactions occur due to effects on the mechanisms through which the body is acted on by drugs, and do not involve a change in drug levels. An example of a pharmacodynamic drug–drug interaction is the interference of the antiparkinsonian effects of a dopamine receptor agonist (such as pramipexole) by a dopamine receptor antagonist (such as risperidone).

Mixed interactions are those that are believed to involve both pharmacologic and pharmacodynamic effects. The apparent enhancement of antidepressant response observed on the combination of fluoxetine and desipramine, for example, may be attributed to the pharmacokinetic elevation of desipramine blood levels due to inhibition of its metabolism by fluoxetine, as well as to putative synergistic pharmacodynamic actions of these two agents at serotonergic and noradrenergic synapses. Finally, idiosyncratic interactions are those that occur sporadically in small numbers of patients in ways that are not yet predicted by the known pharmacokinetic and pharmacodynamic properties of the drugs involved.

Q2 The answer is: (A) Diazepam.

In general, psychotropic drugs have relatively high affinities for plasma proteins (some to albumin, but others, such as antidepressants, to α1-acid glycoproteins and lipoproteins). Most psychotropic drugs are more than 80% protein-bound. A drug is considered highly protein-bound if more than 90% exists in bound form in plasma.

Fluoxetine, aripiprazole, and diazepam are examples of the many psychotropic drugs that are highly protein-bound.

In contrast, venlafaxine, lithium, topiramate, zonisamide, gabapentin, pregabalin, and memantine are examples of drugs with minimal protein-binding, and therefore minimal risk of participating in drug–drug interactions related to protein-binding. A reversible equilibrium exists between bound and unbound drugs. Only the unbound fraction exerts pharmacologic effects. Competition by two or more drugs for protein-binding sites often results in displacement of a previously bound drug, which, in the free state, becomes pharmacologically active. Similarly, reduced concentrations of plasma proteins in a severely malnourished patient or a patient with a disease that is associated with severely lowered serum proteins (such as liver disease or nephrotic syndrome) may be associated with an increase in the fraction of unbound drug potentially available for activity at relevant receptor sites. Under most circumstances, the net changes in plasma concentration of active drugs are, in fact, quite small because the unbound drug is available for redistribution to other tissues and for metabolism and excretion, thereby offsetting the initial rise in plasma levels. Nevertheless, clinically significant consequences can develop when protein-binding interactions alter the unbound fraction of previously highly protein-bound drugs that have a low therapeutic index (e.g., warfarin). For these drugs, relatively small variations in plasma level may be associated with serious untoward effects.

Q3 The answer is: (E) Lorazepam.

Metabolism refers to the biotransformation of a drug to another form, a process that is usually enzyme-mediated and that results in a metabolite that may or may not be pharmacologically active and may or may not be subject to further biotransformations before eventual excretion. Most drugs undergo several types of biotransformation, and many psychotropic drug interactions of clinical significance are based on interference with this process.

Phase 1 reactions include oxidation, reduction, and hydrolysis; metabolic reactions typically result in intermediate metabolites, which are then subject to phase 2 reactions (including conjugation [e.g., glucuronidation and sulfation] and acetylation). Phase 2 reactions typically yield highly polar, water-soluble metabolites suitable for renal excretion.

Most psychotropic drugs undergo both phase 1 and phase 2 metabolic reactions. Notable exceptions include valproic acid and a subset of benzodiazepines (i.e., lorazepam, oxazepam, and temazepam), which skip phase 1 metabolism and undergo phase 2 reactions only. In addition, certain medications, including lithium and gabapentin, do not undergo any hepatic biotransformation before excretion by the kidneys.

Q4 The answer is: (B) False.

The synthesis or activity of hepatic microsomal enzymes is affected by metabolic inhibitors and inducers, as well as by distinct genetic polymorphisms (stably inherited traits). In some circumstances, an inhibitor (such as grapefruit juice) or inducer (e.g., a cruciferous vegetable such as Brussels sprouts) may not be a drug but rather another ingested substance. In some circumstances, a drug is both a substrate of an enzyme but can also inhibit the metabolism of other substrates relying on that enzyme, in which case it is considered an inhibitor as well as a substrate.

Q5 The answer is: (B) False.

Imagine two drugs, drug A and drug B, which are both associated with a metabolic enzyme. Drug B may be an inhibitor or an inducer of that enzyme. Drug A may be normally metabolized by that enzyme and would therefore be called a substrate. If drug B is an inhibitor with respect to the metabolic enzyme, it will impede the metabolism of a concurrently administered substrate (drug A), thereby producing a rise in the plasma levels of that substrate. Whereas if drug B is an inducer of that enzyme, it will enhance the metabolism of the substrate (drug A), resulting in a decline in the plasma levels of that substrate.

Although inhibition is usually immediate, occurring by one or more of a variety of mechanisms including competitive inhibition or inactivation of the enzyme, induction, which requires enhanced synthesis of the metabolic enzyme, is typically a more gradual process. A fall in plasma levels of a substrate may not be apparent for days to weeks following introduction of the inducer. This is particularly important when a patient's care is being transferred to another setting, in which clinical deterioration may be the first sign that drug levels have declined. Reciprocally, an elevation in plasma drug concentrations could reflect the previous discontinuation of an inducing factor (e.g., cigarette smoking or carbamazepine), just as it could reflect the more recent introduction of an inhibitor (e.g., fluoxetine or valproic acid).

Q6 The answer is: (A) True.

The proportion of frankly poor metabolizers with respect to P450 2D6 appears to be higher among whites (approximately 5% to 10%) than among Asian and African Americans (approximately 1% to 3%).

Conversely, approximately 15% to 20% of Asian and African Americans appear to be poor metabolizers with respect to P450 2C19 compared with 3% to 5% of whites.

Most individuals are normal ("extensive") metabolizers with respect to the activity of these isoenzymes. A smaller number are "poor metabolizers" with deficient activity of the isoenzyme. Probably very much smaller numbers are "ultrarapid metabolizers" (who have more than normal activity of the enzyme) and "intermediate metabolizers" (who fall between extensive and poor metabolizers). Individuals who are poor metabolizers with respect to a particular cytochrome P450 isoenzyme are expected to have higher plasma concentrations of a drug that is metabolized by that isoenzyme, thereby potentially being more sensitive to or requiring lower doses of that drug than a patient with normal activity of that enzyme. They may also have higher than usual plasma levels of metabolites of the drug that are produced through other metabolic pathways that are not altered by the polymorphism, thereby potentially incurring pharmacologic activity or adverse effects related to these alternative metabolites. Poor metabolizers are relatively impervious to drug interactions involving inhibition of the particular isoenzyme system for which they are already deficient.

Current understanding of the clinical relevance of genetic polymorphisms in drug therapy in psychiatry remains rudimentary. Commercial genotyping tests for polymorphisms of potential relevance to drug–drug metabolism are increasingly available. Further systematic study of their relevance to the understanding and prediction of drug response is needed before such testing can be meaningfully incorporated into routine psychopharmacologic practice.

Q7 The answer is: (C) Pimozide.

The antipsychotic or neuroleptic drugs include the phenothiazines (e.g., chlorpromazine, fluphenazine, perphenazine, thioridazine, and trifluoperazine), butyrophenones (haloperidol), thioxanthenes (thiothix-ene), indol ones (molindone), diphenylbutylpiperidines (pimozide), dibenzodiazepines (loxapine), and the newer atypical agents (clozapine, olanzapine, risperidone, quetiapine, ziprasidone, and aripiprazole).

As a class, they are generally rapidly, if erratically, absorbed from the gastrointestinal tract after oral administration (peak plasma concentrations range from 30 minutes to 6 hours). They are highly lipophilic and distribute rapidly to body tissues with a large apparent volume of distribution. Protein-binding in the circulation ranges from approximately 90% to 98%, except for molindone and quetiapine, which are only moderately protein-bound.

Q8 The answer is: (A) True.

The lower-potency antipsychotics (including chlorpromazine, mesoridazine, thioridazine, and clozapine) are generally the most sedating and have the greatest anticholinergic, antihistaminic, and α1-adrenergic antagonistic effects, whereas the higher-potency antipsychotics (including haloperidol, loxapine, molin-done, and the piperazine phenothiazines, such as trifluoperazine) are more likely to be associated with an increased incidence of extrapyramidal symptoms, including akathisia, dystonia, and parkinsonism.

Q9 The answer is: (E) Theophylline.

A number of medications are associated with decreased lithium excretion, and therefore increased risk of lithium toxicity. Among the most well studied of these interactions involve thiazide diuretics. These agents decrease lithium clearance, and thereby steeply increase the risk of toxicity. Thiazide diuretics block sodium reabsorption at the distal tubule, producing sodium depletion, which in turn results in increased lithium reabsorption in the proximal tubule. Loop diuretics (e.g., furosemide and bumetanide) appear to interact to a lesser degree with lithium excretion, presumably because they block lithium reabsorption in the loop of Henle, potentially offsetting possible compensatory increases in reabsorption more proximally. The potassium-sparing diuretics (e.g., amiloride, spironolactone, ethacrynic acid, and triamterene) also appear to be somewhat less likely to cause an increase in lithium levels, but close monitoring is indicated when introduced. The potential impact of thiazide diuretics on lithium levels does not contraindicate their combined use, which has been particularly valuable in the treatment of lithium-associated polyuria.

Potassium-sparing diuretics have also been used for this purpose. When a thiazide diuretic is used, a lithium dose reduction and frequent monitoring of lithium levels are required. Monitoring of serum elec-trolytes, particularly potassium, is also important when thiazides are introduced; hypokalemia enhances the toxicity of lithium. Although not contraindicated with lithium, angiotensin-converting enzyme inhibi-tors (e.g., captopril) and angiotensin 2 receptor antagonists (e.g., losartan) can elevate lithium levels, and close monitoring of levels is also required when these agents are introduced. Many of the nonsteroidal antiinflammatory drugs (including ibuprofen, indomethacin, naproxen, and piroxicam) have also been reported to increase serum lithium levels, potentially by as much as 50% to 60% when used at full prescription strength. This may occur by inhibition of renal clearance of lithium by interference with a prostaglandin-dependent mechanism in the renal tubule.

The cyclooxygenase-2 inhibitors may also raise lithium levels. Limited available data suggest that su-lindac, phenylbutazone, and aspirin are less likely to affect lithium levels.

A number of antimicrobials are associated with increased lithium levels, including tetracycline, metro-nidazole, and parenteral spectinomycin. In the event that these agents are required, close monitoring of lithium levels and potential dose adjustment are recommended.

Conversely, a variety of agents can produce decreases in lithium levels, thereby increasing risk of psy-chiatric symptom breakthrough and relapse. The methylxanthines (e.g., aminophylline and theophylline) can cause a significant decrease in lithium levels by increasing renal clearance; close blood level monitoring when coadministration occurs is necessary. A reduction in lithium levels can also result from alkalinization of urine (e.g., with acetazolamide use or with sodium bicarbonate) from osmotic diuretics (e.g., urea or mannitol), or from ingestion of a sodium chloride load, which also increases lithium excretion.

Q10 The answer is: (A) True.

In contrast to other major anticonvulsants (such as carbamazepine and phenobarbital), valproate does not induce hepatic microsomes. Rather, it tends to act as an inhibitor of oxidation and glucuronidation reac-tions, thereby potentially increasing levels of coadministered hepatically metabolized drugs.

A complex pharmacokinetic interaction occurs when valproic acid and carbamazepine are administered concurrently. Valproic acid not only inhibits the metabolism of carbamazepine and its active metabolite, carbamazepine-10,11-epoxide, but also displaces both entities from protein-binding sites. Although the effect on plasma carbamazepine levels is variable, the levels of the unbound (active) epoxide metabolite are increased with a concomitant increased risk of carbamazepine neurotoxicity. Conversely, coadministration with carbamazepine results in a decrease in plasma valproic acid levels.

Q11 The answer is: (E) Venlafaxine.
All of the selective serotonin reuptake inhibitors, as well as nefazodone, are highly protein-bound (95% to 99%) with the exception of fluvoxamine (77%), citalopram (80%), and escitalopram (56%). Mirtazapine and bupropion are moderately protein-bound (85%). The serotonin–norepinephrine reuptake inhibitor duloxetine is highly protein-bound (90%), although venlafaxine is minimally protein-bound (20% to 30%).

Q12 The answer is: (E) Tricyclic antidepressants (TCAs).
Tricyclic antidepressants (TCAs) possess class 1A antiarrhythmic activity, and can lead to depression of cardiac conduction, potentially resulting in heart block or ventricular arrhythmias when combined with quinidine-like agents (including quinidine, procainamide, and disopyramide, as well as the low-potency antipsychotics). The antiarrhythmics quinidine and propafenone, inhibitors of cytochrome P450 2D6, may additionally result in clinically significant elevations of the TCAs; this increases the risk of cardiotoxicity through both pharmacodynamic and pharmacokinetic mechanisms.

The arrhythmogenic risks of a TCA are enhanced in an individual with underlying coronary or valvular heart disease, recent myocardial infarction, or hypokalemia, and in a patient receiving sympathomimetic amines, such as dextroamphetamine.

TCAs also interact with several antihypertensive drugs. TCAs can antagonize the antihypertensive effects of guanethidine, bethanidine, debrisoquine, or clonidine via interference with neuronal reuptake by noradrenergic neurons. Conversely, TCAs can cause or aggravate postural hypotension when coadministered with vasodilator drugs, antihypertensives, and low-potency neuroleptics.

Q13 The answer is: (C) Phentolamine.
Hypertensive crisis is an emergency characterized by an abrupt elevation of blood pressure, severe headache, nausea, vomiting, and diaphoresis; intracranial hemorrhage or myocardial infarction can occur.

Prompt intervention to reduce blood pressure with the α1-adrenergic antagonist phentolamine or the calcium channel-blocker nifedipine may be lifesaving. Potentially catastrophic hypertension appears to be due to release of bound intraneuronal stores of norepinephrine and dopamine by indirect vasopressor substances.

The reaction can therefore be precipitated by the concurrent administration of vasopressor amines, stimulants, anorexiants, and many over-the-counter cough and cold preparations; these include L-dopa, dopamine, amphetamine, methylphenidate, phenylpropanolamine, phentermine, mephentermine, metaraminol, ephedrine, and pseudoephedrine.

By contrast, direct sympathomimetic amines (e.g., norepinephrine, isoproterenol, and epinephrine), which rely for their cardiovascular effects on direct stimulation of postsynaptic receptors rather than on presynaptic release of stored catecholamines, may be somewhat safer when administered to individuals on monoamine oxidase inhibitors, although they are also contraindicated.

Side Effects of Psychotropic Medications

Multiple-Choice Questions

Select the appropriate answer.

Q1   Which of the following is LEAST likely to be a side effect of a tricyclic antidepressant (TCA)?

    A. *Blurred vision*

    B. *Bradycardia*

    C. *Constipation*

    D. *Dry mouth*

    E. *Urinary hesitancy*

Q2   Which of the following is a secondary amine tricyclic antidepressant (TCA)?

    A. *Amitriptyline*

    B. *Clomipramine*

    C. *Doxepin*

    D. *Imipramine*

    E. *Nortriptyline*

Q3   Which of the following receptors is MOST closely linked with sedation?

    A. *Alpha-adrenergic*

    B. *Acetylcholine*

    C. *Beta-adrenergic*

    D. *Dopamine*

    E. *Histamine*

Q4   Which of the following is LEAST likely to be noted in cases of tricyclic antidepressant (TCA) overdose?

    A. *Hypotension*

    B. *Miosis*

    C. *QRS interval widening*

    D. *Sedation*

    E. *Seizures*

Q5   Which of the following is MOST likely to be considered a serotonin–norepinephrine reuptake inhibitor?

    A. *Citalopram*

    B. *Fluoxetine*

C. *Nortriptyline*

D. *Phenelzine*

E. *Venlafaxine*

Q6 Which of the following agents is MOST closely linked with the onset of hypertension?

A. *Citalopram*

B. *Fluoxetine*

C. *Nortriptyline*

D. *Phenelzine*

E. *Venlafaxine*

Q7 Which of the following agents is MOST closely linked with seizures in those with eating disorders, head trauma, or alcohol abuse?

A. *Alprazolam*

B. *Bupropion*

C. *Citalopram*

D. *Fluoxetine*

E. *Trazodone*

Q8 Which of the following foods is LEAST likely to be problematic while taking a monoamine oxidase inhibitor (MAOI)?

A. *Broad bean pods*

B. *Cottage cheese*

C. *Fermented meats*

D. *Pizza*

E. *Soy sauce*

Q9 Which of the following is LEAST likely to induce extrapyramidal symptoms (EPS)?

A. *Aripiprazole*

B. *Chlorpromazine*

C. *Clozapine*

D. *Haloperidol*

E. *Perphenazine*

Chapter 51

Answers

Q1 The answer is: (B) Bradycardia.
Tricyclic antidepressants (TCAs) have a number of common side effects that require careful management. Anticholinergic effects (including dry mouth, blurred vision, urinary hesitancy, constipation, tachycardia, and delirium), which result from the blockade of muscarinic cholinergic receptors, can occur with use of TCAs. In addition, anticholinergic effects can also be dangerous to patients with pre-existing glaucoma (leading to acute angle-closure glaucoma), benign prostatic hypertrophy (leading to acute urinary retention), and dementia (leading to acute confusional states).
    TCAs can also cause sedation, orthostatic hypotension, increased sweating, and weight gain.

Q2 The answer is: (E) Nortriptyline.
Secondary amine TCAs include nortriptyline, desipramine, and protriptyline; tertiary amine TCAs include amitriptyline, doxepin, clomipramine, and imipramine. Side effect clusters are more common with tertiary amine TCAs.

Q3 The answer is: (E) Histamine.
TCAs can cause sedation that results from blockade of histamine H_1 receptors, and orthostatic hypotension that results from blockade of $\alpha 1$ receptors on blood vessels.

Q4 The answer is: (B) Miosis.
Dilated pupils, not constricted pupils, are hallmarks of anticholinergic excess. Adverse effects associated with TCA overdose include the exacerbation of standard side effects (e.g., severe sedation, hypotension, and anticholinergic delirium). Ventricular arrhythmias and seizures can also result from TCA overdose; a characteristic QRS interval widening is often present. TCAs are associated with cardiac conduction disturbances and can lead to prolongation of the PR, QRS, and QT intervals on the electrocardiogram; TCAs have been associated with all manners of heart block.

Q5 The answer is: (E) Venlafaxine.
Venlafaxine and duloxetine are serotonin–norepinephrine reuptake inhibitors, with side effects similar to those of selective serotonin reuptake inhibitors, such as fluoxetine and citalopram. Phenelzine is a monoamine oxidase inhibitor (MAOI), and nortriptyline is a secondary amine TCA.

Q6 The answer is: (E) Venlafaxine.
Increased blood pressure, presumably related to its effects on norepinephrine, can occur with immediate-release venlafaxine. Increased blood pressure has been noted in 7% of patients taking 300 mg per day or less, and 13% of those taking 300 mg or more; this resolves spontaneously in approximately one-half of cases. The extended-release formulation appears to be associated with lower rates of hypertension.
    Use of TCAs and MAOIs commonly leads to hypotension.

Q7 The answer is: (B) Bupropion.
The most serious side effect associated with bupropion use is seizure. The risk of seizure with the immediate-release preparation is 0.1% at doses less than 300 mg/day, and 0.4% at doses from 300 to 400 mg/day; the risk of seizure may be lower with longer-acting preparations, but guidelines to keep the total daily dose at or below 450 mg/day remain. In addition, maximum single doses should not exceed 150 mg for the immediate-release form and 200 mg for the sustained-release form. A new preparation (Wellbutrin XL) can be given as a single dose of up to 450 mg. Because of its increased risk of seizure, bupropion should not be used in those patients with a history of seizures, or in those at increased risk of seizures (e.g., those with eating disorders, head trauma, or alcohol abuse).

Q8 The answer is: (B) Cottage cheese.

Fresh cottage, cream, ricotta, and processed cheese are tolerated. However, all matured or aged cheeses should be avoided.

As a rule, tyramine-containing foods should be avoided by patients taking MAOIs. These foods include pizza, lasagna, and other foods made with cheese; fermented/dried meat (e.g., pepperoni, salami, or summer sausage); improperly stored meat and fish; fava or broad bean pods; banana peels (banana and other fruit are tolerated, but one should not use more than 1/4 pound of raspberries); all tap beers (two or less cans/bottles of beer or 4 oz glass of wine per day); sauerkraut; soy sauce and other soybean products (but soy milk is acceptable); and marmite yeast extract (other yeast extract are acceptable).

Q9 The answer is: (C) Clozapine.

Clozapine causes extrapyramidal symptoms (EPS) infrequently.

In general, second-generation or atypical antipsychotics (aripiprazole) cause fewer EPS than do conventional neuroleptics. Conventional agents that are more potent (e.g., haloperidol) tend to cause more EPS than do low-potency agents (e.g., chlorpromazine).

Natural Medications in Psychiatry

Multiple-Choice Questions

Select the appropriate answer.

Q1 According to a recent National Health Interview Survey, roughly what percent of the general population in the United States used some form of complementary and alternative medicine (including prayer) for health reasons within the past year?

    A. *10% to 15%*

    B. *20% to 25%*

    C. *40% to 45%*

    D. *60% to 65%*

    E. *80% to 85%*

Q2 True or False. The US Food and Drug Administration (FDA) closely regulates natural medications.

    A. *True*

    B. *False*

Q3 Which of the following agents is LEAST likely to improve depressive symptoms when ingested?

    A. *Ginkgo biloba*

    B. *Omega-3 fatty acids*

    C. *S-adenosyl methionine*

    D. *St. John's wort (SJW)*

    E. *Vitamin B_{12}*

Q4 Hyperforin is thought to be the active ingredient in which of the following agents?

    A. *Ginkgo biloba*

    B. *Kava*

    C. *S-adenosyl methionine*

    D. *St. John's wort (SJW)*

    E. *Valerian*

Q5   Which of the following is derived from a root originating in the Polynesian Islands, where it is used as a social and ceremonial herb with mild anxiolytic and hypnotic effects?

A.   *Black cohosh*

B.   *Ginkgo biloba*

C.   *Kava*

D.   *St. John's wort (SJW)*

E.   *Valerian*

Chapter 52

Answers

Q1 The answer is: (D) 60% to 65%.

Complementary and alternative medical (CAM) therapies are made up of a diverse spectrum of practices and beliefs that often overlap with current medical practice. The National Institutes of Health defines CAM as "healthcare practices outside the realm of conventional medicine, which are yet to be validated using scientific methods."

Natural medications are medications that are derived from natural products and are not approved by the US Food and Drug Administration (FDA) for their proposed indication. Natural medications may include a wide variety of types of products, including hormones, vitamins, plants, herbs, fatty acids, amino acid derivatives, and homeopathic preparations. Natural medications have been used in Asia for thousands of years. Their use in the United States has shown a dramatic increase over the past decade and a half. In fact, the National Health Interview Survey conducted in 2002 revealed that 62% of a randomly sampled US population used some form of CAM (including prayer for health reasons) within the past year. When prayer was excluded, 36% of those sampled admitted to using some form of CAM. Moreover, between 1990 and 1997, the prevalence of herbal remedy use increased by 380%, whereas high-dose vitamin use increased by 130%. Between the years 1998 and 2002, use of CAM doubled in the over age 65 years population.

Ethnic considerations seem to be important; African Americans are the least likely US cohort to try natural remedies, and Hispanics are the most prone to their use. Given the considerable portion of the US population trying natural remedies, it is becoming increasingly important to be informed about these medications to provide comprehensive patient care.

Q2 The answer is: (B) False.

The FDA does not routinely regulate natural medications. Consumers often believe that because a remedy is "natural," it is safe. Moreover, because these remedies are most often purchased over-the-counter, there are no clear mechanisms for reports of toxicity to reach those who use them. Another significant problem lies in the limited information regarding the safety and efficacy of combining natural medications with more conventional ones. In cases in which interactions are known, the psychiatrist faces the reality that patients frequently do not disclose their use of CAM therapies to their physicians. In one study, fewer than 40% of CAM therapies used by patients were disclosed to a physician. Asking very specific questions about a patient's use of both prescribed and over-the-counter medications may improve disclosures in this regard. Finally, because natural medications are not regulated as are more conventional ones, significant variability exists among different preparations. Preparations often vary in purity, quality, potency, and efficacy, whereas side effects may vary.

Q3 The answer is: (A) *Ginkgo biloba*.

Numerous natural medications (including omega-3 fatty acids, St. John's wort [SJW], S-adenosyl methionine, folic acid, vitamin B_{12}, and inositol) have been used to treat mood disorders.

Ginkgo biloba, used in Chinese medicine for thousands of years, is a natural medication that comes from the seed of the Gingko tree, and that has been used for the treatment of impaired cognition and affective symptoms in dementing illnesses; however, a possible new role has also emerged in the management of antidepressant-induced sexual dysfunction. As far as its role in cognition is concerned, target symptoms in patients with dementia include memory and abstract thinking. Studies have shown modest but significant improvements in both cognitive performance and social function with doses of 120 mg per day. Evidence suggests that progression of dementia may be delayed by 6 to 12 months, whereas those with mild dementia show greatest improvement, and those with more severe disease may (at best) stabilize. Furthermore, one study of healthy young volunteers taking *Ginkgo biloba* noted significant improvements in speed of information processing, executive function, and working-memory, suggesting that *Ginkgo biloba* may also enhance learning capacity.

Q4 The answer is: (D) St. John's wort (SJW).

SJW (*Hypericum perforatum L.*) is one of the biggest-selling natural medications on the market. It has been shown to be more effective than placebo in the treatment of mild to moderate depression. Studies have further suggested that SJW is as effective as low-dose tricyclic antidepressants (e.g., imipramine 75 mg, maprotiline 75 mg, or amitriptyline 75 mg). When compared with selective serotonin reuptake inhibitors, the efficacy of SJW is more mixed. In other studies, SJW has not shown an advantage over placebo. These mixed results may be explained by more severely depressed study populations in studies with negative outcomes. *Hypericum* is thought to be the main antidepressant ingredient in SJW, whereas polycyclic phenols, pseudohypericin, and hyperforin are also thought to be active ingredients. As far as the mechanisms of action of SJW are concerned, there are several proposed theories. These include the inhibition of cytokines, a decrease in serotonin (5-HT) receptor density, a decrease in reuptake of neurotransmitters, and monoamine oxidase inhibitor activity. Considering that SJW has monoamine oxidase inhibitor activity, it should not be combined with selective serotonin reuptake inhibitors because of the possible development of serotonin syndrome.

Q5 The answer is: (C) Kava.

Kava (*Piper methysticum*) is derived from a root originating in the Polynesian Islands, where it is used as a social and ceremonial herb. Although it is believed to have mild anxiolytic and hypnotic effects, study results have been mixed. The mechanism of action is attributed to kavapyrones, which are central muscle relaxants that are thought to be involved in blockade of voltage-gated sodium ion channels, enhanced binding to $GABA_A$ receptors, diminished excitatory neurotransmitter release, reduced reuptake of noradrenaline (norepinephrine), and reversible inhibition of monoamine oxidase B. The suggested dose is 60 to 120 mg per day. Major side effects include gastrointestinal upset, headaches, and dizziness. Toxic reactions including ataxia, hair loss, respiratory problems, yellowing of the skin, and vision problems that have been seen at high doses or with prolonged use. There have also been more than 35 published reports of severe hepatotoxicity worldwide, including some individuals who have required liver transplantation. For this reason, several countries have pulled kava off the market. In the United States, the FDA has issued a warning regarding the use of kava and is currently investigating its safety.

Although kava appears to be somewhat efficacious in the treatment of mild anxiety, current concerns about safety make cautious use essential.

SECTION 11
SPECIAL TOPICS IN PSYCHIATRY

Chapter 53: The Suicidal Patient

The Suicidal Patient

Multiple-Choice Questions

Select the appropriate answer.

Q1   Which of the following is the MOST common method of committing suicide for both men and women in the United States?

   A.   *Jumping from a height*

   B.   *Poisoning, including drug ingestion*

   C.   *Starvation*

   D.   *Suffocation, including hanging*

   E.   *Use of firearms*

Q2   Which of the following age groups has the HIGHEST suicide rate?

   A.   *Age younger than 15 years*

   B.   *Age 15 to 24 years*

   C.   *Age 25 to 45 years*

   D.   *Age 46 to 65 years*

   E.   *Age older than 65 years*

Q3   Which of the following psychiatric disorders is associated with the HIGHEST rate of suicide?

   A.   *Alcohol and drug abuse*

   B.   *Mood disorders*

   C.   *Panic disorder*

   D.   *Personality disorders*

   E.   *Psychosis*

Q4   Which of the following groups is LEAST likely to commit suicide?

   A.   *Married adults with young children*

   B.   *Single adults*

   C.   *Those who are divorced*

   D.   *Those who are separated*

   E.   *Those who are widowed*

Q5   Which of the following is LEAST accurate?

   A.   *A history of suicide attempts is one of the most powerful risk factors for completed and attempted suicide*

   B.   *Fewer than 30% of people who complete suicide communicated their intent either directly or indirectly*

C. *Hopelessness or negative expectations about the future is a stronger predictor of suicide risk than is depression or suicidal ideation, and may be both a short-term and long-term predictor of completed suicide in patients with major depression*

D. *People who intend to commit suicide may be less likely to communicate their intent to their health care providers than they are to close family and friends*

E. *The lethality of past attempts slightly increases the risk for completed suicide, especially among women with psychiatric illness*

Q6 Which of the following statements is LEAST accurate?

A. *Specific questions concerning potential suicide plans and preparations must follow any admission of suicidal ideation or intent*

B. *The approach to the patient at potential risk for suicide should be nonjudgmental, supportive, and empathic*

C. *The clinician must attempt to identify any possible precipitants for the present crisis in an effort to understand why the patient is suicidal*

D. *The patient should be questioned about suicidal ideation and intent in an open and direct manner*

E. *There is rarely a need to interview the family and friends of the patient at risk for suicide to corroborate gathered information and to obtain new and pertinent data*

Q7 Which of the following statements is LEAST accurate?

A. *A thorough psychiatric, medical, social, and family history of the patient who may be at risk for suicide should be completed to evaluate the presence and significance of potential risk factors*

B. *Conducting a thorough mental status examination adds little to the assessment of a potentially suicidal patient*

C. *The clinician should interview the family and friends of the patient at risk to corroborate gathered information and to obtain new and pertinent data*

D. *The greater the relative risk or lethality and the lesser the likelihood of rescue of a planned attempt, the more serious the potential for a completed suicide*

E. *The patient who carries out a detailed plan, who perceives the attempt as lethal, who thinks that death will be certain, who is disappointed to be alive, and who must face unchanged stressors is likely to be at a continued high risk for suicide*

Q8 Which of the following statements is LEAST accurate?

A. *A patient who is at potential risk for suicide and who threatens to leave before an adequate evaluation is completed must be detained, in accordance with statutes in most states that permit the detention of individuals deemed dangerous to themselves or others*

B. *Appropriate supervision and restraint must be provided only after the evaluation of the patient has been completed, and a decision to hospitalize rendered*

C. *A suicide contract is not a legal contract and it has limited use, if any, if litigation should ensue from a completed suicide*

D. *Potential means for self-harm should be removed from the reach of a patient at risk*

E. *Throughout the evaluation and treatment of the suicidal patient, safety must be ensured until the patient is no longer at imminent risk for suicide*

Answers

Q1 The answer is: (E) Use of firearms.

Use of firearms is the most common method of committing suicide for both men and women in the United States, accounting for between 50% and 60% of suicides annually. Suffocation, including hanging, is the second most common cause of suicide overall in the United States, and the second most common cause in men, accounting for approximately 6500 suicide deaths per year. Poisoning, including drug ingestion, is the third most common cause of completed suicide in the United States, and the second most common cause in women, accounting for approximately 5500 deaths per year. Historically, drug ingestion has accounted for most unsuccessful suicide attempts.

Q2 The answer is: (E) Age older than 65 years.

Suicide rates differ by age. Rates generally increase with age; people older than 65 years are 1.5 times more likely to commit suicide than are younger individuals, whereas white men over age 85 have an even higher rate of suicide. The number of suicides in the elderly is disproportionately high; the elderly appear to make more serious attempts on their lives and are less apt to survive when medical complications from an attempt ensue; and one out of four attempts in this group results in a completed suicide. Although the elderly have the highest suicide rates, suicide in young adults (between ages 15 and 24) rose threefold between 1950 and 1990, becoming the third leading cause of death in this age-group following unintentional injuries and homicide. Since that time, the suicide rate has declined in adolescents.

Q3 The answer is: (B) Mood disorders.

Psychiatric illness is the most powerful risk factor for both completed and attempted suicide. Psychiatric disorders are associated with more than 90% of completed suicides, and with the vast majority of attempted suicides. Mood disorders, including major depressive disorder (MDD) and bipolar disorder, are responsible for approximately 50% of completed suicides, alcohol and drug abuse for 25%, psychosis for 10%, and personality disorders for 5%.

Up to 15% of patients with MDD or bipolar disorder complete suicide, almost always during depressive episodes; this represents a suicide risk 30 times greater than that of the general population. True lifetime risk may be somewhat lower because these estimates (and those for the other diagnoses discussed later) typically derive from hospitalized patient samples. The risk appears to be greater early during a lifetime disorder, early on in a depressive episode, in the first week following psychiatric hospitalization, in the first month following hospital discharge, and in the early stages of recovery. The risk may be elevated by comorbid psychosis.

Approximately 15% to 25% of patients with alcohol or drug dependence complete suicide; comorbidity is common. The suicide risk appears to be greatest roughly 9 years after the commencement of alcohol and drug addiction. The majority of patients with alcohol dependence who commit suicide suffer from comorbid depressive disorders, and as many as one-third have experienced the recent loss of a close relationship through separation or death.

Nearly 20% of people who complete suicide are legally intoxicated at the time of their death. Alcohol and drug abuse are associated with more pervasive suicidal ideation, more serious suicidal intent, more lethal suicide attempts, and a greater number of suicide attempts. Use of alcohol and drugs may impair judgment and foster impulsivity.

Roughly 10% of patients with schizophrenia complete suicide, mostly during periods of improvement after relapse or during periods of depression. The risk for suicide appears to be greater among young men who are newly diagnosed, who have a chronic course and numerous exacerbations, who are discharged from hospitals with significant psychopathology and functional impairment, and who have a realistic awareness and fear of further mental decline. The risk may also be increased with akathisia and with abrupt discontinuation of neuroleptics. Patients who experience hallucinations (that instruct them to harm themselves) in association with schizophrenia, mania, or depression with psychotic features are probably at greater risk for self-harm, and they should be protected.

Between 4% and 10% of patients with borderline personality disorder, and 5% of patients with antisocial personality disorder commit suicide. The risk appears to be greater for those with comorbid unipolar depression or alcohol abuse. Patients with personality disorders often make impulsive suicidal gestures or attempts; these attempts may become more lethal if they are not taken seriously. Even manipulative gestures can turn fatal.

As many as 15% to 20% of patients with anxiety disorders complete suicide, and up to 20% of patients with panic disorder attempt suicide. Although the risk of suicide in patients with anxiety and panic disorders may be elevated secondary to comorbid conditions (e.g., MDD and alcohol or drug abuse), the suicide risk remains almost as high as that of major depression, even after coexisting conditions are considered. The risk for suicide attempts may be elevated for women with an early onset of an anxiety disorder, and with comorbid alcohol or drug abuse.

Q4 The answer is: (A) Married adults with young children.
Widowed, divorced, or separated adults are at greater risk for suicide than are single adults, who are at greater risk than married adults. Married adults with young children appear to carry the lowest risk. Living alone substantially increases the risk for suicide, especially among adults who are widowed, divorced, or separated. Social isolation from family, relatives, friends, neighbors, and coworkers also increases the chance of suicide. Conversely, the presence of social supports is protective against suicide.

Q5 The answer is: (B) Fewer than 30% of people who complete suicide communicated their intent either directly or indirectly.
The communication of present suicidal ideation and intent must be carefully evaluated as a risk factor for completed and attempted suicide. As many as 80% of people who complete suicide communicated their intent either directly or indirectly. Death or suicide may be discussed, new wills or life insurance policies may be written, valued possessions may be given away, or uncharacteristic and destructive behaviors may arise.

Q6 The answer is: (E) There is rarely a need to interview the family and friends of the patient at risk for suicide to corroborate gathered information and to obtain new and pertinent data.
The clinician should interview the family and friends of the patient at risk to corroborate gathered information and to obtain new and pertinent data. The family may provide information that a patient is hesitant to provide, and that may be essential to the patient's care. A patient who refuses to discuss an attempt or insists that the entire event was a mistake may speak in an open and honest manner only when confronted with reports from his or her family. The evaluation of suicidal risk and the protection of the patient at risk are emergency procedures, which may take precedence over the desire of the patient for privacy and the maintenance of confidentiality in the physician-patient relationship. Concern over a life-or-death situation may obviate obtaining formal consent from the patient before speaking to family and friends.

Specific questions concerning potential suicide plans and preparations must follow any admission of suicidal ideation or intent. The patient should be asked when, where, and how an attempt would be made, and any potential means should be evaluated for feasibility and lethality. An organized and detailed plan involving an accessible and lethal method may place the patient at higher risk for suicide. The seriousness of the wish or the intent to die must also be assessed. The patient who has begun to carry out the initial steps of a suicide plan, who wishes to be dead, and who has no hopes or plans may be at greater risk. The last-mentioned domain (plans for the future) may be assessed by asking questions such as "What do you see yourself doing five years from now?" or "What things are you still looking forward to doing or seeing?"

The approach to the patient at potential risk for suicide should be nonjudgmental, supportive, and empathic. The initial establishment of rapport may include an introduction, an effort to create some degree of privacy in the interview setting, and an attempt to maximize the physical comfort of the patient for the interview. The patient who senses interest, concern, and compassion is more likely to trust the examiner, and to provide a detailed and accurate history. Often ambivalent about their thoughts and plans, suicidal patients may derive significant relief and benefit from a thoughtful and caring evaluation.

The clinician must attempt to identify any possible precipitants for the present crisis in an effort to understand why the patient is suicidal. The patient who must face the same problems and stressors following the evaluation or who cannot or will not discuss potential precipitants may be at greater risk for suicide. The clinician must also assess the social support in place for a given patient. A lack of outpatient care providers, family, or friends may elevate potential risk.

The patient should be questioned about suicidal ideation and intent in an open and direct manner. Patients with suicidal thoughts and plans are often relieved and not offended when they find someone with whom they can speak about the unspeakable. Patients without suicidal ideation do not have the thoughts planted in their mind, and do not develop a greater risk for suicide. General questions concerning suicidal thoughts can be introduced in a gradual manner, while obtaining the history of present illness. Questions such as "Has it ever seemed like things just aren't worth it?" or "Have you had thoughts that life is not worth living?" may lead to a further discussion of depression and hopelessness. "Have you gotten so depressed that you've considered killing yourself?" or "Have you had thoughts of killing yourself?" may open the door to a further evaluation of suicidal thoughts and plans.

Q7 The answer is: (B) Conducting a thorough mental status examination adds little to the assessment of a potentially suicidal patient.

A careful mental status examination allows the clinician to detect psychiatric difficulties and to assess cognitive capacities. Important aspects to evaluate in the examination include level of consciousness, appearance, behavior, attention, mood, affect, language, orientation, memory, thought form, thought content, perception, insight, and judgment. A psychiatric review of systems also aids in the detection of psychiatric disease.

A thorough psychiatric, medical, social, and family history of the patient who may be at risk for suicide should be completed to evaluate the presence and significance of potential risk factors. Attention should be paid to the presence of MDD, alcohol or drug abuse, psychotic disorders, personality disorders, and anxiety disorders. The presence of multiple significant risk factors may confer an additive risk.

The clinician should interview the family and friends of the patient at risk to corroborate gathered information and to obtain new and pertinent data. The family may provide information that a patient is hesitant to provide, and that may be essential to the patient's care. A patient who refuses to discuss an attempt or insists that the entire event was a mistake may speak in an open and honest manner only when confronted with reports from his or her family. The evaluation of suicidal risk and the protection of the patient at risk are emergency procedures, which may take precedence over the desire of the patient for privacy and the maintenance of confidentiality in the physician–patient relationship. Concern over a life-or-death situation may obviate obtaining formal consent from the patient before speaking to family and friends.

Many clinicians have addressed the issues of lethality and intent by means of the risk/rescue ratio. The greater the relative risk or lethality and the lesser the likelihood of rescue of a planned attempt, the more serious the potential for a completed suicide. Although often useful, the risk/rescue ratio cannot be applied as a simple formula; instead, one must examine and interpret the beliefs of a given patient. For example, a patient may plan an attempt with a low risk of potential harm but may sincerely wish to die and believe that the plan will be fatal; the patient may thus have a higher risk for suicide. Conversely, a patient may plan an attempt that carries a high probability of death, such as an acetaminophen overdose, but may have little desire to die and little understanding of the severity of the attempt; the patient may thus have a lower risk.

The patient who carries out a detailed plan, who perceives the attempt as lethal, who thinks that death will be certain, who is disappointed to be alive, and who must face unchanged stressors is likely to be at a continued high risk for suicide. The patient who makes a calculated, premeditated attempt may also be at a higher risk for a repeat attempt than the patient who makes a hasty, impulsive attempt (out of anger, a desire for revenge, or a desire for attention), or the patient who is intoxicated.

Q8 The answer is: (B) Appropriate supervision and restraint must be provided only after the evaluation of the patient has been completed, and a decision to hospitalize rendered.

Appropriate supervision and restraint must be provided at all times for a patient at risk for suicide. Frequent supervision, constant one-to-one supervision, physical restraints, and medications may be used alone or in combination to protect a patient at risk. The least restrictive means that ensures the safety of the patient should be used.

A patient who is at potential risk for suicide and who threatens to leave before an adequate evaluation is completed must be detained, in accordance with statutes in most states that permit the detention of individuals deemed dangerous to themselves or others. Patients who attempt to leave nonetheless should be contained by locked environments or restraints.

A suicide contract is not a legal contract and it has limited use, if any, if litigation should ensue from a completed suicide. Safety contracts or suicide prevention contracts, although intended to manage risk, are generally overvalued and of limited use. Specifically, suicide contracts depend on the subjective beliefs of the psychiatrist and the patient and not on objective data; they have never been shown to be clinically efficacious. Many suicide attempters and completers have had suicide contracts in place at the time of the suicidal act.

Potential means for self-harm should be removed from the reach of a patient at risk. Sharp objects (such as scissors, sutures, needles, glass bottles, and eating utensils) should be removed from the immediate area. Open windows, stairwells, and structures to which a noose could be attached must be blocked. Medications or other dangerous substances that patients may have in their possession must be secured by staff in a location out of the patient's access.

Throughout the evaluation and treatment of the suicidal patient, safety must be ensured until the patient is no longer at imminent risk for suicide. Appropriate intervention and the passage of time may aid in the resolution of suicidal ideation and intent.

SECTION 12

PSYCHOSOMATIC MEDICINE

Chapter 54

Psychiatric Consultation to Medical and Surgical Patients

Multiple-Choice Questions

Select the appropriate answer.

Q1   True or False. Although the consultee's question must be kept in mind throughout the interview, consultees often misidentify psychopathology, and the consultation question should be taken only as a *suggestion*.

    A. *True*

    B. *False*

Q2   True or False. Assessment of attention begins with simple observation of the patient during the interview while watching for distraction by extraneous internal or external stimuli.

    A. *True*

    B. *False*

Q3   True or False. Impairment in clock-drawing and Luria hand maneuvers suggests that the patient will have an aprosodia.

    A. *True*

    B. *False*

Q4   Which of the following individuals is MOST closely linked with the technique called the "life narrative"?

    A. *Ned Cassem*

    B. *Thomas Hackett*

    C. *Milton Viederman*

    D. *Avery Weisman*

    E. *Thomas Wise*

Q5   True or False. Consulting psychiatrists should refrain from touching and performing a physical examination on patients in the general hospital.

    A. *True*

    B. *False*

Q1 The answer is: (A) True.
Although the consultee's question must be kept in mind throughout the interview, consultees often mis-identify psychopathology, and the consultation question should be taken only as a *suggestion*. At the same time, the psychiatrist should not function as the local "biopsychosocial expert," for whom just about anything in the patient's life is worthy of attention.

Q2 The answer is: (A) True.
Attention and concentration refer to the abilities to engage appropriate stimuli without distraction by sensory inputs. Assessment of attention begins with simple observation of the patient during the interview while watching for distraction by extraneous internal or external stimuli.

Forward digit span is the gold standard for quantitatively testing attention at the bedside. Backward digit span or backward recitation of overlearned information (e.g., days of the week or months of the year) uses information that is less determined by education or culture than is a spelling or a mathematical task.

Q3 The answer is: (B) False.
Errors on clock-drawing, cognitive estimations, Luria hand maneuvers, alternating figures, word-list generation, and the go/no-go task suggest disruption of the brain's frontal-subcortical circuitry, particularly the dorsolateral prefrontal circuit. Such disruptions can occur through functional or anatomic lesions that affect the cortex, basal ganglia, thalamus, or the intervening white matter. Such errors do not herald an impairment of the ability to interpret emotional tonality or to convey a variety of affects with spoken language (which occur with aprosodia).

Q4 The answer is: (C) Milton Viederman.
Although a hospital unit may not be a suitable venue for exploratory, insight-oriented psychotherapy, it may be an appropriate place for brief, supportive psychotherapy. A patient in the midst of a protracted hospitalization for a complicated illness may benefit greatly from acknowledgment of his or her suffering; support in bearing it; bolstering of adaptive coping mechanisms; and opportunities for ventilation and catharsis. Even when family, friends, and other supportive associates are plentiful, the psychiatrist may be the only resource available to the patient for such emotional release and relief. For some patients, it can be appropriate to offer limited interpretations of their illness experiences against the backdrop of their biographical themes and events. Viederman's "life narrative" is one such technique that sees certain aspects of the hospitalized patient's vulnerability (e.g., regression and self-examination) as opportunities for empathic intervention.

Q5 The answer is: (B) False.
The taboo against psychiatrists touching their patients, although arguably categorically obsolete, certainly has no place in consultation psychiatry. The consulting psychiatrist should be able to perform a competent neurologic examination, and at least a serviceable and targeted physical examination. There are several reasons for this. First, many psychiatric presentations, including many well described neuropsychiatric ones, are associated with non-idiopathic causes. Second, psychiatric patients are at greater risk for somatic illnesses, yet often get medical short shrift, particularly when they have atypical complaints. The consulting psychiatrist may need to advocate for such patients and will lack both information and credibility if concerns are not backed up by action.

Chapter 55

Life-Threatening Conditions in Psychiatry: Catatonia, Neuroleptic Malignant Syndrome, and Serotonin Syndrome

Multiple-Choice Questions

Select the appropriate answer.

Q1 Which of the following is generally considered to have first named and defined the syndrome of catatonia?

A. *Alois Alzheimer*

B. *Eugen Bleuler*

C. *Karl Kahlbaum*

D. *Emil Kraepelin*

E. *Richard Sternbach*

Q2 Which of the following is NOT a characteristic feature of catatonia?

A. *Excessive motor activity*

B. *Extreme mutism or negativism*

C. *Immobility*

D. *Myoclonic jerking*

E. *Peculiarities of movement*

Q3 Which of the following features is LEAST commonly associated with neuroleptic malignant syndrome?

A. *Autonomic dysfunction*

B. *Creatine phosphokinase elevation*

C. *Fever*

D. *Leukopenia*

E. *Rigidity*

Q4　Which of the following interventions is MOST likely to lead to rapid improvement of catatonia?

A. *Empathic interviewing*

B. *Intravenous diphenhydramine*

C. *Intravenous lorazepam*

D. *Oral fluoxetine*

E. *Intravenous physostigmine*

Q5　Which of the following class of agents when combined with a selective serotonin reuptake inhibitor is MOST likely to result in a serotonin syndrome?

A. *A benzodiazepine*

B. *A monoamine oxidase inhibitor (MAOI)*

C. *An anticholinergic*

D. *An antipsychotic*

E. *A tricyclic antidepressant*

Q1 The answer is: (C) Karl Kahlbaum.
Catatonia was first named and defined in 1847 by Karl Kahlbaum, who published a monograph that described 21 patients with a severe psychiatric disorder. This was among the first studies in the area of mental illness to use the symptom-based approach of Sydenham to diagnose disorders without a known etiopathogenesis.

Kahlbaum believed that patients with catatonia passed through several phases of illness: a short stage of immobility (with waxy flexibility and posturing), a second stage of stupor or melancholy, a third stage of mania (with pressured speech, hyperactivity, and hyperthymic behavior), and finally, after repeated cycles of stupor and excitement, a stage of dementia.

Kraepelin, who was influenced by Kahlbaum, included catatonia in the group of deteriorating psychotic disorders named "dementia praecox." Bleuler adopted Kraepelin's view that catatonia was subsumed under severe idiopathic deteriorating psychoses, which he renamed "the schizophrenias."

Alois Alzheimer identified the plaques and tangles of what became known as Alzheimer dementia.

Richard Sternbach has been a prominent investigator of serotonin syndrome.

Q2 The answer is: (D) Myoclonic jerking.
Catatonia, whether a consequence of medical illness, major depression, mania, a mixed affective disorder, or schizophrenia, is diagnosed when the clinical picture includes at least two of the following five features: immobility (as evidenced by catalepsy [including waxy flexibility] or stupor); excessive motor activity (that is apparently purposeless and not influenced by external stimuli); extreme mutism or negativism (that is characterized by an apparently motiveless resistance to all instructions or by the maintenance of a rigid posture against attempts to be moved); peculiarities of voluntary movement (such as the voluntary assumption of an inappropriate or bizarre posture, stereotyped movement, prominent mannerism, or grimace); or echolalia (or echopraxia). Fever and creatine phosphokinase elevation may also be present, but myoclonic jerking is not characteristic of the syndrome.

Q3 The answer is: (D) Leukopenia.
A variety of clinical features have been associated with neuroleptic malignant syndrome; these include altered mental status, autonomic dysfunction, creatine phosphokinase elevation, fever, leucocytosis, and rigidity. Leukopenia is not a feature of neuroleptic malignant syndrome.

Q4 The answer is: (C) Intravenous lorazepam.
Intravenous lorazepam has been found to be effective in catatonia secondary to medical illness, and it has become a first-line treatment for catatonia, regardless of etiology.

Catatonia has also responded to use of electroconvulsive therapy, dopaminergic agents (e.g., bromocriptine and amantadine), and muscle relaxants (e.g., dantrolene), as well as calcium-channel blockers, carbamazepine, anticholinergics, lithium, thyroid medications, stimulants, and corticosteroids (in anecdotal reports).

Q5 The answer is: (B) A monoamine oxidase inhibitor (MAOI).
The most common drug interactions associated with serotonin syndrome include monoamine oxidase inhibitor (MAOI)–selective serotonin reuptake inhibitor, MAOI–tricyclic antidepressant, and MAOI–venlafaxine combinations. In general, when a selective serotonin reuptake inhibitor is used in combination with an MAOI, a serotonin syndrome is more likely to occur.

Psycho-Oncology: Psychiatric Comorbidities and Complications of Cancer and Cancer Treatments

Multiple-Choice Questions

Select the appropriate answer.

Q1 True or False. Panic disorder and other anxiety disorders occur among cancer patients at about the same rate as they do in the general population.

   A. *True*

   B. *False*

Q2 Which of the following agents is MOST likely to reduce conditioned vomiting?

   A. *Dexamethasone*

   B. *Doxepin*

   C. *Doxorubicin*

   D. *Fluoxetine*

   E. *Phenytoin*

Q3 Which of the following is the MOST commonly reported symptom in people with cancer?

   A. *Anxiety*

   B. *Depression*

   C. *Fatigue*

   D. *Nausea*

   E. *Pain*

Q4 Which of the following is MOST closely associated with the syndrome of inappropriate antidiuretic hormone secretion?

   A. *Hypercalcemia*

   B. *Hypernatremia*

   C. *Hypocalcemia*

   D. *Hypoglycemia*

   E. *Hyponatremia*

Q5   Which of the following is a hormonal agent for the treatment of cancer?

A.   *Interferon-alpha*

B.   *Interleukin-2*

C.   *Procarbazine*

D.   *Tamoxifen*

E.   *Vincristine*

Chapter 56
Answers

Q1 The answer is: (A) True.
Panic disorder and other anxiety disorders occur among cancer patients at about the same rate as they do in the general population. However, specific cancer-related symptoms (such as embarrassment related to unexpected diarrhea) can contribute to anticipatory anxiety and agoraphobia.

Q2 The answer is: (A) Dexamethasone.
Many chemotherapy agents and radiation treatments cause nausea and vomiting. Even in this era of advanced antiemetics, highly and moderately emetogenic chemotherapy is associated with nausea in 60% and vomiting in 36% of patients. Nausea significantly compromises quality of life even more than does vomiting. As a result of vomiting during chemotherapy, patients can develop conditioned nausea and anxiety associated with the smells and sights linked with treatment and develop nausea and vomiting even before arriving at the hospital for treatment. Conditioned nausea morphs into anticipatory anxiety, insomnia, and aversion to treatment. Hypnosis, cognitive-behavioral techniques, and antianxiety agents (e.g., alprazolam or lorazepam) can reduce phobic responses and anticipatory nausea and vomiting (both during and after chemotherapy).

The best antiemetic drugs make conditioned vomiting less likely, but patients still vomit after doxorubicin, cisplatin, or carboplatin (even when a 5-hydroxytryptamine-3 receptor antagonist and dexamethasone are employed). Some patients who develop anticipatory anxiety avoid the hospital and its routine smells long after cancer treatment has ended. Anticipatory nausea and vomiting are more likely to occur in younger patients, in those who have had more emetic treatments, and in those who have trait anxiety.

Q3 The answer is: (C) Fatigue.
Fatigue is the most commonly reported symptom in people with cancer, and the symptom that causes the most functional impairment in people with cancer; it can often be confused with major depressive disorder.

The prevalence (estimated at 60% to 90%) of fatigue in people affected by cancer varies widely because of differing measures of fatigue and heterogeneous populations studied.

Q4 The answer is: (E) Hyponatremia.
Hyponatremia is a common in-hospital metabolic abnormality that often results from the syndrome of inappropriate antidiuretic hormone secretion that occurs as a result of paraneoplastic syndrome (especially from small cell carcinoma, but also from non–small cell lung cancer, mesothelioma, pancreatic cancer, duodenal cancer, lymphoma, endometrial cancer, and leukemia). The syndrome of inappropriate antidiuretic hormone secretion is associated with lung infections, cerebral tumors, brain injury, and complications of many psychotropic medications (e.g., phenothiazines, selective serotonin reuptake inhibitors, carbamazepine, and tricyclic antidepressants). If the sodium level is less than 125 mmol/L or if it falls rapidly, it may cause agitation, confusion, and hallucinations; chronic hyponatremia is associated with falls and with inattention in the elderly.

Q5 The answer is: (D) Tamoxifen.
Anti-estrogen hormonal treatments for cancer include tamoxifen, toremifene, anastrazole, letrozole, vorozole, exemestane, raloxifene, and goserelin. Androgen blockers include leuprolide, flutamide, bicalutamide, and nilutamide.

Biologicals include interferon-alpha, interferon-beta, and interleukin-2.

Chemotherapy agents include vincristine, vinblastine, vinorelbine, procarbazine, asparaginase, cytarabine, fludarabine, 5-fluorouracil, capecitabine, methotrexate, pemetrexed, gemcitabine, etoposide, carmustine (brand name BCNU), thiotepa, ifosfamide, cisplatin, carboplatin, oxaliplatin, paclitaxel, and docetaxel.

Psychiatric Aspects of HIV Infection and AIDS

Multiple-Choice Questions

Select the appropriate answer.

Q1 With regard to the worldwide pandemic of HIV infection, what is the epicenter of the pandemic?

A. *Africa, especially the sub-Saharan region*

B. *Asia, especially Southeast Asia*

C. *Europe, especially Scandinavia*

D. *North America, especially the New York metropolitan area*

E. *South America*

Q2 Which of the following groups in the United States accounts for the HIGHEST proportion of new cases of HIV infection?

A. *African Americans*

B. *Hemophiliacs*

C. *Injection drug users*

D. *Men who have sex with men*

E. *Women, mostly through heterosexual contact*

Q3 What type of virus causes infection with HIV?

A. *Cytomegalovirus*

B. *Enterovirus*

C. *Influenza*

D. *Papillomavirus*

E. *Retrovirus*

Q4 Which of the following is the MOST common response during the first weeks after HIV infection?

A. *CD4+ T-lymphocyte count decreases*

B. *CD4+ T-lymphocyte count increases*

C. *Kaposi sarcoma develops*

D. *Opportunistic infections (OIs) arise*

E. *Viral load in the blood decreases*

Q5   According to the Centers for Disease Control and Prevention, what is the CD4 count that defines AIDS (unless there is an AIDS-defining condition)?

A. *200*

B. *400*

C. *600*

D. *800*

E. *1000*

Q6   Which of the following conditions is NOT an AIDS-defining condition?

A. *Candidiasis*

B. *Kaposi sarcoma*

C. *Pneumocystis carinii pneumonia*

D. *Trichinosis*

E. *Toxoplasmosis (cerebral)*

Q7   Which of the following is NOT a commonly used term associated with the cognitive impairment associated with HIV infection?

A. *AIDS dementia complex*

B. *HIV-associated dementia*

C. *HIV-associated dementia complex (HADC)*

D. *HIV-related encephalopathy*

E. *Viral-associated cortical impairment*

Q8   Which of the following is the MOST common neurologic complication of HIV infection?

A. *Cerebellar dysfunction*

B. *Distal sensory polyneuropathy (DSP)*

C. *Ischemic cerebrovascular disease*

D. *Spinal stenosis*

E. *Syncope*

Chapter 57

Answers

Q1 The answer is: (A) Africa, especially the sub-Saharan region.
At the end of 2005, nearly 40 million people worldwide were living with HIV infection. Although the prevalence rate of infection has plateaued, the absolute number of people with HIV continues to rise. Africa, especially the sub-Saharan region, remains the epicenter of the pandemic, followed by the Caribbean.

Q2 The answer is: (D) Men who have sex with men.
In the United States, at the end of 2005, more than 1 million people were living with HIV infection. Approximately 40,000 new infections occur yearly. Of these, in 2004, the largest proportion occurred in men who have sex with men; 27% occurred in women, mostly through heterosexual contact; and half occurred among African Americans. New cases of and deaths due to AIDS declined sharply in 1996, owing largely to highly active antiretroviral therapy (HAART). The sharpest declines were in the men who have sex with men and injection-drug-using populations. Between 2000 and 2004, however, while AIDS deaths decreased by 8%, new AIDS cases increased by the same amount.

Q3 The answer is: (E) Retrovirus.
HIV is a retrovirus—a virus containing ribonucleic acid and the enzyme, reverse transcriptase, for replication—that affects the immune system and the central nervous system (CNS), gaining entry to cells (e.g., T-lymphocytes, monocytes, and macrophages) that express the CD4 receptor on their membranes. All of the currently available antiretroviral medications target the three key steps and enzymes in this process: fusion of the virus with the host cell membrane; reverse transcriptase; and protease.

Q4 The answer is: (A) CD4+ T-lymphocyte count decreases.
During the first weeks after infection, the population of CD4+ T-lymphocytes (i.e., the CD4 count) decreases as the amount of virus in the blood (i.e., the viral load) increases. Following a weak and short-lived rebound, the CD4 count steadily declines. At the same time, the viral load oscillates around a "set-point" until ultimately viral replication intensifies and peripheral viremia surges. Administration of HAART, when effective, halts this process. Opportunistic infections (OIs), neoplasms, and neuropsychiatric conditions occur with increasing frequency as the immune deficiency worsens; prophylaxis for certain OIs (e.g., *Pneumocystis carinii* pneumonia and toxoplasmosis) is instituted during infection according to the CD4 count.

Q5 The answer is: (A) 200.
According to the Centers for Disease Control and Prevention, AIDS is defined by a CD4 count less than 200 cells/μL (or less than 14% of total lymphocytes) or the presence of an AIDS-defining condition. This 1993 revised classification established nine possible categories of illness. The introduction of HAART has diminished the clinical use of this taxonomy.

Q6 The answer is: (D) Trichinosis.
Trichinosis, the disease that results from ingestion of raw or inadequately cooked meat (especially pork), is not an AIDS-defining condition.

However, the following are AIDS-defining conditions: candidiasis; cervical cancer, invasive; coccidioidomycosis; cryptococcosis; cryptosporidiosis; cytomegalovirus disease or retinitis; encephalopathy, HIV-related; herpes simplex virus infection; histoplasmosis; isosporiasis; Kaposi sarcoma; lymphoma (Burkitt, immunoblastic, or primary CNS); mycobacterial infection (*Mycobacterium avium complex*, *M. kansasii*, *M. tuberculosis*, or other species); *Pneumocystis carinii* pneumonia; pneumonia, recurrent; progressive multifocal leukoencephalopathy; *Salmonella* septicemia, recurrent; toxoplasmosis, cerebral; and wasting syndrome, HIV-related.

Q7 The answer is: (E) Viral-associated cortical impairment.
Cognitive complaints and problems are common in HIV-infected patients, with the brain being invaded by HIV shortly after infection. Before HAART, most patients developed cognitive problems, including a

late-stage subcortical dementia termed HIV-associated dementia complex (HADC) by the American Academy of Neurology AIDS Task Force (other terms include AIDS dementia complex, HIV-associated dementia, and—the Centers for Disease Control and Prevention term—HIV-related encephalopathy). Although the incidence of HADC has declined since the introduction of HAART, its prevalence is likely to increase over the coming years as patients survive longer. A less severe variant of HADC that is otherwise clinically similar has been termed minor cognitive/motor disorder. Some patients have irreversible deficits (accrued in the absence of HAART during times of prolonged and high viremia and poor immune function), whereas newly diagnosed patients might recover substantially if treated with HAART, even if they have HADC. Some cohorts might have other pathophysiological processes adding insult to injury. For example, the hepatitis C virus has been shown to be neurotropic, and past or current significant drug use can further impair brain function.

As a subcortical dementia, HADC is characterized by disturbances of mood, memory, and motor function. Impairments in attention, new learning, processing speed, and executive functions cause significant disability. Depression and anxiety are often present in HADC and can eclipse the cognitive problems. Motor and cognitive slowness can be pronounced. Behavioral problems ranging from apathy to hypomania and disinhibition can greatly complicate management, particularly if judgment is impaired.

Any HIV-infected patient should be carefully assessed for cognitive problems, particularly if there were periods of high viremia and low CD4 counts in the past. It is useful to screen for cognitive problems with the HIV Dementia Scale or its modified form, supplemented by other bedside tests (e.g., Luria hand maneuvers and verbal forms of the Trail Making Tests A and B). The Folstein Mini-Mental State Examination is not sensitive for subcortical dementias, particularly if mild, and includes no timed tasks, so it is relatively poor at detecting the psychomotor slowing that is the hallmark of HADC. Comprehensive neuropsychological testing should be ordered in unclear diagnostic situations, for longitudinal assessments, and to delineate further the nature and severity of detected or suspected deficits.

Recognition of cognitive impairment is important because patients with executive dysfunction and poor memory, left to their own devices, may be unable to participate in their HIV treatment and to adhere optimally to HAART, thus setting up a vicious cycle of exacerbated brain dysfunction. Any treatment recommendations must take these limitations into account, and enough support provided to compensate for those deficits.

Q8 The answer is: (B) Distal sensory polyneuropathy (DSP).

One peripheral neurologic complication—distal sensory polyneuropathy (DSP)—deserves special mention, as it has emerged as a significant long-term problem. The most common neurologic complication of HIV disease, it affects about one-third of all HIV-infected patients. The etiology of DSP is often a mixture of macrophage-driven nerve damage and mitochondrial dysfunction caused by nerve-toxic nucleoside reverse transcriptase inhibitors (the dideoxynucleosides or "d drugs": ddI, d4T, and ddC), resulting in an axonal neuropathy. Many patients bear the burden of additional toxins (e.g., alcoholism, OI prophylaxis, or past treatment with vincristine for HIV-related cancers). A lower CD4 count is one recognized risk factor; others include older age, lower hemoglobin, and higher viral set point. Thus DSP encompasses two phenotypically identical neuropathies: HIV-associated DSP and antiretroviral toxic neuropathy.

As the most common neurologic condition, DSP is important for psychiatrists for two reasons: (1) many long-term patients suffer from it, resulting in a chronic pain syndrome that can be excruciating, leading to depressive overlay, disability, and reduced quality of life; and (2) CNS-active medications are often required to treat the pain, adding iatrogenic morbidity (e.g., fatigue).

DSP is a pure sensory neuropathy with symptoms typical of sensory neuropathies (i.e., tingling, analgesic pain, and burning on the soles of the feet). In addition, ankle reflexes are often absent.

The diagnosis can be suspected on clinical grounds in the right setting and with typical symptoms. Nerve conduction studies demonstrate an axonal neuropathy. In unclear situations, particularly when severe symptoms are not supported by signs, an outpatient biopsy can clarify the situation. In patients with DSP, the intraepidermal nerve fiber density is reduced.

Treatment involves removal of toxic agents; if the offending agents can be discontinued, the neuropathy might resolve. Considering that most HAART medications do not cause neuropathy, regimens that do not contain the "d drugs" can usually be found. Treatment of confounding conditions (e.g., alcoholism and diabetes) must be optimized. In many cases, symptomatic treatment will be necessary. Treatments include pain medications, antiepileptic drugs, and tricyclic antidepressants. Carbamazepine is difficult to use in this population because of a higher rate of rashes and leukopenia.

Chapter 58

Organ Transplantation: Pretransplant Assessment and Posttransplant Management

Multiple-Choice Questions

Select the appropriate answer.

Q1 True or False. Solid organ transplantation is an accepted, successful, and commonly employed treatment option for patients with end-organ failure.

- A. *True*
- B. *False*

Q2 True or False. In recent years, transplant centers have attempted to expand the donor pool by harvesting organs from persons who have been declared dead secondary to cardiac arrest (i.e., non–heart-beating donors) in addition to harvesting organs from persons who have been declared dead by neurologic criteria (i.e., brain death).

- A. *True*
- B. *False*

Q3 Which of the following organizations in the United States regulates the allocation and distribution of donor organs?

- A. *AMA*
- B. *APA*
- C. *NIH*
- D. *NIMH*
- E. *UNOS*

Q4 True or False. There are universally accepted guidelines for the psychiatric evaluation of potential candidates for organ transplantation.

- A. *True*
- B. *False*

Q5 True or False. Most young patients require transplantation due to congenital disorders, and are not held responsible for their disease.

- A. *True*
- B. *False*

Chapter 58
Answers

Q1 The answer is: (A) True.

Solid organ transplantation is an accepted, successful, and commonly employed treatment option for patients with end-organ failure. The introduction of cyclosporine in 1980 marked the beginning of successful immunosuppression; this drug allowed for the prevention of graft rejection, thereby dramatically improving recipient survival. Transplant patients (e.g., those who have received a heart, kidney, liver, pancreas, lung, or small intestine) now live longer with an overall improved quality of life.

However, several factors have limited the success of organ transplantation. First is the ever-present potential for allograft rejection. Unfortunately, the side effects of immunosuppressive medications that are used to manage rejection can be debilitating, disfiguring, or life-threatening. Finally, immunocompromised hosts are vulnerable to infection by bacteria, viruses, or fungi not considered pathogenic in the normal population.

Q2 The answer is: (A) True.

Unfortunately, the scarcity of cadaveric organs creates a mismatch between the number of patients who need transplantation and the number who can undergo transplantation. Currently, there are over 93,000 persons on the waiting list for a solid organ transplantation, but there were only 17,000 transplants done between January and July 2006. Some European countries follow the doctrine of "presumed consent" for postmortem donation, but the United States does not.

In recent years, transplant centers have attempted to expand the donor pool by harvesting organs from persons who have been declared dead secondary to cardiac arrest (i.e., non–heart-beating donors) in addition to harvesting organs from persons who have been declared dead by neurologic criteria (i.e., brain death). In response to this problem, the Institute of Medicine created a committee to study ways in which the supply of transplantable organs can be increased. The committee's report, released in May 2006, recommended the following: vigorous public education about organ donation; provision of more opportunities for registration as an organ donor; easier access to state donor registries; and renewed attention to improvement of organ procurement systems.

Q3 The answer is: (E) UNOS.

In the United States, the United Network for Organ Sharing (UNOS), a non-profit organization, endowed by Congress but reporting to the Department of Health and Human Services, regulates the allocation and distribution of donor organs. UNOS has two branches: the Organ Procurement and Transplant Network and the Scientific Registry. The Organ Procurement and Transplant Network divides the country into 11 distinct geographic regions, and each region has its own waiting list. The length of time spent on the waiting list can differ among regions. Determination of priority is organ-specific.

Q4 The answer is: (B) False.

There are no universally accepted guidelines for the psychiatric evaluation of potential candidates for organ transplantation, and there are few reliable or predictive data regarding "suitability for transplantation." Some centers routinely offer a face-to-face clinical interview with a mental health provider, whereas other centers require formal psychological testing or rely on a structured or a semistructured interview. Transplant centers differ in their determination of who is an "acceptable" candidate, and what degree of risk the candidate is willing to assume.

Common psychosocial and behavioral exclusion criteria include active substance abuse, active psychotic symptoms, suicidal ideation (with intent or plan), dementia, or a felony conviction. Relative contraindications include poor social supports with inability to arrange for pretransplant or posttransplant care, personality disorders that interfere with a working relationship with a transplant team, non-adherence to a medication regimen, and neurocognitive limitations.

Q5 The answer is: (A) True.

Pediatric transplant patients differ from adult transplant patients in a number of ways. Among these differences are the following: a parent or an appointed legal guardian makes the medicolegal decisions; the children (infants, toddlers, and school-age children) are not responsible for the decision to proceed with transplant or for pretransplant and posttransplant care; and most young patients require transplant due to congenital disorders (such as biliary atresia, cardiac malformations, or pulmonary atresia), and are not held responsible for their disease.

Chapter 59

Approaches to Collaborative Care and Primary Care Psychiatry

Multiple-Choice Questions

Select the appropriate answer.

Q1   Which of the following is NOT a major goal of collaborative care?

A.   *To improve access to care*

B.   *To improve communication*

C.   *To improve outcomes*

D.   *To improve reimbursement*

E.   *To improve treatment*

Q2   Which of the following statements is LEAST accurate?

A.   *Managed care organizations often carve out "behavioral health care" to managed behavioral health organizations that may have limited referral networks not inclusive of the primary care physician's (PCP's) psychiatric colleagues*

B.   *Outcomes are no better for seriously depressed primary care patients treated collaboratively by their PCP and a psychiatrist*

C.   *Primary care patients frequently seek treatment for somatic complaints, rather than psychiatric symptoms*

D.   *Some PCPs fear that their patients will leave their practice if asked about mental health issues*

E.   *The psychiatrically disordered population experiences increased physical health care use, work absenteeism, unemployment, subjective disability, and mortality*

Q3   Which of the following is MOST closely associated with service that maintains separate records, requires the patient to be seen in the psychiatric clinic, and develops some means of ongoing, clinically relevant communication with the primary care provider?

A.   *Collaborative management*

B.   *Psychiatric consultation service*

C.   *Psychiatric teleconsultation service*

D.   *Specialty psychiatric clinic*

E.   *Three-Component Model*

Chapter 59

Answers

Q1 The answer is: (D) To improve reimbursement.
Now that clinically proven and effective treatments exist, access and quality of care remain significant issues, best addressed through the collaboration of psychiatry and primary care. The four major goals of collaboration are to improve access, treatment, outcomes, and communication; enhanced reimbursement is not a goal of collaborative care.

Q2 The answer is: (B) Outcomes are no better for seriously depressed primary care patients treated collaboratively by their PCP and a psychiatrist.
Several studies have demonstrated better outcomes for seriously depressed primary care patients treated collaboratively by their primary care physician (PCP) and a psychiatrist. Cost offset, however, is difficult to demonstrate because of the hidden costs of psychiatric disability. Nonetheless, there is some evidence for a decrease in total health care spending when mental health problems are adequately addressed. Even if this were not so, the case for cost-effectiveness could be made. That is, care for the patient's psychiatric problem is more cost-effective than spending the same amount of money addressing the often non-responsive, somatic complaints of high-maintenance, high-cost medical patients.

Q3 The answer is: (D) Specialty psychiatric clinic.
Specialty psychiatric clinics often maintain separate records, require the patient to be seen in the psychiatric clinic, and develop some means of ongoing, clinically relevant communication with the primary care provider.

In collaborative management, the patient alternates visits between the psychiatrist and the PCP in the primary care setting during initiation of treatment (i.e., the first 4 to 6 weeks). The PCP then assumes responsibility for the patient's continued psychopharmacologic treatment. This model was developed as a research protocol for the treatment of depressed, primary care patients (and has been extended to the treatment of panic disorder and patients with persistent depressive symptoms). Patients are referred by the PCP, usually after an initial ineffective trial of medication. This intensive program of care has been cost-effective for more severely depressed primary care patients.

Consultation psychiatrists may render a one-visit opinion in the primary care clinic (sometimes patients are sent to the consultant psychiatrist's office, just as with other specialty consultations). This model is similar to the consultation model used in the inpatient medical setting. The consultation should be written or transcribed into the primary care record. Immediate verbal communication, in person whenever possible, or by telephone, e-mail, or voice mail, greatly enhances the use of such consultations. The consultant generally does not initiate treatment but makes practical recommendations.

Psychiatric teleconsultation is a service with experienced consultation psychiatrists available for immediate telephone consultation to PCPs. This service, which is not accessible to patients, can provide general psychiatric information, consultation about pharmacologic or behavioral management, or triage and referral functions. Computer technology is used to maintain a database, promote timely referrals, and generate follow-up letters to PCPs.

The Three-Component Model, supported by the MacArthur Initiative on Depression in Primary Care, is a formalized system of consultative care that promotes the primary care treatment of depression as a chronic disease, with regular measures of adherence and outcome to guide the evidence-based protocol of medication and other treatment adjustments. Educational modules exist for PCPs, consultant psychiatrists, telephone-based care managers, and patients. The Patient Health Questionnaire-9, a 10-item, 1-page, self-administered tool that quantifies the patient's neurovegetative symptoms of depression, is repeatedly used to track the patient's progress. Multiple measures of symptoms and treatment adherence are recorded on a standard form that facilitates consultation, communication, and organized treatment review, planning, and adjustment.

Chapter 60

Psychiatric and Ethical Aspects of Care at the End of Life

Multiple-Choice Questions

Select the appropriate answer.

Q1 Which of the following was a Florida woman in a minimally conscious state who died in 2005 after a protracted legal battle between her husband and her parents about whether her feeding tube should be removed?

A. *Linda Ganzini*

B. *Jimmie Holland*

C. *Karen Ann Quinlan*

D. *Elisabeth Kübler-Ross*

E. *Theresa Schiavo*

Q2 Which of the following is the BEST approximation of the meaning of the term *primum non nocere* (which is a basic tenet of medical care)?

A. *Don't get too involved*

B. *First, do no harm*

C. *Primary care is fundamental*

D. *Relieve suffering*

E. *Think before you speak*

Q3 Which of the following stages, according to Kübler-Ross, is the FIRST stage of a transformational process in a patient who is dying?

A. *Acceptance*

B. *Anger*

C. *Bargaining*

D. *Denial*

E. *Depression*

Q4 True or False. Severely depressed patients make MORE restricted advance directives when they are depressed.

A. *True*

B. *False*

Q5 True or False. Competent patients with a reversible illness have the right to refuse any treatment, including lifesaving treatments.

A. *True*

B. *False*

Q6   True or False. Under the Oregon Death with Dignity Act, euthanasia is legal.

    A.   *True*

    B.   *False*

Answers

Q1 The answer is: (E) Theresa Schiavo.

Recent attention regarding end-of-life issues has focused on physician-assisted suicide, and on legal cases that surround withdrawal of life-sustaining treatments (such as the case of Theresa Schiavo, a Florida woman in a minimally conscious state who died in 2005 after a protracted legal battle between her husband and her parents about whether her feeding tube should be removed).

Linda Ganzini, Jimmie Holland, and Elisabeth Kübler-Ross are health care providers who have contributed to our understanding of end-of-life care and medical ethics.

Karen Ann Quinlan was a 21-year-old woman who in 1976 fell into an irreversible coma while at a party. Her case became a legal battle between the right of Quinlan's mother (who as her guardian wished to withdraw life-sustaining treatment from her daughter and allow her daughter to die with dignity) and the state's interest in preserving life. In the end, the Supreme Court of New Jersey decided that (if it was believed to a reasonable degree that the coma was irreversible) life-sustaining treatment (e.g., with a respirator) could be removed. Now, more than 30 years later, the standard medical recommendation in the case of irreversible coma is to stop all treatment, including nutrition and hydration. This judgment is made on the principle of the inevitability of death, and the futility of any treatments to prevent this.

Q2 The answer is: (B) First, do no harm.

End-of-life care may create tension between two essential medical principles: first, do no harm (*primum non nocere*) and to relieve suffering. Caring for patients at the end of life is further complicated when the medically ill also suffer from psychiatric comorbidities (such as major depression and anxiety), which can greatly increase suffering. One should remember that end-of-life decisions occur in a dynamic societal and legal context.

Q3 The answer is: (D) Denial.

According to Kübler-Ross, patients who are dying go through a transformational process (which include stages of denial, anger, bargaining, guilt/depression, and eventual acceptance). These stages may occur in a unique order, may occur simultaneously, and may last variable amounts of time. Psychiatrists and other physicians may assist the dying patient in the transition through these often difficult stages toward the end of acceptance.

Q4 The answer is: (A) True.

Ganzini documented that severely depressed patients made more restricted advance directives when depressed, and they changed them after their depression remitted. At Memorial Sloan Kettering Cancer Center, Breitbart and Holland compared terminally ill patients with cancer and AIDS and with suicidal ideation to similar patients without suicidal ideation. The primary difference was the presence of depression in the patients with suicidal thoughts. Thus aggressive treatment of depression is a cornerstone of care, as it dramatically decreases suffering and improves quality of life.

Q5 The answer is: (A) True.

Competent patients with a reversible illness have the right to refuse any treatment, including lifesaving treatments.

However, challenges emerge when a patient is not able to make or to voice a decision regarding his or her wishes. In these situations, the state has a recognized legal interest in preserving life, and it may be difficult to ascertain whether the patient had a countervailing autonomy interest.

Q6 The answer is: (B) False.

Active killing of a patient, even when requested by the patient, is euthanasia. Euthanasia is illegal in all 50 states and all US districts and territories. Unlike euthanasia, physician-assisted suicide has become legal in the state of Oregon and has survived numerous legal challenges in the US Supreme Court. Physician-assisted suicide allows physicians to help patients acquire the means to end their lives but does not permit the physician to actually administer those means.

Under the Oregon Death with Dignity Act, physicians in Oregon are permitted to write prescriptions for lethal doses of medications for patients who request to die and meet the other requirements of the state law. From 1998 to 2004, there were 208 deaths by ingestion in Oregon (with 325 prescriptions written). Although Oregon has legalized the practice, organized medicine (and psychiatry) opposes the practice. The debate over physician-assisted suicide will no doubt continue as other states consider passing laws that authorize physician-assisted suicide.

SECTION 13

PSYCHIATRIC EPIDEMIOLOGY AND STATISTICS

Psychiatric Epidemiology
Multiple-Choice Questions

Select the appropriate answer.

Q1 Which of the following terms BEST defines the number of new events that develop in a population over a specified period of time?

    A. *Cumulative incidence (CI)*

    B. *Incidence*

    C. *Incidence density*

    D. *Point prevalence*

    E. *Prevalence*

Q2 Which of the following is the number of events (outcomes) in proportion to the population at risk for the event?

    A. *Cumulative incidence (CI)*

    B. *Incidence*

    C. *Incidence density*

    D. *Point prevalence*

    E. *Prevalence*

Q3 Which of the following is the proportion of individuals who have a particular disease or outcome at a point in time?

    A. *Cumulative incidence (CI)*

    B. *Incidence*

    C. *Incidence density*

    D. *Lifetime prevalence*

    E. *Point prevalence*

Q4 Which of the following is the degree to which an assessment instrument produces consistent or reproducible results when used by different examiners at different times?

    A. *Reliability*

    B. *Sensitivity*

    C. *Specificity*

    D. *Statistical significance*

    E. *Validity*

Q5 Which of the following expresses the degree to which the results of a measurement instrument actually measures what it purports to measure?

    A. *Reliability*

    B. *Sensitivity*

C. *Specificity*

D. *Statistical significance*

E. *Validity*

Q6   Which of the following is the extent to which the measurement can predict or agree with constructs external to the construct being measured?

A. *Construct validity*

B. *Criterion validity*

C. *Reliability*

D. *Sensitivity*

E. *Statistical significance*

Q7   Which of the following refers to the extent to which the measure assesses the underlying theoretical construct that it intends to measure?

A. *Construct validity*

B. *Criterion validity*

C. *Reliability*

D. *Sensitivity*

E. *Statistical significance*

Q8   Which of the following is the proportion of true cases (known as true-positive cases), as identified by the criterion instrument?

A. *Reliability*

B. *Sensitivity*

C. *Specificity*

D. *Statistical significance*

E. *Validity*

Q9   Which of the following study designs is the WEAKEST of all study designs?

A. *Case-controlled studies*

B. *Cohort studies*

C. *Cross-sectional studies*

D. *Descriptive studies*

E. *Randomized controlled trials*

Q10 Which of the following study designs is the gold standard of all study designs?

A. *Case-controlled studies*

B. *Cohort studies*

C. *Cross-sectional studies*

D. *Descriptive studies*

E. *Randomized controlled trials*

Chapter 61

Answers

Q1 The answer is: (B) Incidence.

Incidence refers to the number of new events that develop in a population over a specified period of time $(t_0$ to $t_1)$.

Q2 The answer is: (A) Cumulative incidence (CI).

The incidence rate is described as the number of events (outcomes) in proportion to the population at risk for the event; it is called the cumulative incidence (CI), and is calculated by the following equation:

$$CI = \frac{\text{Number of new cases, } t_0 \text{ to } t_1}{\text{Population at risk at } t_0}$$

The denominator equals the total number of persons at risk for the event at the start of the time period (t_0) without adjustment for reduction in the cohort size for any reason, for example, loss to follow-up, death, or reclassification to "case" status. Therefore, CI is best used to describe stable populations in which there is little reduction in cohort size for any reason. An example would be a study of the incidence of major depressive disorder (MDD) in a residential program. If at the beginning of the study, 8 of the 100 residents have MDD, and of the 92 remaining patients, 8 develop MDD over the next 12 months, the CI for MDD would be $(8/92 \times 100) = 8.7\%$ for this period (i.e., 1 year). Note that the denominator does not include those in the population with the condition at t_0 because they are not at risk for newly experiencing the outcome.

Q3 The answer is: (E) Point prevalence.

Prevalence is the proportion of individuals who have a particular disease or outcome at a point or period in time. In most psychiatric studies, prevalence refers to the proportion of the population that has the outcome at a particular point in time; it is called the point prevalence:

$$\text{Point prevalence} = \frac{\text{Number of existing cases at } t_0}{\text{Population at } t_0}$$

Q4 The answer is: (A) Reliability.

Reliability is the degree to which an assessment instrument produces consistent or reproducible results when used by different examiners at different times. Lack of reliability may be the result of divergence between observers, imprecision in the measurement tool, or instability in the attribute being measured. Inter-rater reliability is the extent to which different examiners obtain equivalent results in the same subject when using the same instrument; test-retest reliability is the extent to which the same instrument obtains equivalent results in the same subject on different occasions.

Reliability is not sufficient for a measurement instrument—it could, for example, consistently and reliably give results that are neither meaningful nor accurate. However, it is a necessary attribute because inconsistency would impair the accuracy of any tool. The demonstration of the reliability of an assessment tool is thus required before its use in epidemiologic studies. The use of explicit diagnostic criteria, trained examiners to interpret data uniformly, and a structured assessment that obtains the same types of information from all subjects can enhance the reliability of assessment instruments.

Q5 The answer is: (E) Validity.

Validity is a term that expresses the degree to which the results of a measurement instrument actually measures what it purports to measure. However, when translating a theoretical concept into an operational instrument that purports to assess or measure it, several aspects of validity need to be accounted for.

Q6 The answer is: (B) Criterion validity.

Criterion validity is the extent to which the measurement can predict or agree with constructs external to the construct being measured. Two types of criterion validity are generally distinguished: predictive validity and concurrent validity. Predictive validity is the extent to which the instrument's measurements can predict an external criterion. For instance, if we devise an instrument to measure math ability, we might postulate that math ability should be correlated to better grades in college math courses. A high correlation between the measure's assessment of math ability and college math course grades would indicate that the instrument can correctly predict as it theoretically should and has predictive validity. Concurrent validity refers to the extent to which the measurement correlates to another criterion at the same point in time. For example, if we devise a measure relying on visual inspection of a wound to determine infection, we can correlate it to a bacteriologic examination of a specimen taken at the same time. A high correlation would indicate concurrent validity and suggest that our new measure gives valid results for determining infection.

Q7 The answer is: (A) Construct validity.

Construct validity refers to the extent to which the measure assesses the underlying theoretical construct that it intends to measure. This concept is the most complex, and both content and criterion validity point to it. An example of a measure lacking construct validity would be a test for assessing algebra skills using word problems that inadvertently assesses reading skills rather than factual knowledge of algebra. Construct validity also refers to the extent that the construct exists as theorized and can be quantified by the instrument. In psychiatry, this is especially difficult because there are no gold standard laboratory (e.g., chemical, anatomic, or physiological) tests, and the criteria, if not the existence, of many diagnoses are disputed. To establish the validity for any diagnosis, certain requirements have been proposed, and include an adequate clinical description of the disorder that distinguishes it from other similar disorders, and the ability to correlate the diagnosis to external criteria such as laboratory tests, familial transmission patterns, and consistent outcomes (including response to treatment).

Q8 The answer is: (B) Sensitivity.

Sensitivity is the proportion of true cases, as identified by the criterion instrument, that are identified as cases by the new instrument (also known as the true-positive rate).

Specificity is the proportion of non-cases, as identified by the criterion instrument, that are identified as non-cases by the new instrument (also known as the true-negative rate).

For any given instrument, there are trade-offs between sensitivity and specificity, depending on where the threshold limits are set to distinguish "case" from "noncase." For example, for the Hamilton Depression Scale instrument, the cutoff value for the diagnosis of MDD (often set at 15) would determine whether an individual would be identified as "case" or "non-cases." If the value were instead set at 5, which most clinicians would consider "normal" or not depressed, the Hamilton Depression Scale would be an unusually sensitive instrument (e.g., using a structured clinical interview as the criterion instrument), because any person evaluated with even a modicum of depressive thinking would be considered a "case," as would anyone typically considered to have major depression. However, the test would not be especially specific because it would be poor at identifying those without depression. Conversely, if the cutoff value were set at 25, sensitivity would be low, but the specificity would be high.

Q9 The answer is: (D) Descriptive studies.

Descriptive studies are the weakest of all study designs; these studies simply describe the health status of a population or of a number of subjects. Case series are an example of descriptive studies, and are simply descriptions of cases, without a comparison group. They can be useful for monitoring unusual patients, and in generating hypotheses for future study. Case series can also be misleading, as in the early 1980s when physicians began describing male homosexuals with depressed immune systems. The use of amyl nitrate-based sexual stimulants was suspected, and studies on the effects of amyl nitrates on the immune system were underway when HIV was discovered.

Ecological studies study groups of individuals, and the overall occurrence of disease (outcome) is correlated with the aggregate level of exposure to a risk factor. The groups being studied can be differentiated by geographic region or by other criteria, such as school, workplace, or clinic. Data are usually collected at different times for different reasons, and do not include data on individuals. Ecological studies are helpful for generating hypotheses and are generally inexpensive and not time-consuming (because they are often based on data that are routinely published, such as death and disease rates, per capita income, religious affiliation, or food consumption). However, these studies are limited in showing causality because of the lack of individual data, the temporal ambiguity of the data (it is not known if a given risk factor precedes the outcome, for example), and problems with using data in an aggregate form to generalize about individuals.

Cross-sectional studies examine individuals and determine their case status and risk factor exposures at the same time. Outcome rates between those with exposure can then be compared with those without. Data are collected by surveys, laboratory tests, physical measurements, or other procedures, and there is no follow-up or other longitudinal component. Cross-sectional studies are also called prevalence studies (more precisely, they are point prevalence studies) and, as with ecological studies, are relatively inexpensive and are useful for informing future research. They also aid in public health planning (e.g., determining the number of hospital beds needed) and generating more specific hypotheses around disease etiology by looking at specific risk factors.

In case-control studies, subjects are selected based on whether they have the outcome (case) or not (control), and their exposures are then determined by looking backward in time. For this reason, they are also called retrospective studies because they rely on historical records or recall. This type of study design is appropriate for rare diseases or for those with long latencies, and they can also be used to study possible risk factors. Problems with case-control studies include recall bias (which occurs if cases and controls recall past exposures differently) and difficulty in selecting controls. Ideally, one wants controls who are exactly matched to the cases in all other exposures except for the risk factor in question. Thus controls should be matched for a variety of factors, for example, sex, socioeconomic status, smoking status (unless that is what is being studied), and alcohol use. For case-control studies, an odds ratio is used to determine whether the outcome is more likely in those with the exposure or in those without one, and it approximates their relative incidence rates.

In cohort studies, a group of healthy individuals are identified and followed over time to see who develops the outcomes (diseases) of interest and who does not. Exposure to risk factors are assessed over time, and so the sequence between exposure and outcome can be determined, as well as the relationship between different exposures and outcomes. Because neither the subjects nor the researchers know whether and who will develop which outcomes, bias in measuring exposure is avoided. Disadvantages include high cost (both in terms of manpower and time), potential for loss to follow-up, and inefficiency in studying rare diseases. In cohort studies, the association between outcome and exposure is expressed as relative risk, the ratio between the incidence rates in those with the risk factor and those without.

Q10 The answer is: (E) Randomized controlled trials.

A randomized controlled trial is a type of cohort study in which the exposure is controlled by the researchers. Like standard cohort studies, a population who has yet to develop the outcome(s) of interest is defined; then, unlike standard cohort studies, the subjects are randomly assigned to different exposures. In these trials, the exposure is usually a treatment, such as a medication, or an intervention, such as counseling or a behavioral program. Those randomized to non-exposure may receive a placebo, or treatment-as-usual for the community. Multiple outcomes can be studied, from cessation of psychosis, reduction of depressive or anxious symptoms, to side effects or other adverse outcomes. Randomized controlled trials, also known as experimental studies, are the gold standard of epidemiologic research.

Chapter 62

Statistics in Psychiatric Research

Multiple-Choice Questions

Select the appropriate answer.

Q1 Which of the following terms BEST describes the simple count of things (e.g., the populations of towns or the amount of grain produced by a town)?

A. *Descriptive statistics*

B. *Inferential statistics*

C. *Psychometrics*

D. *P value*

E. *Standard deviation*

Q2 True or False. You can tell that a psychiatric researcher is reporting on inferential statistics when you see *P* values and asterisks denoting statistical significance.

A. *True*

B. *False*

Q3 True or False. Without inferential statistics and their computed probability values, the researcher cannot generalize any positive findings beyond the group being studied.

A. *True*

B. *False*

Q4 Which of the following is the optimal test of significance for comparing continuous variables that are obtained through repeated measurements of the same subjects?

A. *Analysis of covariance*

B. *Analysis of variance (ANOVA)*

C. *Analysis of variance (ANOVA) with repeated measure(s)*

D. *Chi-square test*

E. *Cluster analysis*

Q5 Which of the following is used to statistically reduce the number of variables needed to explain or to describe a larger set of original variables, based on the correlation matrix?

A. *Analysis of covariance*

B. *Canonical correlation*

C. *Chi-square*

D. *Cluster analysis*

E. *Factor analysis*

Q6 Which of the following reflects the chance of a result of a statistical test being a false positive (i.e., the probability of a spurious finding)?

A. *Chi-square*

B. *Confidence interval*

C. *Correlation matrix*

D. *Dependent t test*

E. *P value*

Q7 True or False. Reliability is the degree of usefulness of a rating scale for a purpose.

A. *True*

B. *False*

Q8 True or False. Inferential statistics include the mean, median, standard deviation, variance, estimates of effect size, proportions, percentages, mean differences, and odds ratios.

A. *True*

B. *False*

Chapter 62

Answers

Q1 The answer is: (A) Descriptive statistics.

Three classes of statistics are commonly used in psychiatric research: statistics assessing the reliability and validity of diagnostic interviews or rating scales, statistics used to describe these clinical variables and demographic variables, and statistics used to make probabilistic statements about these descriptive statistics.

The word "statistics" derives from a term used for "numbers describing the *state*;" that is, the original statistics were numbers used by rulers of states to better understand their population. Thus, the first statistics were simply counting of things (such as the population of towns, or the amount of grain produced by a town). Today, we call these kinds of simple counts or averages "descriptive statistics," and these are used in almost every research study to describe the demographic and clinical characteristics of the participants in a study.

Q2 The answer is: (A) True.

Psychiatric researchers study relatively small samples of subjects, usually with the intent to generalize their findings to the larger population from which their sample was drawn. This is the realm of inferential statistics, which is based on probability theory. Researchers are reporting inferential statistics when you see the tell-tale P values and asterisks denoting statistical significance in the text and tables of the "Results" sections.

Q3 The answer is: (A) True.

All three kinds of statistics (descriptive, psychometric, and inferential) are present in most published papers in psychiatry research, and are considered in a particular order for the following reasons. First, without reliable and valid measures, neither of the other kinds of statistics will be meaningful. For example, if we rely solely on clinicians' judgments of patient improvement, but the study clinicians rarely agree on whether a patient has improved, then any additional statistics will be meaningless. Likewise, a measure can be very reliably measured, as with a patient's cell phone number, but this measure is not reliable for any of the purposes of the study. Second, descriptive statistics are needed to summarize the many individual subjects' scores into summary statistics (such as counts, proportions, averages [or means], and standard deviations) that can then be compared between groups. Inferential statistics would be impossible without first having these summary statistics. Third, without inferential statistics and their computed probability values, the researcher cannot generalize any positive findings beyond the particular group being studied (and this is, after all, the usual goal of a research study).

Q4 The answer is: (C) Analysis of variance (ANOVA) with repeated measure(s).

An "analysis of variance (ANOVA) with repeated measure(s)" is the optimal test of significance for comparing continuous variables that are obtained through repeated measurements of the same subjects (because each subject's scores are usually correlated; the regular ANOVA would give results that are "too significant"). An experimenter may select a repeated-measures design because these are generally more sensitive to treatment effects (i.e., they have high power) because score differences between subjects are ignored.

An "analysis of covariance" is a form of ANOVA that tests the significance of differences between group means by adjusting for initial differences among the groups on one or more covariates. As an example, a psychologist interested in studying the effectiveness of a behavioral weight loss program versus self-dieting includes pretreatment weights as a covariate. An ANOVA is an optimal test of significance of difference among means from independent groups. If a medical researcher wants to compare the effects of three or more different drugs on a single dependent measure, he or she would compute a one-way ANOVA. The more complex, factorial ANOVA also tests for interaction effects between multiple factors. For example, if the two factors being tested were "drug/placebo" and "male/female," the ANOVA interaction test may find that the drug is more effective than the placebo in the female subjects only. The significance of the ANOVA is tested by the F-statistic.

A "contingency table analysis by chi-square" is a test to determine whether the frequencies in each cell of a contingency table are different from the proportions expected by chance. It is most commonly used on a 2×2 contingency table, represented as four cells forming a square. A common use is to answer the question, "Is there a difference between the occurrence of a given side effect in the drug versus a placebo group?" In this case, the table is arranged with *drug versus placebo* as the two rows, and *side effect versus no side effect* as the two columns. As the (squared) difference between the observed and expected frequencies in each cell increases, the chi-square statistic also increases; the higher those increases, the more significant the result becomes. If all cells contain exactly the frequencies that would be expected by chance, then the chi-square statistic is zero. If the frequencies differ greatly from chance, the chi-square statistic gets larger and larger. The size of the chi-square statistic is based on the number of cells in the contingency table (because df = (number of rows—1) $\times$ (number of columns—1), a 2×2 table always has a single degree of freedom).

A "cluster analysis" is a data reduction technique used to group subjects together into subgroups (or "clusters") based on their similarities or differences on a set of variables. This technique answers questions such as, "Do my subjects fall into subgroups?" or "What variables give a profile that distinguishes subgroups of my subjects?" A simple rule of thumb is "cluster analysis groups people, while factor analysis groups variables." It is considered a multivariate statistical procedure because many intercorrelated variables are analyzed simultaneously.

Q5 The answer is: (E) Factor analysis.

A "factor analysis" is used to statistically reduce the number of variables needed to explain or to describe a larger set of original variables based on the correlation matrix. For example, the 10 subscale scores of the Minnesota Multiphasic Personality Inventory personality test were derived from the 567 items that make up the questionnaire. As a rule of thumb, "factor analysis groups variables, while cluster analysis groups people." It is considered a multivariate statistical procedure because many intercorrelated variables are analyzed simultaneously.

A "canonical correlation" is a generalization of multiple regressions to the case of multiple independent variables and multiple dependent variables. It is rarely used today, except in neuroimaging studies with hundreds or thousands of correlated measurements. It is considered a multivariate statistical procedure because many intercorrelated variables are analyzed simultaneously.

Q6 The answer is: (E) *P* value.

The "*P* value" reflects the chance of a result of a statistical test being a false positive (i.e., the probability of a spurious finding). If a finding is almost certainly a spurious finding, which would not be reproducible in another sample, the *P* value will be near 1.00. However, if the finding almost certainly represents a "true" finding, the *P* value will be near zero (small *P* values are represented by several zeros after the decimal point, e.g., $P < 0.0001$; the *P* value should never be listed as 0.00, as this is impossible).

Most journals require $P < 0.05$ for significance. If many statistical tests are performed in a study, a more conservative *P* value can be used to minimize experiment-wise error. One should not be overly impressed by very low *P* values. Remember that all this tells you is the chance that the difference is probably not zero. Also, remember that given enough subjects, this is easy to prove. Thus a very low *P* value does not necessarily indicate a large clinical effect, but instead represents that it is a very reliable effect. One should check the effect size (the correlation coefficient squared, or the size of the t-statistic) to get an idea of the magnitude of the difference or relation.

Q7 The answer is: (B) False.

Reliability is the dependability of a score, or the degree to which we can be certain that a measurement can be depended on (i.e., how reproducible is the score?). For self-rated scales, such as paper-and-pencil questionnaires, because there is no rater error to consider, the main source of unreliability to assess is the difference in the person's self-rating over time. For example, if a patient completes a depression questionnaire at 3 PM, how close would his or her score be on the same questionnaire if he or she were to take the same scale at 4 PM, assuming no change in his or her depression? If the scores were identical, and this was the case for all patients, the correlation coefficient would be a perfect 1.00 (in this case the correlation coefficient is referred to as the "reliability coefficient").

Validity is the degree of usefulness of a rating scale for a particular purpose. It is also the degree to which the test measures what it is supposed to be measuring. The determination of validity usually requires independent, external criteria of whatever the test is designed to measure. For example, if an investigator develops a single question that he or she purports to be a good screening instrument for clinical depression, patients' responses to this question should relate well to gold-standard measures of clinical depression, such as structured interviews and well-established rating scales for depression. There is no real rule of thumb for validity because there is no one measure. As a bare minimum, however, the scale should at least be significantly correlated with gold-standard measures for that characteristic.

Q8 The answer is: (B) False.
Descriptive statistics include the mean, median, standard deviation, variance, estimates of effect size, proportions, percentages, mean differences, and odds ratios.

Inferential statistics include the t-statistic, F-statistic, chi-square, and confidence intervals.

Psychometric statistics include the test-retest reliability coefficient, intraclass correlation, kappa coefficient, sensitivity, and specificity.

GENETICS AND PSYCHIATRY

Chapter 63: Genetics and Psychiatry

Chapter 63

Genetics and Psychiatry

Multiple-Choice Questions

Select the appropriate answer.

Q1 Which of the following letters denotes the long arm of a chromosome?

A. *p*

B. *q*

C. *r*

D. *s*

E. *t*

Q2 True or False. The prototypic Mendelian disorder is one in which mutations or alterations in a single gene cause a disease according to classical Mendelian patterns of inheritance (e.g., recessive, dominant, or X-linked) and are often highly penetrant (that is, the risk of illness in those carrying the genetic liability is high).

A. *True*

B. *False*

Q3 True or False. One index of the strength of familiality is the "recurrence risk ratio" for first-degree relatives ($\lambda 1$), defined as the ratio of the risk of the disorder in a first-degree relative of an affected individual to the prevalence in the general population.

A. *True*

B. *False*

Q4 True or False. The observation that a trait aggregates in families does NOT establish that genes influence the phenotype.

A. *True*

B. *False*

Q5 True or False. Heritability refers to the strength of genetic influences in an individual, NOT in a population.

A. *True*

B. *False*

Q6 True or False. Linkage studies address the question of where in the genome (i.e., in which chromosomal region) a disease mutation or susceptibility locus may reside.

A. *True*

B. *False*

Q7   True or False. Numerous family studies have demonstrated that attention-deficit/hyperactivity disorder (ADHD), autism, Tourette syndrome (TS), and Alzheimer disease (AD) run in families.

A. *True*

B. *False*

Q8   Which of the following conditions is MOST closely associated with an extra X chromosome?

A. *DiGeorge syndrome*

B. *Klinefelter syndrome*

C. *Prader-Willi syndrome (PWS)*

D. *Smith-Magenis syndrome*

E. *Turner syndrome*

Q9   Which of the following conditions is associated with gonadal dysgenesis and a missing copy of the X chromosome?

A. *DiGeorge syndrome*

B. *Prader-Willi syndrome (PWS)*

C. *Smith-Magenis syndrome*

D. *Turner syndrome*

E. *Williams syndrome*

Q10 Which of the following syndromes is a genetic condition MOST often due to microdeletion on the paternal copy of chromosome 15q11-13 and MOST closely associated with hyperphagia and obesity that develops in later childhood?

A. *DiGeorge syndrome*

B. *Fragile X syndrome (FRX)*

C. *Prader-Willi syndrome (PWS)*

D. *Smith-Magenis syndrome*

E. *Williams syndrome*

Q11 Which of the following conditions is the MOST common inherited cause of intellectual disability, occurring in approximately 1 in 4000 boys?

A. *DiGeorge syndrome*

B. *Fragile X syndrome (FRX)*

C. *Prader-Willi syndrome (PWS)*

D. *Smith-Magenis syndrome*

E. *Williams syndrome*

Chapter 63

Answers

Q1 The answer is: (B) q.
The human genome comprises the full sequence of DNA found in the nucleus of each nucleated human cell (mature erythrocytes and platelets lack nuclei, and thus do not contain a copy of the genome). The DNA sequence is distributed over 23 pairs of chromosomes, long strands of DNA that include the 22 autosomes and two sex chromosomes. One of each pair of the autosomes and the sex chromosomes is inherited from each parent. The autosomes are numbered 1 through 22 in order of size, and most consist of two arms divided by a region called the centromere.

The longer arm of a chromosome is denoted by the letter "q," and the short arm is denoted by the letter "p." Thus the long arm of chromosome 1 is referred to as 1q. Subdivisions of chromosomes, originally identified on the basis of chromosome staining, are referred to by numbers (e.g., 1q31.2).

Q2 The answer is: (A) True.
Genetic disorders are often categorized as either "Mendelian" or "complex" phenotypes. The prototypic Mendelian disorder is one in which mutations or alterations in a single gene cause a disease according to classical Mendelian patterns of inheritance (e.g., recessive, dominant, or X-linked) and are often highly penetrant (that is, the risk of illness in those carrying the genetic liability is high).

In contrast, complex phenotypes, which include common medical and psychiatric disorders, reflect the additive or interactive influence of multiple genes and environmental influences. In some cases, single major genes may contribute along with several other genes (oligogenic disorders) or many other genes (polygenic disorders). Most common medical and psychiatric disorders are believed to have multifactorial etiologies, involving both genetic and environmental (and possibly epigenetic) factors. As more is learned about the genetic basis of single gene disorders, the distinction between complex and Mendelian disorders is increasingly difficult to draw.

Q3 The answer is: (A) True.
A higher prevalence among relatives of affected probands is evidence that the disorder aggregates in families. The risk to relatives of affected probands is referred to as the recurrence risk. One index of the strength of familiality is the recurrence risk ratio for first-degree relatives (λ_1), defined as the ratio of the risk of the disorder in a first-degree relative of an affected individual to the prevalence in the general population. It is important to bear in mind that the size of these risk ratios depends on both the risk to relatives (numerator) and the base rate of the disorder (denominator). Even when the relative risk of a disorder is high, the absolute risk to a first-degree relative may be relatively low if the base rate of the disorder is low.

Q4 The answer is: (A) True.
The observation that a trait aggregates in families does not, in itself, establish that genes influence the phenotype. Traits and disorders may run in families for non-genetic reasons. For example, shared environmental experiences may produce the disorder in multiple family members. Twin and adoption studies can be used to separate the contribution of genetic and environmental causes of familial aggregation.

Q5 The answer is: (B) False.
Heritability refers to the strength of genetic influences in a population, not a particular individual, and heritability estimates may differ depending on the population studied. A heritability of 60% says nothing about the contribution of genes to an individual's risk of a phenotype. Also, because the heritability is defined as the ratio $V_G/V_p + V_E$, as the environmental variance increases, the genetic component (heritability) decreases. Put another way, if the genetic homogeneity of a population increases, the apparent heritability of a trait will decrease.

Heritability refers to the additive sum of all genetic influences on a trait in a population. Thus a heritability of 0.80 (80%) suggests that genes contribute more to trait variance in the population than does a heritability of 40%. However, heritability provides no information regarding how many genes are involved, how strong the effect of any given gene is, or how easy it will be to identify contributing genes.

Heritability does not illuminate the genetic architecture of a trait, although a heritability greater than 0 does imply that genes play a role.

The magnitude of heritability is not a strong predictor of the potential impact of environmental interventions. A classic illustration is the case of phenylketonuria, a recessively inherited disorder owing to a mutation in the gene encoding phenylalanine hydroxylase that results in a toxic accumulation of phenylalanine. Untreated, phenylketonuria can result in progressive brain damage with seizures and intellectual disability. However, these devastating outcomes can be minimized by entirely environmental interventions: avoidance of dietary phenylalanine and supplementation with tyrosine.

Q6 The answer is: (A) True.

Linkage studies address the question of where in the genome (i.e., in which chromosomal region) a disease mutation or susceptibility locus may reside. Linkage analysis examines the degree to which alleles at two or more genetic loci are coinherited (cosegregate) within families (thus deviating from Mendel's law of independent assortment of loci). The likelihood that two loci on a chromosome will cosegregate is inversely proportional to the distance between them. This principle is because of the phenomenon of recombination between homologous chromosomes that occurs during gamete formation (meiosis). During meiosis, the two members of each chromosomal pair (comprising a maternal and a paternal chromosome) align and undergo crossovers that result in an exchange of chromosomal segments (recombination). The closer two loci are on a chromosome, the less likely it is that they will be separated by a recombination event.

In linkage analyses, if individuals affected with a disorder within a family tend to inherit the same alleles at a marker locus, this implies that the marker locus is linked to (i.e., is physically close to) a gene that influences the disorder. In classical (parametric) linkage analysis, the strength of the evidence in favor of linkage is calculated as a logarithm of the odds score. The logarithm of the odds score compares the likelihood of obtaining the observed genotypes and phenotypes when linkage is present with the likelihood assuming no linkage.

Q7 The answer is: (A) True.

Numerous family studies have demonstrated that attention-deficit/hyperactivity disorder (ADHD) runs in families.

First-degree relatives (parents and siblings) of ADHD probands have a two- to eight fold higher risk of the disorder than relatives of controls. Family studies also suggest that ADHD and depression share familial determinants, and that ADHD with conduct disorder or bipolar disorder may be a distinct familial subtype. Most twin studies have shown significantly higher concordance rates for monozygotic (MZ) as compared with dizygotic (DZ) twins.

The risk of autism to siblings of affected children is approximately 2% to 7%, which is 50 to 100 times higher than the general population prevalence. When the "broader autism phenotype" (including autism spectrum disorders and milder abnormalities of social and language function) is considered, the risk to first-degree relatives may be as high as 10% to 45%. Concordance rates for MZ twins are markedly higher (70% to 90%) than those for DZ twins (5% to 10%), and the heritability has been estimated to exceed 90%.

Familial aggregation studies have found an approximately 5- to 15-fold increased risk in first-degree relatives of Tourette syndrome (TS) probands compared with the general population (7% to 18% vs. 1% to 2%, respectively). There is evidence for variable expression of the genetic liability for TS; for example, relatives of probands with TS have a higher risk of obsessive-compulsive disorder and chronic motor or vocal tics. Concordance rates in MZ twins (50% to 70%) are significantly greater than rates in DZ twins (9%).

The familiality of early-onset (before age 60 to 65 years) Alzheimer disease (AD) has been well established, and three specific genes influencing early-onset AD have been identified. Inheritance of early-onset AD follows an autosomal dominant pattern, but the early-onset form is rare, with a prevalence under 0.1%. Late-onset AD is far more common and has a more complex etiology. Having an affected first-degree relative is associated with an approximately 2.5-fold increased risk of AD. Twin studies have estimated the heritability of late-onset AD at 48% to 60%.

Q8 The answer is: (B) Klinefelter syndrome.

Klinefelter syndrome refers to a group of disorders occurring in males with at least one additional X chromosome, classically 47, XXY, and secondary to failure of the sex chromosomes to separate during meiosis. The incidence of this disorder is approximately 1 per 600 live male births. Men with Klinefelter syndrome are typically tall, with long legs. In contrast to previous reports, they have a male distribution of body fat and hair, although gynecomastia may be present, and body hair may be sparse. A diagnosis of Klinefelter syndrome is often made at puberty, when hypogonadism becomes apparent. The testes and penis remain small, and secondary sexual changes fail to occur. Testosterone levels are low, and follicle-stimulating hormone and luteinizing hormone are elevated. Men with Klinefelter syndrome may have normal sexual function, especially when treated with testosterone supplementation, but are infertile. Developmentally, boys with Klinefelter syndrome may have some minor motor and verbal delays and increased rates of learning disorders. Individuals with Klinefelter syndrome have also been described as shyer and more immature and lacking in confidence than peers. There are increased rates of ADHD in this population, and possibly depression, but major psychopathology has not been commonly reported. Recently, increased interest in the relationship between smaller cortical brain volumes seen on magnetic resonance imaging in patients with Klinefelter syndrome and underlying cognitive deficits and psychiatric symptoms has resulted in exploration of schizophrenia-spectrum findings in these men; two studies have reported results that raise the possibility of increased rates of auditory hallucinations and other psychosis-spectrum findings. The diagnosis of Klinefelter syndrome is made by karyotype examination of chromosomes.

Q9 The answer is: (D) Turner syndrome.

Turner syndrome is a genetic condition that occurs in women, and is due to missing one copy of the X chromosome, designated as 45, X. This condition occurs in approximately 1 per 3000 female births, but, paradoxically, is also a common cause of miscarriage. Females with this condition are short, with a broad flat chest, and may have a webbed neck (due to congenital lymphedema). Increased rates of congenital heart disease, including coarctation of the aorta and bicuspid aortic valve, are noted. Minor problems with hearing and vision are also reported, as are renal abnormalities. Women with Turner syndrome have gonadal dysgenesis, and for this reason fail to develop secondary sexual characteristics and are infertile. Hypothyroidism is also seen. Developmentally, intelligence is normal in more than 90% of patients, but specific learning deficits, especially in visual-spatial areas, are seen. Performance IQ may be lower than verbal IQ, and may manifest as problems in math and multitasking. ADHD is reported at increased rates in this population. Immaturity, problems reading social cues, and difficulties with peer relationships may occur. In adults, increased rates of depression have been measured. The diagnosis of Turner syndrome is made by karyotype analysis of chromosomes.

Q10 The answer is: (C) Prader-Willi syndrome (PWS).

Prader-Willi syndrome (PWS) is a genetic condition most often owing to a microdeletion on the paternal copy of chromosome 15q11-13 (chromosome 15, long arm band 11-13). Genes in this region undergo imprinting, resulting in silencing of copies of the gene on the maternal chromosome, leaving a lack of expressed genes in this region in those with a paternal deletion. Additional genetic mechanisms including a defect in the imprinting control region ($\approx$1% to 2% of cases) and maternal uniparental disomy (having both copies of chromosome 15 be from the mother, in $\approx$30% cases) may also result in PWS. PWS is associated with prominent hypotonia in infancy and initial failure to thrive. The characteristic hyperphagia and obesity develop in later childhood and may be manageable with behavioral techniques. Physical findings include fair coloring, small hands and feet, and hypogonadism. Facial features include almond-shaped eyes and a small down-turned mouth with a thin upper lip. Developmentally, patients with PWS tend to show motor and verbal delays, as well as intellectual disability, usually in the mild to moderate range. Behaviorally, patients with PWS often exhibit tantrums and stubbornness and may have difficulty with change. Increased rates of obsessive-compulsive symptoms, some of which may be centered on food, and other rituals are also described. Some skin-picking is noted. Mood disorders are also seen, as well as increased rates of psychosis. Testing for PWS involves a combination of methylation analysis, microsatellite profiling, and deletion testing.

Q11 The answer is: (B) Fragile X syndrome (FRX).

Fragile X syndrome (FRX) is the most common inherited cause of mental retardation, occurring in about 1 in 4000 boys. The disorder is owing to dysfunction of the *FMR-1* gene, located at Xq27.3. This region contains an area of repetitive DNA, which involves a trinucleotide repeat, CGG. The number of repeats in the region is significant for the onset of disease. Repeat length may be normal (5 to 44 CGG repeats), intermediate (45 to 58 repeats, which are prone to expand during transmission), premutation (59 to 200 repeats, which are likely to expand to a full mutation with the next generation), and full (greater than 200 repeats). Because this disorder is X-linked, classically it has been described in males. However, females with full mutation–length repeats may be unaffected, mildly affected, or as severely affected as their male counterparts. Furthermore, premutation-length alleles are associated with premature ovarian failure in woman and fragile X tremor ataxia syndrome in males. Physical findings in males with FRX include hypotonia, a long face with a prominent jaw and forehead, large ears, and large testicles. Of note, some changes may not be apparent until after puberty. Verbal and motor delays are common, and intellectual disability is present, which may be in the moderate to severe range. Seizures occur at increased rates. Psychiatric comorbidities include ADHD and pervasive developmental disorder–spectrum disorders. Testing for FRX is aimed at detecting the number of CGG repeats and methylation status (methylation leads to gene inactivation when repeat length exceeds 200), most often through Southern blot techniques.

SECTION 15
SOCIAL AND COMMUNITY PSYCHIATRY

Serious Mental Illness

Multiple-Choice Questions

Select the appropriate answer.

Q1 True or False. In 1998, the number of people in psychiatric hospitals in the United States was only 10% of what it had been in the 1950s.

  A. *True*

  B. *False*

Q2 The prevalence of schizophrenia or mania in homeless adults is roughly how many times greater than it is in matched housed samples?

  A. *3*

  B. *10*

  C. *30*

  D. *100*

  E. *300*

Q3 True or False. Patients with schizophrenia have a life expectancy that is nearly 20% shorter than the life expectancy of people without mental illness.

  A. *True*

  B. *False*

Q4 True or False. The prevalence of obesity, diabetes mellitus (DM), cigarette smoking, and infectious diseases (e.g., hepatitis B and C) is higher in those with chronic mental illness than it is in the general population.

  A. *True*

  B. *False*

Q5 True or False. According to data from the Epidemiologic Catchment Area Study, nearly half of those with schizophrenia have met criteria for substance abuse or dependence.

  A. *True*

  B. *False*

Chapter 64

Answers

Q1 The answer is: (A) True.

By 1903, 144,000 people were housed in public mental hospitals in the United States, and by 1955, this number had grown to 559,000. However, it was in the 1950s when newly created antipsychotic medications led to significant changes in psychiatric treatment that care could more easily be provided to chronically mentally ill patients in the community. New commitment laws and legal proceedings that restricted involuntary commitment and that endorsed patients' rights to access care in the least restrictive setting led to more dramatic changes in hospitalization practices. In addition, there was a growing belief that treatment in the community would be more humane, and that hospitalization may contribute to the withdrawal and apathy associated with chronic mental illness. All these factors contributed to a period of deinstitutionalization in which thousands of patients were released from mental hospitals to live and receive treatment in the community. In 1998, there were just over 57,000 people in psychiatric hospitals in the United States, a decrease of nearly 90% as compared to 1955.

Q2 The answer is: (C) 30.

One unfortunate effect of inadequate housing and access to treatment has been high rates of homelessness among the chronically mentally ill. Homeless adults have approximately 30 times the prevalence of schizophrenia or mania compared with matched housed samples; about one-fourth of the homeless population report a history of psychiatric hospitalization. In addition, the prevalence of schizophrenia is three times higher in jails than it is in the general population. These psychiatrically ill patients become institutionalized through the criminal justice system, which does not provide either the best opportunity or the environment for treatment.

Q3 The answer is: (A) True.

Compelling evidence reveals that individuals with serious mental illness have higher rates of medical morbidity and mortality when compared with those in the general population. Patients with schizophrenia have a life expectancy (57 years for men and 65 years for women) that is nearly 20% shorter than the life expectancy of people without mental illness.

The Massachusetts Department of Mental Health review of client mortality from the year 2000 revealed a mortality rate for patients with severe mental illness that was three times higher than the age-matched comparison group. Cardiovascular disease was the most significant contributor to the increase in deaths, followed by respiratory illnesses. The difference in mortality between the two populations was most notable for individuals in the 25 to 44 year age-group. In this age-group, cardiac deaths were more than six fold higher than in age-matched comparison samples.

Q4 The answer is: (A) True.

Although the prevalence of obesity in the United States has increased dramatically over the past 20 years, individuals with severe mental illness are even more likely than those in the general population to be overweight or obese. Among the atypical antipsychotic medications, clozapine and olanzapine are associated with the most clinically significant weight gain, quetiapine and risperidone convey a moderate risk, and aripiprazole and ziprasidone are least likely to cause weight gain. Certain mood stabilizers and antidepressants (notably, amitriptyline, mirtazapine, paroxetine, valproic acid, and lithium) are also associated with weight gain.

Patients with chronic mental illness are at higher risk for developing type 2 diabetes mellitus (DM) than are those in the general population. A recent New York State study found that the prevalence of DM was 14.2% (between 2001 and 2002) among a cohort of 436 outpatients with schizophrenia. This is nearly double the prevalence (7.7%) among the general New York State population during the same period. Accumulating data link treatment with atypical antipsychotic drugs to an increased incidence of DM. Clozapine and olanzapine have the highest association, followed by quetiapine and risperidone.

The prevalence of cigarette smoking is estimated to be as high as 85% in patients with schizophrenia and 60% to 70% with bipolar disorder as compared to a rate of 23% in the general population. Patients with schizophrenia are also more likely to be classified as a heavy smoker (defined as more than 25 cigarettes per day). One theory is that the high prevalence of smoking among patients with schizophrenia is due to self-medication with nicotine as a way to address the deficits in attention and cognition that are present in schizophrenia (considering that nicotine has been shown to improve sustained attention, memory, and information processing).

Patients with chronic mental illness are also at higher risk for contracting infectious diseases (including hepatitis B and C, tuberculosis, and HIV infection). Studies of mentally ill outpatients have found an HIV-seropositivity rate of 3%, which is elevated nearly eight times the overall rate in the United States population. Rates of hepatitis B and C were elevated 5- and 11-fold, respectively. Risk factors among this population include a high incidence of drug use, impulsivity, high-risk sexual activity, homelessness, and poor knowledge about HIV transmission.

Q5 The answer is: (A) True.
According to data from the Epidemiologic Catchment Area Study, about 47% of people with schizophrenia have met criteria for substance abuse or dependence (33.7% with an alcohol disorder and 27.5% for another drug disorder) as compared to a rate of 17% for those in the general population. Alcohol is the most commonly used substance among those with schizophrenia; cocaine abuse and cannabis abuse are also frequent.

Chapter 65

Aggression and Violence

Multiple-Choice Questions

Select the appropriate answer.

Q1 True or False. The prevalence of violence in those with schizophrenia and other psychotic conditions is similar to that seen in people with bipolar disorder and major depression.

    A. *True*

    B. *False*

Q2 Which of the following personality disorders is MOST closely linked with violence and aggressive behavior?

    A. *Antisocial personality disorder*

    B. *Avoidant personality disorder*

    C. *Borderline personality disorder*

    D. *Paranoid personality disorder*

    E. *Schizotypal personality disorder*

Q3 Which of the following is LEAST likely to herald escalation of tension that leads to violence?

    A. *Agitation*

    B. *Avoiding direct gaze*

    C. *Invasion of personal space*

    D. *Pacing*

    E. *Verbal threats*

Q4 Which of the following is LEAST likely to be a risk factor for violent behavior?

    A. *Alcoholism in the family*

    B. *Impaired impulse control*

    C. *Panic disorder*

    D. *Physical or sexual abuse*

    E. *Prior violent behavior*

Q5 True or False. The evaluation of the potentially violent patient is rarely facilitated by the accrual of information from ancillary sources.

    A. *True*

    B. *False*

Chapter 65
Answers

Q1 The answer is: (A) True.
The prevalence of violence in those with schizophrenia and other psychotic conditions is similar to that seen in people with bipolar disorder and major depression; of note, however, the prevalence is approximately five times higher than it is in those without an Axis I disorder. Individuals with paranoia who suffer from delusions of persecution may interpret individuals within their immediate environment as threatening, and therefore act in a violent manner. Command hallucinations substantially increase the risk of both self-inflicted violence and violence toward others. Disorganized thought and behavior may also increase the risk of violent acts.

Q2 The answer is: (A) Antisocial personality disorder.
The personality disorder most commonly associated with violence and aggressive behavior is antisocial personality disorder; affected individuals often have co-occuring substance abuse and dependence diagnoses, which increase the likelihood of impulsive and aggressive behavior. Patients with borderline personality disorder often act violently toward themselves, that is, with self-mutilatory behavior. If individuals with a paranoid personality disorder perceive a threat, they will often act violently toward that threat. Developmental disorders, as well as other causes (including head trauma) of poor impulse control, may lead to violent behavior.

Q3 The answer is: (B) Avoiding direct gaze.
Before the examiner can interview the potentially violent patient, a safe environment must be secured. All potentially dangerous materials should be removed from the patient and from the interview room. Objects that can be used as weapons (e.g., pens, needles, and telephones) should be scrutinized before and during the interview. The interview room should allow for possible escape and should be highly visible. The ideal room for such an interview should contain an emergency call-button and the inability to lock the door from within.

   The physician should pay careful attention to the patient's behavior for signs of imminent danger. Behaviors that convey escalation include verbal threats or gestures, rapid movements, agitation, pacing, knocking over furniture, slamming doors, invasion of personal space, clenching of the jaw, and signs of muscular tension.

   At this time, the examiner's interventions are designed to direct the patient to regain the locus of control. If the examiner's attempts to redirect the patient fail to decrease the patient's level of agitation and increase his or her level of self-control, tranquilization and emergency restraints may be necessary to regain control and to ensure the safety of all involved.

Q4 The answer is: (C) Panic disorder.
Risk factors for violent behavior include demographics (e.g., youth, sex, poor education, lower socioeconomic status, a legal history, and being a member of a gang), historical factors (e.g., a history of previous violent behavior, physical or sexual abuse, exposure to violence, a chaotic/violent family, a father being arrested, drug abuse in the patient or in the father, alcoholism in the family, access to guns or lethal weapons, verbalization of intent to harm others, impaired impulse control, risk-taking, and reckless behavior), psychosocial factors (e.g., financial stress, difficult interpersonal relationships, and ill health), medical conditions (e.g., delirium, traumatic brain injury, dementia, and states involving disturbed central nervous system function), and psychiatric conditions (e.g., substance use disorders, conduct disorder, antisocial personality disorder, intermittent explosive disorder, schizophrenia, bipolar disorder, depression with psychotic features, and intellectual impairment).

Q5 The answer is: (B) False.
Collecting information from as many ancillary sources as possible (including family members, victims, court records, medical records, and previous treaters) can be crucial to the evaluation.

   Assessment for violence is one of the most difficult tasks for the medical and psychiatric professional. The best indicator of future violence remains a history of violence. Therefore, seeking a history of violence by a patient is an integral part of the interview. Given the nature of violent perpetrators, it is difficult to elicit an accurate account. The best approach is indirect questioning for previous violent behaviors.

Questions about prior violence may include the following: At what age did violent acts begin? How frequently did those acts occur? What was the most recent act? How severe were the actions? Has there been a recurring pattern of escalation preceding violence? Have there been common precipitants surrounding the acts? Have any violent actions resulted in legal recourse, or incarceration? Has there been a history of recklessness, suicidality, arrests, or impulsivity? Does the patient have a family history of violence, abuse, or gang involvement?

Screening questions include the following: Do you ever think of harming anyone else? Have you ever seriously injured another human being? (Tell me about the most violent thing that you have ever done.) It is also useful to ask about prior evaluations and treatments related to violent behavior, including medical workups, diagnostic tests, and old records.

Chapter 66

Culture and Psychiatry

Multiple-Choice Questions

Select the appropriate answer.

Q1   Which of the following features is LEAST likely to be involved in a cultural formulation of a patient?

    A.   *Determination of cultural explanations*

    B.   *Determination of cultural identity*

    C.   *Determination of handedness*

    D.   *Determination of psychosocial function*

    E.   *Determination of the relationship between the clinician and the patient*

Q2   True or False. African Americans are frequently misdiagnosed as having schizophrenia when instead they have bipolar disorder or a psychotic depression.

    A.   *True*

    B.   *False*

Q3   True or False. A non-psychotic patient may admit to hearing voices of her ancestors.

    A.   *True*

    B.   *False*

Q4   True or False. Culture-bound syndromes ONLY occur in the country or region of their origin.

    A.   *True*

    B.   *False*

Q5   True or False. Patients typically feel comfortable revealing personal issues or conflicts to interpreters from their own community.

    A.   *True*

    B.   *False*

Q6   True or False. In general, Asians are MORE likely to be poor metabolizers (i.e., those with little enzyme activity) for CYP2D6 isoenzymes than are whites.

    A.   *True*

    B.   *False*

Q7 Which of the following culture-bound syndromes deals with genital retraction?

A. *Amafufanyane*

B. *Koro*

C. *Latah*

D. *Piblokto*

E. *Qi-gong*

Q1 The answer is: (C) Determination of handedness.

A cultural formulation contains several components; these include the following:

Determination of cultural identity. Ethnic or cultural references and the degree to which individuals are involved with their culture of origin and their host culture are important. It is crucial to listen for clues about culture and to ask specific questions concerning a patient's cultural identity. For instance, an Asian-American man who grew up in the Southern United States may exhibit patterns, behaviors, and views of the world more consistent with those of a white southerner. Attention to language abilities and preferences must also be addressed.

Determination of cultural explanations. How an individual understands distress or the need for support is often communicated through symptoms (e.g., nerves, possession by spirits, somatic complaints, and misfortune); therefore, the meaning and severity of an illness in relation to one's culture, family, and community should be determined. This explanatory model may be helpful when developing an interpretation, a diagnosis, and a treatment plan. Many patients from non-Western cultures are unfamiliar with the concepts and terminologies used by mental health professionals, leading to misunderstanding and avoidance of mental health services. Careful elicitation of a patient's explanatory model and using it as a common platform for communication frequently facilitates disclosure of a patient's diagnosis and treatment negotiation.

Determination of psychosocial function. Cultural factors can have a significant impact on the psychosocial environment and on function. Cultural interpretations of social stress, support, and one's level of disability and function must also be addressed. It is the physician's responsibility to determine the level of disability and to help the patient and his or her family adjust to role changes caused by illness.

Determination of the relationship between the clinician and the patient. Cultural aspects of the relationship between the individual and the clinician need to be considered. Moreover, cultural differences and their impact on the treatment must not be ignored. Language difficulties, difficulties eliciting symptoms or understanding their cultural significance, difficulties negotiating the appropriate relationship, and difficulties determining whether a behavior is normal or pathological are common barriers to care. In the hospital, the psychiatrist must also attend to the environment in which the patient is receiving treatment. An intervention of this nature may improve the comfort of patients and their health care providers and the quality of the care provided.

Handedness is least likely to reflect an individual's ethnic and cultural beliefs.

Q2 The answer is: (A) True.

In the United States, race and ethnicity have a significant impact on psychiatric diagnosis and treatment. Moreover, the need to reduce disparities in the mental health care of racial and ethnic minorities was recently underscored by the US Surgeon General.

African Americans are frequently misdiagnosed as having schizophrenia when instead they have bipolar disorder or a psychotic depression. African-American patients are also more likely to receive higher doses of antipsychotics, to receive depot preparations, to have higher rates of involuntary psychiatric hospitalizations, and to have significantly higher rates of seclusion and restraints while in psychiatric hospitals. The tendency is to oversedate such patients to reduce their "risk of violence," despite, in some cases, little evidence that the patient has ever been violent.

Depression is frequently underrecognized and undertreated among Asian Americans, as they tend to underreport their affective symptoms. Moreover, treatment approaches and responses often differ depending on the diagnosis.

The reasons for misdiagnosis are complicated. They include the fact that individuals from some ethnic or cultural backgrounds may present to the medical system later in the course of their illness than do white individuals; this results in the perception of a more severe illness. The late presentation may, in part, be related to mistrust of the health care system, lack of familiarity with what mental health services are about, and fear of stigma associated with mental illnesses. Physician biases also play a major role in misdiagnosis.

Psychiatric diagnoses are often established by eliciting symptoms from patients that are then interpreted by the psychiatric expert. Many disorders have overlapping symptoms and can be used to support one diagnosis or to disregard another. In the case of African Americans, affective symptoms are frequently ignored, and psychotic symptoms are emphasized. This pattern has also been seen in other ethnic populations, including Hispanics, some Asian populations, and the Amish (in the United States).

Q3 The answer is: (A) True.

From a cross-cultural perspective, evaluating the meanings of bizarre delusions, hallucinations, and psychotic-like symptoms remains a clinical challenge. A non-psychotic patient may admit to hearing voices of her ancestors (a feature that is culturally appropriate in certain cultural groups).

In many traditional, non-Western societies, spirits of the deceased are regarded as capable of interacting with and possessing those still alive. It is difficult to determine whether symptoms are bizarre enough to yield a diagnosis of schizophrenia without an adequate understanding of a patient's sociocultural and religious background. However, caution must be taken not to assume that bizarre symptoms are culturally appropriate when in fact they are a manifestation of psychosis. The use of bicultural and bilingual interpreters, along with the search for information from other sources (such as family, community leaders, or religious officials), may help to determine whether an individual's experience is culturally appropriate or acceptable.

Q4 The answer is: (B) False.

In the past, it was believed that culture-bound syndromes only occurred in the country or region of their origin. However, with significant population movements and the tendency for immigrants to remain within their culture (although they have moved to a new country), culture-bound syndromes have been observed in other parts of the world.

A culture-bound syndrome is a collection of signs and symptoms that is restricted to a limited number of cultures by reason of certain psychosocial features. Culture-bound syndromes are usually restricted to a specific setting, and they have a special relationship to that setting. Culture-bound syndromes are classified based on common etiology (e.g., magic, evil spells, or angry ancestors); clinical pictures may vary.

Q5 The answer is: (B) False.

Quite the contrary. Patients often feel uneasy about revealing personal issues or conflicts to individuals from their own community. As most ethnic communities are small and close-knit, patients may fear that the interpreter will divulge their private information to those in the community. Patients are more likely to open up if they feel reassured that what they share with the clinician and interpreter would be kept in strict confidence. If possible, the same interpreter should be used with a given patient repeatedly to help build trust and continuity of care for the patient.

Q6 The answer is: (B) False.

The incidence of "poor metabolizers" (i.e., those individuals with little enzyme activity) at the CYP2D6 is roughly 3% to 7% in whites, 0.5% to 2.4% in Asians, 4.5% in Hispanics, and approximately 1.9% in African Americans. Individuals from these backgrounds are at great risk for toxicity, even when medications are used at low doses. For instance, a woman who develops hypotension and a change in mental status several days after starting 20 mg of nortriptyline may be found to have toxic blood levels and require cardiac monitoring.

Recently, a genetic variation of the extensive metabolizer gene that decreases activity at the CYP2D6 enzymes by approximately 50% ("slow metabolizer") was discovered. This group appears to have enzyme activity levels that are intermediate between poor and extensive metabolizers. Approximately 18% of Mexican Americans, 37% of Asians, and 33% of African Americans have this gene variation. This may explain ethnic differences in the pharmacokinetics of neuroleptics and antidepressants. Although these individuals are not as likely to experience toxicity at extremely low doses (e.g., poor metabolizers), they are likely to experience significant side effects at lower doses. These individuals may quickly be classified as the "difficult patients" because they complain of side effects at unexpectedly low doses.

Q7 The answer is: (B) Koro.

Amafufanyane involves sleep paralysis (in the Zulu population of Southern Africa), *koro* involves genital retraction (among inhabitants of China and Malaysia), *latah* involves startle reactions (among those living in Malaysia and Indonesia), *piblokto* involves running (in Eskimos), and *qi-gong* involves psychotic reactions (in China).

Chapter 67
Community Psychiatry
Multiple-Choice Questions

Select the appropriate answer.

Q1 Which of the following terms BEST defines a community mental health service area with a population of 75,000 to 200,000 people?

A. *Borough*

B. *Catchment area*

C. *Neighborhood*

D. *Town*

E. *Zone*

Q2 Which of the following terms BEST defines the sociopolitical, economic trend to discharge long-term psychiatric inpatients to live and receive services in the community?

A. *Dehospitalization*

B. *Deinstitutionalization*

C. *Downsizing*

D. *Primary prevention*

E. *Transinstitutionalization*

Q3 Which of the following terms BEST describes measures to decrease the new onset (incidence) of disease (e.g., causative agent eradication, risk-factor reduction, host resistance-enhancement, and disease transmission-disruption)?

A. *Deinstitutionalization*

B. *Managed care*

C. *Primary prevention*

D. *Secondary prevention*

E. *Tertiary prevention*

Q4 Which of the following terms is BEST described as a cost-containment strategy that manages payment for care of a population through monitoring of services allocated to members of the specified population?

A. *Care management*

B. *Community mental health*

C. *Managed care*

D. *Moral treatment*

E. *Primary prevention*

Q5   Which of the following advanced the concept that physical work and fresh air would return the mentally ill to a state of mental health and well-being?

A. *Ben Franklin*

B. *John F. Kennedy*

C. *Sigmund Freud*

D. *Adolf Meyer*

E. *Philippe Pinel*

Answers

Q1 The answer is: (B) Catchment area.
Community mental health, as defined by the Community Mental Health Center (CMHC) Acts of 1963 (Public Law 88-164) and 1965 (Public Law 89-105), was envisioned to be an inclusive, multidisciplinary, systemic approach to publicly funded mental health services provided for all in need, residing in a given geographic locale (i.e., a catchment area), without consideration of ability to pay. Catchment is a term borrowed from sanitation engineering (i.e., a cistern into which the sewage of a defined area is dumped) that refers to a community mental health service area with a population of 75,000 to 200,000.

Q2 The answer is: (B) Deinstitutionalization.
Deinstitutionalization was a sociopolitical, economic trend to discharge long-term psychiatric inpatients to live and receive services in the community. It has been argued that this should have been called dehospitalization (or transinstitutionalism) because patients were maintained in non-hospital, but still institutional, settings. (Although the point is well taken, the former term has wide recognition.) There is also evidence of this trend long before the term (and such associated terms as policy, or movement) ever appeared in the psychiatric literature, which suggests the convergence of multiple precipitants but no formal, purposeful, or driving policy.

Q3 The answer is: (C) Primary prevention.
Primary prevention is concerned with measures to decrease the new onset (incidence) of disease (e.g., causative agent eradication, risk-factor reduction, host resistance-enhancement, and disease transmission-disruption). Such measures, although highly effective in the realms of infectious disease, toxins, deficiency states, and habit-induced chronic illnesses (e.g., lung and heart diseases), are less obviously efficacious in the realm of psychiatry because the outcome without intervention is less predictable. Nonetheless, putative programs and clinical activities of primary prevention include anticipatory guidance (e.g., for parents with young children), enrichment and competence-building programs (e.g., Head Start or Outward Bound), social support or self-help programs for at-risk individuals (e.g., bereavement groups), and early or crisis intervention following trauma (e.g., onsite student counseling after a classmate's suicide).

Secondary prevention is concerned with measures to decrease the number of disease cases in a population at a given point in time (prevalence) by early discernment (case-finding) and timely treatment to shorten the course and to avoid or lessen residual disability. An educational campaign and screening for peripartum depression would be a psychiatric example of secondary prevention.

Tertiary prevention is concerned with measures to decrease the prevalence and severity of residual disease-related defect or disability. Because optimal function in the setting of serious psychiatric illness is so allied with adherence to treatment, examples of tertiary prevention in psychiatry would include case management and other measures to promote continuous care and treatment.

Q4 The answer is: (C) Managed care.
Managed care is primarily a cost-containment strategy that manages payment for care of a population through monitoring of services allocated to members of the specified population. Prior authorization, primary care provider specialty referral (i.e., a gate-keeper system), and concurrent (or utilization) review are strategies commonly employed to manage health care expenditure. Managed care organizations have proliferated to provide this service for public and private insurers. Contracts between insurers and managed care organizations may include penalties for exceeding the service budget or financial incentives to hold service payments within a fixed budget. Health care costs have long been a concern of both providers and recipients of health care, but managed care has imposed the payer's interests into the doctor–patient relationship. Although critics believe this has negatively affected the therapeutic process, proponents believe it has led to greater transparency, standardization, and evidence-based care (which may also have paved the way for the current explosion of pay-for-performance initiatives).

Case, or care, managers (usually social workers or mental health clinicians) assist in the patient's negotiation of a fragmented and complex system of (often disconnected) agencies, providers, and services, with the goal of care continuity and coordination through better interprovider communication. Obviously, patients with more, and more complex, needs will also require more intensive care management, and the greater the intensity of the management needs, the fewer cases a manager can adequately handle. Care managers are the members of the treatment-planning team who follow the patient through all care levels (e.g., inpatient, aftercare, and residential), types (e.g., mental health, substance abuse, and physical health), and agencies or services (e.g., housing, welfare, and public entitlements).

Moral treatment began in the 18th century; it rested in the concept that physical work and fresh air would return the mentally ill to a state of mental health and well-being.

Q5 The answer is: (E) Philippe Pinel.

The "first psychiatric revolution" occurred late in the 18th century, when a French alienist (i.e., a psychiatrist), Philippe Pinel, advanced the concept that physical work and fresh air would return the mentally ill to a state of mental health and well-being. Moral treatment dawned as Pinel released the insane from their shackles. By the early 19th century, the movement had found its way to the United States, where Dorothea Dix promoted the development of village-style asylums for the mentally ill to retreat from the stresses of daily living. Government funds were used to build institutions for the behaviorally deviant and mentally ill.

Ben Franklin, a noted US statesman and inventor, led a commission that found no basis for the efficacy of hypnosis and for magnetism as its mechanism.

Spurred by the urbanization of the Industrial Revolution, the preventive, public health movement grew out of the necessity for sanitation and infection control. Parallel to this was the mental hygiene movement, promoted by Adolf Meyer, and his writings on prevention and the social context of mental illness. In 1908, the deplorable living conditions inside mental institutions were exposed in Clifford Beers's first-person account of his time living in one. Beers joined forces with Meyer and William James to create the National Association for Mental Health in 1909. The mental hygiene movement advocated for smaller hospitals and the establishment of community-based outpatient evaluation clinics. These clinics (variously viewed as the forerunners or beginnings of community psychiatry) were less stigmatizing than the large state hospitals, and they concentrated on evaluation, prevention, and differentiation between persistent and acute disorders. They also emphasized interdisciplinary training, affiliation with medical school and mainstream medicine, and the use of applied psychodynamic theory and principles.

Sigmund Freud is the father of psychoanalysis.

By 1963, the political and social optimism were ripe for the first-ever presidential address to congress regarding mental health and retardation. In this address, President Kennedy voiced his opposition to the prevailing institutional system and his conviction (in opposition to that of the Joint Commission) that more funding for this system would not improve the quality of mental health care. He called for a "bold new approach" that relied on new pharmacology and knowledge to treat the mentally ill in their home communities, in which they would be "returned to a useful place in society." Kennedy foresaw a "new type of health facility," the CMHC, as part of a comprehensive community care system, that would both improve quality and "return mental health care to the mainstream of American medicine." Within weeks of his signing the CMHC Act, President Kennedy was assassinated.

Chapter 68

Managed Care and Psychiatry

Multiple-Choice Questions

Select the appropriate answer.

Q1 During which of the following time frames did private health insurers grow in both size and number, with the number of covered individuals rising by a factor of seven?

   A. *During the Civil War*

   B. *During the Revolutionary War*

   C. *During the War of 1812*

   D. *During World War I*

   E. *During World War II*

Q2 In which of the following years was Medicare established?

   A. *1925*

   B. *1935*

   C. *1945*

   D. *1955*

   E. *1965*

Q3 In which year did all states start to participate in Medicaid?

   A. *1952*

   B. *1962*

   C. *1972*

   D. *1982*

   E. *1992*

Q4 True or False. When an individual has copays for care, his or her utilization of medical services will decrease without a similar decrease in health outcome.

   A. *True*

   B. *False*

Q5 True or False. Insurance plans with slightly better benefits have significantly higher utilization of mental health care benefits.

   A. *True*

   B. *False*

Chapter 68

Answers

Q1 The answer is: (E) During World War II.

During World War II, when the government allowed employers to offer health insurance in lieu of wage increases, private health insurers grew in both size and number, with the number of covered individuals rising from 20.6 million to 142 million between 1940 and 1950. Coverage expanded even further when in 1954 the Internal Revenue Service ruled that employer-based health insurance would not be considered as tax-deductible income. Although coverage was expanded for general medical care, mental health care coverage was substantially more limited. Insurance policies did not include mental health services until after World War II, when insurers began covering some hospital-based psychiatric care.

Q2 The answer is: (E) 1965.

Medicare was established in 1965 in response to the country's growing number of senior citizens. Financed through federal payroll taxes, subsidized premiums, and general tax revenues, Medicare was designed to cover both inpatient (sometimes referred to as Part A) and outpatient (Part B) care. All individuals above age 65 were covered by Part A (regardless of income). Although there have been some changes in which treatments Medicare pays for and how it pays for them, its basic structure and benefits have stayed relatively consistent.

Q3 The answer is: (D) 1982.

Medicaid was enacted through the same federal legislation that saw the enactment of Medicare. However, its mission and structure were quite different from those of Medicare. One major difference was that Medicaid was designed to provide medical care to categorically eligible low-income children and adults as opposed to the elderly, who were covered by Medicare. Funding also differs between Medicaid and Medicare, with Medicaid being funded in part by states with the federal government matching state contributions. Although Medicaid enrollment is optional for states, all states have participated since 1982. Within broad federal guidelines, states have a significant amount of control over eligibility, as well as what services are covered. Medicaid offers enrollees a somewhat richer mental health benefit than Medicare does.

The creation of Medicaid and Medicare had the practical effect of shifting a large number of elderly state mental hospital patients into federally financed general hospitals and nursing homes, thereby accelerating deinstitutionalization.

Q4 The answer is: (A) True.

One economic concept, referred to as "moral hazard," states that individuals who obtain a product or service at no cost will consume more of it than if they paid a price for it. Much as the person who overeats at an all-you-can-eat buffet, this behavior affects the use of health care services (i.e., without any cost to themselves for health care services, individuals will use more than may be appropriate or necessary).

The RAND health experiment in the 1970s showed that when individuals had copays for care, their utilization of medical services decreased without a similar decrease in health outcome. These results proved the existence of moral hazard and led to the development of copay mechanisms that continue in use today.

Evidence from the RAND study showed that individuals tended to decrease use of psychotherapy services at roughly twice the rate of other medical services when faced with copayments; this suggested that the relative value of additional psychotherapy sessions was less than that of health-related services.

Q5 The answer is: (A) True.

Adverse selection-related incentives are particularly strong in mental health care. Numerous studies have shown that insurance plans with slightly better benefits have significantly higher utilization of mental health care benefits, implying that people with mental illness seek out plans with better benefits. Evidence indicates that those with prior mental health service use are likely to have higher health spending in future years and tend to use other medical services at higher rates compared with otherwise similar individuals. Given that insurance companies lose money on such "high-utilizers" who cost more per person than they pay into a plan, a strong incentive exists to offer plans that have limited mental health benefits to discourage this particular group of high-utilizers from joining their plans.

Adverse selection occurs because individuals are usually more aware of their health status than insurers are. If an individual thinks that he is buying more insurance than he needs given his good health, he will choose to move to plans with lower benefits at a lower cost. As more healthy people leave a given plan, the average cost of insuring the (less healthy) people remaining in that plan becomes higher, thus making insurance premiums more expensive, causing yet more people to leave, ending in what economists have referred to as a "death spiral."

SECTION 16

SECTION 16

CHILD PSYCHIATRIC DISORDERS

Chapter 69

Child and Adolescent Psychiatric Disorders

Multiple-Choice Questions

Select the appropriate answer.

Q1 During which of the following age ranges is healthy separation anxiety typically seen?

A. *2 to 4 months*

B. *4 to 6 months*

C. *8 to 10 months*

D. *12 to 14 months*

E. *36 to 40 months*

Q2 Which of the following is MOST closely linked with pediatric autoimmune neuropsychiatric disorders associated with streptococcal infection (PANDAS)?

A. *Attention-deficit/hyperactivity disorder (ADHD)*

B. *Generalized anxiety disorder*

C. *Obsessive-compulsive disorder (OCD)*

D. *Oppositional defiant disorder*

E. *Separation anxiety disorder*

Q3 Which of the following disorders is MOST likely present when anxiety, dissociative symptoms, persistent re-experiencing of a trauma, and avoidance of stimuli that raise recollections of the trauma occurs within days of a traumatic event?

A. *Acute stress disorder (ASD)*

B. *Dissociative identity disorder*

C. *Generalized anxiety disorder*

D. *Posttraumatic stress disorder (PTSD)*

E. *Separation anxiety disorder*

Q4 Which of the following conditions is MOST closely linked with tics?

A. *Acute stress disorder (ASD)*

B. *Bipolar disorder*

C. *Generalized anxiety disorder*

D. *Obsessive-compulsive disorder (OCD)*

E. *Oppositional defiant disorder*

Q5 Which of the following conditions in childhood is MOST likely to be associated with an extremely irritable or explosive mood?

    A. *Acute stress disorder (ASD)*

    B. *Bipolar disorder*

    C. *Obsessive-compulsive disorder (OCD)*

    D. *Oppositional defiant disorder*

    E. *Posttraumatic stress disorder (PTSD)*

Q6 Which of the following medications is specifically approved by the US Food and Drug Administration to treat bipolar disorder in children younger than age 12 years?

    A. *Carbamazepine*

    B. *Lithium carbonate*

    C. *Olanzapine*

    D. *Valproic acid*

    E. *None of the above*

Q7 Which of the following conditions is LEAST common in childhood?

    A. *Attention-deficit/hyperactivity disorder (ADHD)*

    B. *Major depression*

    C. *Obsessive-compulsive disorder (OCD)*

    D. *Schizophrenia*

    E. *Tourette disorder*

Chapter 69

Answers

Q1 The answer is: (C) 8 to 10 months.

In separation anxiety, the predominant disturbance is a developmentally inappropriate excessive anxiety on separation from familial surroundings. A certain level of separation anxiety is an expected and healthy part of normal development that occurs in all children to varying degrees between infancy and age 6 years.

Healthy separation anxiety is typically seen around age 8 to 10 months, when an infant becomes anxious when meeting strangers (stranger anxiety). Children also may become mildly anxious around age 18 to 24 months, when they are increasingly exploring their world but wanting to return to their caregiver frequently for security. In contrast, approximately 2% to 5% of children will experience separation anxiety disorder at some point with separation worries that are excessive and overwhelm the child for even brief separations (such as leaving to go to school, going to sleep, or staying behind at home when a parent runs an errand). The child's fears usually appear to be irrational (such as a fear that the parent may suddenly die or become ill).

People with separation anxiety disorder often go to great extremes to avoid being apart from their home or caregivers. They may protest leaving a parent's side, refuse to play with friends, or complain about physical illness at the time of separating. When separation occurs or is even anticipated, the child may experience severe anxiety to the point of panic. It may develop during the preschool age, but more commonly appears in elementary school-age children.

Q2 The answer is: (C) Obsessive-compulsive disorder (OCD).

Interest has grown in a syndrome that resembles both obsessive-compulsive disorder (OCD) and tic disorders called pediatric autoimmune neuropsychiatric disorders associated with streptococcal infection (PANDAS). Investigators recently have studied plasma exchange, intravenous immunoglobulin, and penicillin to treat OCD/tics associated with PANDAS. These treatments appear to be effective only for those patients (<10%) in whom OCD/tics were associated with streptococcal infections.

Q3 The answer is: (A) Acute stress disorder (ASD).

Acute stress disorder (ASD) develops within days of a traumatic event, and is manifest by anxiety, dissociative symptoms, persistent re-experiencing of the trauma, and avoidance of stimuli that raise recollections of the trauma. This disorder is likely to be observed in pediatric patients or their parents after acute injuries. The severity, duration, and proximity to the trauma are factors that influence the development of ASD, and approximately 15% to 33% of individuals in severe accidents or observing significant harm to others develop an ASD. In addition to the nature (e.g., burns, self-injurious behaviors, or abuse) and extent of the injuries, pre-existing psychiatric illness increases the risk of ASD.

If the stressful symptoms surrounding the trauma last beyond 1 month, the diagnosis changes to post-traumatic stress disorder (PTSD). PTSD may occur following a traumatic event that continues to haunt a person months later, beyond the "acute" reaction to a trauma. Children, like adults, may experience nightmares months to years after a traumatic event, as well as flashbacks or distressing recollections sometimes suppressed successfully for years. Sometimes patients will not have symptoms immediately following the traumatic event, but months or years later. Events resembling a past trauma may rekindle the trauma, culminating in anxiety symptoms, or sometimes a person will experience a PTSD reaction when reaching a developmental point related to the trauma. For example, when children reach high school or college, have their own children, or experience the loss of someone, their distress may emerge as the trauma is re-experiencing from a different role (e.g., older sibling or parent instead of child). Although ASD and PTSD are not genetic disorders, vulnerabilities to anxiety reactions do have genetic components; in addition, some individuals live in more dangerous or chaotic environments, as do their children, so that PTSD may occur more commonly in some families. Approximately 8% of Americans have experienced PTSD at some point in their lives, although susceptibility to traumatic events increases one's risk of developing PTSD.

Q4 The answer is: (D) Obsessive-compulsive disorder (OCD).

Perhaps as many as 15% of boys between ages 8 and 12 years have transient tics, often excessive eye-blinking or facial grimacing. These tics usually wax and wane over several years, and manifest most frequently when the child is anxious or fatigued.

Tics, however, can intensify and become conspicuous, such that the child may feel ostracized or distressed, and thus necessitating treatment. Perhaps the best-known persisting tic disorder is Tourette syndrome (TS), a childhood-onset neuropsychiatric disorder afflicting up to 3 per 1000 children that usually begins with motor tics around age 6 years; it is manifest by both multiple motor and phonic tics and is accompanied by other behavioral and psychological symptoms. TS is commonly associated with OCD (in about 30% of cases) and attention-deficit/hyperactivity disorder (ADHD) (in about 50% of cases). It is noteworthy that in many cases it is not the tics but the comorbid disorders that are the major source of distress and disability. Some interesting associations include the findings that ADHD appears earlier in life than tics, and stimulants may exacerbate tics. For many patients with tics and ADHD, the symptoms of ADHD appear to be associated with the most severe impairment.

Q5 The answer is: (B) Bipolar disorder.

Prepubertal mania is often preceded by ADHD, and these patients have extreme hyperactivity, impulsivity, and aggression, which may improve on ADHD medications, although mood symptoms, particularly lability, may become prominent. In children, bipolar disorder commonly manifests as an extremely irritable or explosive mood with associated poor psychosocial function that is often devastating to the child and family. Children with prepubertal mania appear to be much more likely to experience ultrarapid mood changes, rather than discrete episodes of mania for several days followed by depressive symptoms for weeks to months. Rather, within a day, these children are often crying for several hours, then giddy or silly, then explosively angry at the seemingly smallest provocation. These children often overreact to the environment (mood reactivity). In milder conditions, additional symptoms consistent with mania include temper tantrums, unmodulated high energy, such as decreased sleep, overtalkativeness, racing thoughts, increased goal-directed activity (e.g., social, work, school, and sexual), and poor judgment (such as seeking out reckless activities).

Although the juvenile symptom complex of mania should be differentiated from ADHD, conduct disorder, depression, trauma, substance use/abuse, and psychotic disorders, these disorders commonly co-occur with childhood mania. A family history of bipolar disorder increases the risk of the child developing bipolar disorder, and treatment for these comorbidities may unmask underlying or evolving bipolar disorder. The clinical course of juvenile mania appears most frequently chronic and mixed with co-occurring manic and depressive features.

Q6 The answer is: (E) None of the above.

There are no medications specifically approved to treat bipolar disorder in children younger than age 12 years. For patients with bipolar disorder between ages 12 and 17 years, lithium is the only US Food and Drug Administration–approved medication. However, investigators have noted that early-onset bipolar disorder appears to be less responsive to lithium. Therefore, children and adolescents with bipolar disorder are often treated with antipsychotic medications, anticonvulsants, or combinations of lithium, anticonvulsants, and/or atypical antipsychotic mood stabilizers. If is the patient does not respond to an adequate trial (in dose and time) of a single agent or cannot tolerate the medication, subsequent trials with alternative medication(s) are recommended. In manic or mixed presentations with psychotic symptoms, additional antipsychotic treatment is recommended. In bipolar disorder with prominent symptoms of depression, combined treatment with a mood stabilizer and an antidepressant is indicated. One must be mindful of the potential destabilizing effects of selective serotonin reuptake inhibitors in the treatment of bipolar depression in children and adolescents.

Q7 The answer is: (D) Schizophrenia.

Childhood-onset schizophrenia is rare, occurring in less than 1 in 10,000 children, and less than 1% of patients with schizophrenia are diagnosed in childhood. More often, childhood psychosis is seen in pediatric patients having major depression, bipolar disorder, or severe dissociative states, such as PTSD.

ADHD is a common psychiatric condition present in 3% to 10% of school-age children. The classic triad of impaired attention, impulsivity, and excessive motor activity characterizes ADHD, although up to one-third of children may only manifest the inattentive aspects of ADHD. With developmental variations, ADHD affects children of all ages, sometimes as early as age 3 years, and it persists throughout adolescence and into adulthood about half of the time.

Major depression increases in prevalence with age. Epidemiologic studies from community and clinical samples estimate the prevalence of major depressive disorder as approximately 0.3% of preschoolers, 2% of children, and between 1.5% and 9% of adolescents. By the end of adolescence, the cumulative incidence of major depressive disorder has been estimated as high as 20%. Although the sex ratio appears to be equal in children, by age 14 years girls appear to be twice as likely to experience depression as boys. Depressive disorders commonly co-occur with anxiety, ADHD, conduct, and substance use disorders in older children and adolescents.

OCD often develops early in life; nearly one-third of adults with obsessions report the onset of their symptoms before age 15 years, and cases of the disorder have been described as early as age 3 years. However, less than 25% of patients with OCD seek treatment or admit having OCD before adulthood.

Perhaps as many as 15% of boys between ages 8 and 12 years have transient tics, often excessive eye-blinking or facial grimacing. These tics usually wax and wane over several years, and manifest most frequently when the child is anxious or fatigued. Tics, however, can intensify and become conspicuous, such that the child may feel ostracized or distressed, and thus necessitating treatment. Perhaps the best-known persisting tic disorder is TS, a childhood-onset neuropsychiatric disorder afflicting up to 3 per 1000 children that usually begins with motor tics around age 6 years; it is manifest by both multiple motor and phonic tics, and is accompanied by other behavioral and psychological symptoms.

Psychiatric and Substance Use Disorders in Transitioning Adolescents and Young Adults

Multiple-Choice Questions

Select the appropriate answer.

Q1 Which of the following is NOT true regarding the care of young adults with psychiatric illness?

A. *Psychiatric illness often begins in late adolescence or young adulthood*

B. *Much of the disease burden in those aged 15 to 24 years is related to mental health and substance use disorders (SUDs)*

C. *Parents should not be involved in the care of young adults*

D. *Substance use and abuse often complicates the mental health evaluation and the treatment of young adults*

Q2 Which of the following typically begins between the ages of 16 and 26 years?

A. *Bipolar disorder*

B. *Bulimia nervosa*

C. *Major depression*

D. *Schizophrenia*

E. *All of the above*

Q3 Which of the following is TRUE regarding substance use disorders (SUDs) in transitional aged youth (TAY)?

A. *SUD occurs in at least half of all TAY*

B. *SUD does not generally begin until the third decade of life*

C. *Poor emotional self-regulation may predispose one to SUD*

D. *Attention-deficit/hyperactivity disorder (ADHD) or conduct disorder reduces the likelihood of SUD in TAY*

Chapter 70

Answers

Q1 The answer is: (C) Parents should not be involved in the care of young adults.

Although individuals over the age of 18 years are considered (legally) as adults, the involvement of parents with proper proactive disclosure and consent of such involvement is recommended for the treatment of young adults. Many young adults still are very involved in their nuclear families through living arrangements, financial subsidy, and/or interpersonal support, and thus have an ongoing and active relationship with their parents. Conversely, parents often feel relegated to providing for their "young" adult children, particularly if a psychiatric or substance use disorder (SUD) is identified.

Emerging data suggest that psychiatric disorders often begin during childhood or the young adult years. Although some young adults have lived with a disorder throughout childhood, others note the onset of their disorder during their college years and may suffer for many years before seeking treatment for their disorders. Data also suggest that the total mental health (largely depression) and substance use burden on those aged 15 to 24 years constitutes almost half of the total "disease burden" in this age group. Three-quarters of cases with substance use reveal high rates of psychiatric comorbidities.

Q2 The answer is: (E) All of the above.

Research indicates that the heterogeneous group of eating disorders (including bulimia, anorexia, binge-eating) often emerges during early adolescence, and shows a rapid increase in its incidence during the transitional years. For instance, Hudson and coworkers in the National Comorbidity Survey Replication (N = 2980) reported a steep increase in the cumulative prevalence of eating disorders during the transitional aged youth (TAY) years. From a prospective analysis of 8594 women, Fields and colleagues found that the prevalence of eating disorders increased substantially until early adulthood, with up to 22% of the sample manifesting an eating disorder. Furthermore, Stice and associates examined the peak periods for onset of the various eating disorders and found that the peak periods for onset was between ages 17 and 18 years for bulimia nervosa and binge-eating disorder and was between ages 18 and 20 years for purging disorder.

Mood disorders, such as dysthymia and major depressive disorder (MDD), are common and highly disabling in TAY. In the National Comorbidity Survey, Kessler and colleagues found that the lifetime prevalence of minor depression in those aged 15 to 18 years was 11%, and was 14% for MDD. Zisook and colleagues reported that over half of all cases of depression had their onset during childhood or TAY years. Consistent with the work of Zisook and colleagues, others have shown an elevated risk for mood disorders that begin in the early teens and rises in a linear fashion throughout the TAY years, with rates of up to 25% by late adolescence. Longitudinally derived data indicate that having a mood disorder or having prominent mood dysregulation in childhood increases the likelihood for a mood disorder in adolescence and adulthood. It is not surprising then that the rates of depression reported during the TAY years approximates those in adult samples, suggesting that the peak onset of the disorders are during the TAY years. Similarly, the majority of adults with bipolar disorder develop their disorder in childhood and the TAY years, and at least one-third of adults with bipolar disorder had their bipolar disorder begin before the age of 12 years. For example, Perlis and associates reported on 1469 subjects from a large multicenter systematic treatment enhancement program for bipolar disorder and found that the mean age of onset of bipolar disorder was 16.7 years.

Schizophrenia frequently has its beginning in the TAY years. In a Swedish family study of 270 schizophrenic probands, Sham and associates found that for both men and women there was a rapid increase in onset of schizophrenia in the late teens and early 20s, followed by a rapid decline in the late 20s. Similar results were found by Hafner and coworkers who studied 267 patients with schizophrenia and found that the onset of the disorder showed an early and steep increase in adolescents until the age of 25 years; 47% of the women and 62% of the men had their first symptoms of schizophrenia before the age of 25 years.

Q3 The answer is: (C) Poor emotional self-regulation may predispose one to SUD.

SUDs are now conceptualized as having their developmental roots in childhood (with the vast majority beginning during adolescence or young adulthood). For instance, data indicate that 1 in 10 adolescents have a SUD, and up to 25% of adults will have a lifetime prevalence of a SUD. Compton and coworkers showed that in those with a drug use disorder, over half had the onset of the disorder before their 18th birthday, with roughly 80% having an onset prior to age 25 years. As with other disorders (such as depression, bipolar disorder, attention-deficit/hyperactivity disorder [ADHD], or conduct disorder), the ability of TAY to manage their own emotions may be an important factor within the context of youths with a SUD. Not surprisingly, deficits in self-monitoring and regulation of mood and anxiety frequently found in TAY (particularly with underlying psychopathology) are related to the continuation of a SUD. SUDs may serve as a coping mechanism for negative affect, avoidance of depression, or substance withdrawal, whereas excessive affect (such as mania or agitation) may drive SUD.

Data suggest that up to three-quarters of TAY with SUDs also have psychiatric comorbidity. Among disorders comorbid with a SUD, conduct disorder, ADHD, mood disorder, and anxiety disorder are most frequently encountered. One of the most robust risk factors for SUD is delinquency in childhood, often referred to as conduct disorder. One of the most common disorders seen in association with early-onset a SUD is ADHD. Follow-up studies of children with ADHD report their risk for SUD to be almost twice that of those without ADHD, with those with concurrent conduct disorder (delinquency) to be at highest risk. Moreover, almost one-quarter of adults with an addiction have ADHD with higher rates in adolescent SUD. The greatest time for risk for a SUD in individuals with ADHD starts around the time of separation from the family (e.g., age 18 years), although it is earlier in the context of conduct disorder or bipolar disorder.

Long-standing interest in mood disorders in early-onset and TAY SUD exists. High rates of low-level long-standing (dysthymia) and more severe episodic depressions (i.e., MDD) are found in TAY with a SUD. Longitudinal data indicate that having a depressive disorder in childhood increases the likelihood for a later SUD, although SUD does not appear to be the cause of a new mood disorder.

Likewise, frank manic behavior, poor judgment, severe mood swings, and dysregulation indicative of bipolar disorder in youth are also highly linked with SUD. Pediatric-onset bipolar disorder occurs in 3% of youth, and places one at a high risk for cigarette smoking and SUDs. For example, one-third of young adolescents with bipolar disorder have a SUD, compared to 4% of controls, with the SUD rate climbing to over 50% in college-aged students with bipolar disorder.

As expected, during the TAY years, one disorder may influence the emergence of, or complicate, another disorder. For instance, mood disorder, psychotic disorder, and personality disorders are linked to a two-fold increase in the likelihood of transitioning from using substances to having a SUD. SUD in general, and marijuana smoking in particular, may increase the risk for other psychiatric disorders. For instance, a growing literature supports the notion that excessive marijuana use may heighten the risk for psychosis in vulnerable youth.

SECTION 17

GERIATRIC PSYCHIATRY

Chapter 71: Geriatric Psychiatry

Geriatric Psychiatry

Multiple-Choice Questions

Select the appropriate answer.

Q1   True or False. The risk for depression in the poststroke period is LOWER than the risk for depression in Alzheimer disease.

    A. *True*

    B. *False*

Q2   True or False. The rate of suicide in the elderly is HIGHER than that of adolescents.

    A. *True*

    B. *False*

Q3   Which of the following MOST closely approximates the prevalence of the elderly population that has a problem with alcoholism?

    A. *1%*

    B. *10%*

    C. *15%*

    D. *25%*

    E. *50%*

Q4   Which of the following MOST closely approximates the prevalence of Alzheimer disease in those over age 85 years?

    A. *Less than 2%*

    B. *5% to 8%*

    C. *15% to 20%*

    D. *25% to 50%*

    E. *More than 50%*

Chapter 71

Answers

Q1 The answer is: (B) False.

The risk for depression in the poststroke period is high, with 25% to 50% developing depression within 2 years of the event. Alzheimer disease carries an increased risk of depression; approximately 20% to 30% (either before or at time of diagnosis) are diagnosed with depression; delusions are also prominent in depression associated with dementia. Recent research confirms the association of depression with the increased risk of developing late-onset Alzheimer disease.

Fifty percent of patients with Parkinson disease develop depression or have a history of depression with anxiety, dysthymia, or frontal lobe dysfunction.

Q2 The answer is: (A) True.

The rate of suicide in those older than age 65 years is nearly double that of the rate for the US population in general, and the group with the highest suicide rate of any age-group is those whose age is 65 years and older. In 1998, suicide ranked as the 16th leading cause of death among those aged 65 years; this group represented 13% of the population, but it accounted for 19% of all suicides. Suicide disproportionately affects the elderly; the suicide rate among those aged 65 to 69 years was 13.1 per 100,000 (all of the following rates are per 100,000 population), and the rates increased as age increased (i.e., it was 15.2 among those aged 70 to 74 years; it was 17.6 among those aged 75 to 79 years; it was 22.9 among those aged 80 to 84 years; and it was 21.0 among those aged 85 years or older). Firearms (71%), overdose (11%), and suffocation (11%) were the three most common methods of suicide used by persons aged 65 years or older.

Risk factors for suicide among the elderly differ from those among the young. In addition to a higher prevalence of depression, older persons are more socially isolated, and they more frequently use highly lethal methods. They also make fewer attempts per completed suicide, have a higher male-to-female ratio than other groups, have frequently visited a health care provider before their suicide, and have more physical illnesses. Approximately 20% of elderly (i.e., over age 65 years) persons who commit suicide have visited a physician within 24 hours of their death, 41% visited within 1 week of their suicide, and 75% were seen by a physician within 1 month of their suicide. Of every 100,000 people aged 65 years and older, 14.3 died by suicide in 2004. This figure is higher than the national average of 10.9 suicides per 100,000 people in the general population. White men aged 85 years or older had an even higher rate, with 17.8 suicide deaths per 100,000. Suicide rates among the elderly are highest for those who are divorced or widowed. Among men aged 75 years and older, the rate for divorced men was 3.4 times that of married men, and for widowed men it was 2.6 times that for married men. In the same age-group, the suicide rate for divorced women was 2.8 times that of married women, and for widowed women it was 1.9 times the rate among married women. Several factors (including growth in the size of that population; health status; availability of, and access to, services; and attitudes about aging and suicide) relative to those over age 65 years will play a role in future suicide rates among the elderly.

Q3 The answer is: (A) 1%.

Symptoms of problem drinking include insomnia, memory loss, confusion, anxiety, and depression, as well as somatic complaints that may mimic medical illness, further delaying accurate diagnosis.

Roughly 1% of the elderly population has a problem with alcoholism; the prevalence of alcoholism in the Epidemiological Catchment Area study was 1.5% to 3.7%. Although cross-sectional studies have suggested that the percentage of alcoholism declines after age 60 years, longitudinal studies propose a stable pattern of lifelong alcohol abuse.

Women drink less than men at all ages, but older widowed women are at risk for increasing their intake. Studies note that the prevalence of alcohol problems in women is on the rise. Older adults with alcohol dependence also have a high prevalence of comorbid nicotine dependence.

Q4 The answer is: (D) 25% to 50%.

Alzheimer disease typically affects 1% of those aged 60 years, 5% to 8% of those over age 65 years, 15% to 20% of those over age 75 years, and 25% to 50% of those over age 85 years; its course is that of a steady decline over approximately 8 to 10 years.

SECTION 18
NEUROPSYCHIATRY

Neuroanatomic Systems Relevant to Neuropsychiatric Disorders

Multiple-Choice Questions

Select the appropriate answer.

Q1 Which of the following is thought to have coined the term *limbic system* in 1878?

A. *Broca*

B. *Brodmann*

C. *MacLean*

D. *Nauta*

E. *Papez*

Q2 Which of the following brain territories is the portion of the cerebral hemisphere that is located anterior to the central sulcus?

A. *Cerebellum*

B. *Frontal lobe*

C. *Occipital cortex*

D. *Parietal lobe*

E. *Temporal lobe*

Q3 Which of the following areas is MOST closely linked with the inferior frontal gyrus of the left hemisphere?

A. *Basal ganglia (BG)*

B. *Brodmann area 17*

C. *Brodmann area 25*

D. *Brodmann area 44*

E. *Wernicke area*

Q4 Which of the following brain regions is generally considered to be located at the highest point of a sensorimotor pyramid, starting with the sensory cortices and ending at the primary motor cortex?

A. *Basal ganglia (BG)*

B. *Hippocampus*

C. *Occipital cortex*

D. *Prefrontal cortex (PFC)*

E. *Thalamus*

Q5   Which of the following was a respected railroad construction foreman who sustained damage to most of his prefrontal cortex (PFC) in a work accident?

   A.   *Brodmann*

   B.   *Gage*

   C.   *MacLean*

   D.   *Nauta*

   E.   *Papez*

Q6   Which of the following brain structures consists of the following four structures: the neostriatum (or striatum), the globus pallidus, the substantia nigra, and the subthalamic nucleus?

   A.   *Amygdala*

   B.   *Basal ganglia (BG)*

   C.   *Hippocampus*

   D.   *Hypothalamus*

   E.   *Prefrontal cortex (PFC)*

Q7   Which of the following structures is an almond-shaped group of cells located deep within the medial temporal lobe, and is comprised of several nuclei that have further subdivisions that are named partly based on their relative anatomic locations in the medial temporal lobe?

   A.   *Amygdala*

   B.   *Basal ganglia (BG)*

   C.   *Hippocampus*

   D.   *Hypothalamus*

   E.   *Reticular activating system*

Chapter 72

Answers

Q1 The answer is: (A) Broca.

The term *limbic system* was initially coined in 1878 by the French anatomist Paul Pierre Broca, who used the name the "grand lobe limbique," which means the lobe on the *margin* or *rim,* to refer to the fact that many of the cortical regions involved in emotional function are located on the medial edge or rim of the cortical mantle.

The concept has subsequently undergone many revisions since it was first described in detail in the classic paper of James Papez in 1937, and expanded and popularized by Paul MacLean in the 1950s.

The most restrictive definition of the limbic system includes only the gyrus fornicatus (the cingulate gyrus, retrosplenial cortex, and parahippocampal gyrus), the hippocampus, and the amygdala; based on a range of experimental data gathered in animals and humans (many completed by the neuroanatomist Walle Nauta), these regions were initially deemed to represent the neural substrate of emotion. Because of the observation that emotional responses are tightly linked with endocrine and autonomic functions that are largely controlled at the central nervous system level by the hypothalamus, additional regions (including the anterior thalamus, septum, substantia innominata, and piriform cortex) that have significant connections with the hypothalamus were subsequently included in the limbic system concept. Later the limbic system concept was expanded further to include telencephalic and midbrain targets of the descending fibers of the medial forebrain bundle, the "limbic forebrain-midbrain circuit," with the addition of the habenular complex, the ventral tegmental area, and dorsal raphe nuclei, among other areas. Also, because the ventral striatum receives projections from the amygdala, ventral tegmental area, and the anterior cingulate gyrus, the ventral striatum has been referred to as the "limbic striatum." Thus, in general, a region has been included in the limbic system if it appears to be involved in the generation of emotions and/or it is separated from the hypothalamus by only one or two synapses. However, it has been argued that many of the regions included in this designation are not primarily involved in emotion generation (e.g., the hippocampus participates in episodic memory processes and spatial navigation, but not directly in emotional responses). Also, distinct networks of regions may be involved in the production of different types of emotions, such as fear, joy, or sadness. However, the general concept of the limbic system has been largely retained by the majority of neuroscientists, for convenience, to indicate regions that are involved in the integration of highly processed information from the cerebral cortex with data about the state of the organism's internal milieu, to serve the overall purpose of selecting survival-promoting behaviors.

For purposes of definition, anatomists recognize and still use the nomenclature proposed by the German neuroanatomist Korbinian Brodmann.

Q2 The answer is: (B) Frontal lobe.

The portion of the cerebral hemisphere anterior to the central sulcus is termed the *frontal lobe.* A large and heterogeneous mantle of cerebral cortex covers the frontal lobe, and this cortical expanse has been the focus of intense investigation by neuroscientists. The frontal cortex is expanded significantly in primates, especially in humans, with an apparent diversification of cortical areas within it. For purposes of definition, anatomists recognize the primary motor cortex on the precentral gyrus and distinguish this area from the rest of the frontal cortex, which is termed the *prefrontal cortex* (PFC).

Q3 The answer is: (D) Brodmann area 44.

The dorsolateral prefrontal cortex (DLPFC) includes the entire cortex lying on the dorsolateral surface of the frontal lobe, bounded anteriorly by the frontal pole, posteriorly by motor areas, dorsally by the dorsomedial convexity, and ventrally by the ventrolateral convexity. It covers a large expanse in humans, typically on three gyri termed the *superior, middle,* and *inferior frontal gyri.* Almost all of the cortical areas within the DLPFC are six-layered, well-differentiated cortex.

One region of special interest is the inferior frontal gyrus of the left hemisphere, also known as Broca's area (Brodmann areas 44, 45, and some of 47). It has strong connections with the superior temporal cortex (Wernicke's area), and projections to premotor areas.

The relationship between the medial prefrontal cortex (mPFC) and subcortical brain areas related to the autonomic nervous system deserves special comment. In primates, the mPFC provides the only major cortical input to the hypothalamus, the periaqueductal gray (PAG), as well as dopaminergic, serotonergic, and noradrenergic brainstem nuclei (although there are lighter projections to these areas from the agranular and dysgranular insula, the orbitofrontal cortex [OFC], and the temporal pole). The mPFC projections to the hypothalamus and PAG are organized topographically. For example, the ventral mPFC (particularly Brodmann area 25) projects to the ventromedial nucleus of the hypothalamus and the dorsolateral PAG, whereas the anterior cingulate cortex projects to the dorsal hypothalamus and the lateral PAG. This is important because different regions within the hypothalamus and the PAG are associated with distinct functions (such as aggression, feeding, sexual behavior, thermoregulation, and antinociception).

Q4 The answer is: (D) Prefrontal cortex (PFC).

The PFC is a large and complex brain region that is best conceptualized as being located at the highest point of a sensorimotor pyramid, starting with the primary sensory cortices and ending at the primary motor cortex.

Highly processed information from sensory association areas converges onto the PFC, which then integrates the information with existing priorities, leading to the construction of adaptive behavioral plans based on this input. Different PFC sectors receive different sensory information and project to different effector areas, but the pattern is consistent. The DLPFC contains its own sensorimotor transfer machinery, whereas the OFC and mPFC are located in the same sensorimotor circuit (with OFC receiving sensory inputs, transferring relevant information to the mPFC, which then generates appropriate reactions).

Q5 The answer is: (B) Gage.

The best-known example of the consequences of PFC lesions in humans is the 19th-century story of Phineas Gage, a respected railroad construction foreman who sustained damage to most of his PFC in a work accident. After the accident, Gage became impulsive and socially inappropriate. Despite apparently having sustained no focal neurologic deficits and possessing all of his intellectual faculties, he lost his job, strained his family ties, and was left a changed person. More recently, the experience with iatrogenic PFC lesions (as a result of frontal leucotomy) has shown that humans with these procedures experience a loss of emotional regulation that manifests itself either in apathy toward emotional stimuli or in disinhibition and inappropriate intrusiveness.

Brodmann, MacLean, Nauta, and Papez were all neuroanatomists.

Q6 The answer is: (B) Basal ganglia (BG).

The basal ganglia (BG) consist of a collection of heterogeneous, tightly interconnected nuclei that reside beneath the cortical mantle. Although the BG have long been known for their role in motor function, over recent decades it has become clear that the BG nuclei are also involved in the cognitive and affective processes that drive movements. Although the precise role that the BG have in each of these domains is incompletely understood, its overall function has been inferred from knowledge of the BG anatomic connections, results of neurophysiological studies in monkeys, neuroimaging studies in humans, and studies of patients with BG disorders and lesions. These data suggest that the BG integrate a diverse range of information received from widespread areas of cortex (e.g., sensory input from the environment, memories of personal events, accumulated knowledge about the world, and current motivational states) to select and initiate goal-oriented behaviors.

The BG include four structures: the neostriatum or "striatum," the globus pallidus, the substantia nigra, and the subthalamic nucleus. The striatum, which is the major input nucleus of the BG, is divided into a medial part, the *caudate nucleus*, and a lateral part, the *putamen*, by perforating fibers of the internal capsule. Although the caudate nucleus and the putamen receive inputs from different cortical regions, their overall pattern of connections and cellular composition are the same. The division of the striatum by the internal capsule is incomplete; below the ventral border of the internal capsule lies the nucleus accumbens, which in humans does not have a distinct border with the caudate nucleus or the putamen, merging imperceptibly with these overlying structures. Also, the cellular composition of the nucleus accumbens is virtually identical to the composition of the caudate nucleus and the putamen. (The olfactory tubercle is also considered to be part of the striatum, although this structure is very small in humans.) The two main output structures of the BG are the *globus pallidus* and *substantia nigra*. The globus pallidus, or pallidal complex, is divided into an internal segment; an external segment; and the ventral pallidum (which lies ventral to the anterior commissure). The substantia nigra is comprised of the substantia nigra pars reticulata, which contains gamma-aminobutyric acid (GABA)–ergic neurons, and the substantia nigra pars compacta, which contains primarily dopaminergic neurons and is part of a larger complex of dopaminergic cell groups in the midbrain.

Q7 The answer is: (A) Amygdala.

The amygdala is an almond-shaped group of cells located deep within the medial temporal lobe, anterior and superiorly adjacent to the hippocampus depending on the rostrocaudal level. It is not a unitary structure, as it is composed of several nuclei that have further subdivisions and that are named partly based on their relative anatomic locations in the medial temporal lobe. The main medially located nuclei are the cortical, medial, and amygdalocortical transition areas (including amygdalohippocampal and amygdala pyriform transitions areas). In humans, the central amygdala is centrally and dorsally located, whereas the lateral nucleus forms the most lateral border of the amygdala.

Information flowing through the amygdala generally proceeds in a lateral-to-medial direction, from the lateral, basolateral, and basomedial nuclei to the central, medial, cortical, and transition areas. For example, no nuclei give significant back projections to the lateral nucleus, but the lateral nucleus projects to essentially all other amygdala nuclei. The basolateral nucleus also projects to most other amygdala nuclei but does not give reciprocal projection to the lateral nucleus. The basomedial nucleus does not project back to the basolateral or lateral nuclei but does project to most other amygdala nuclei (including the central nucleus). In contrast, the central nucleus projects only to the medial, cortical transition area nuclei, but not back to the basomedial, basolateral, or lateral nuclei.

The Neurologic Examination

Multiple-Choice Questions

Select the appropriate answer.

Q1 Which of the following is the interpretation and recognition of tactile sensory information?

A. *Apoptosis*

B. *Autognosis*

C. *Graphesthesia*

D. *Praxis*

E. *Stereognosis*

Q2 Which of the following is the acquired inability to perform a complex or skilled motor act in the absence of impairments of arousal, attention, language, comprehension, motivation, or sensorimotor function?

A. *Apoptosis*

B. *Apraxia*

C. *Autognosis*

D. *Graphesthesia*

E. *Stereognosis*

Q3 Which of the following cranial nerves is MOST closely associated with the sense of smell?

A. *Cranial nerve I*

B. *Cranial nerve II*

C. *Cranial nerve III*

D. *Cranial nerve IV*

E. *Cranial nerve V*

Q4 Which of the following cranial nerves control eye movements and lid elevation?

A. *Cranial nerves I, II, and III*

B. *Cranial nerves II, III, and IV*

C. *Cranial nerves III, IV, and VI*

D. *Cranial nerves VII, VIII, and IX*

E. *Cranial nerves X, XI, and XII*

Q5 Which of the following is characterized by involuntary, non-rhythmic, brief, sometimes repetitive muscle contractions that are irregular in frequency and amplitude?

A. *Asterixis*

B. *Chorea*

C. *Fasciculations*

D. *Myoclonus*

E. *Tics*

Q6 Which of the following reflexes is LEAST likely to be considered a primitive or atavistic reflex?

A. *Glabellar*

B. *Palmomental*

C. *Plantar*

D. *Snout*

E. *Suck*

Q7 In which of the following conditions is the Argyll Robertson pupil found?

A. *Brain herniation*

B. *Horner syndrome*

C. *Neurosyphilis*

D. *Progressive supranuclear palsy*

E. *Wilson disease*

Chapter 73

Answers

Q1 The answer is: (E) Stereognosis.
Stereognosis is the interpretation and recognition of tactile sensory information. Astereognosis is the inability to recognize objects by touch. This can be tested by placing common objects (such as coins, keys, paper clips, or safety pins) in the patient's hands and asking the patient to name the objects with his or her eyes closed. Characteristics (such as size and shape) can be described by the patient. Often, people can identify the denomination of coins.

Q2 The answer is: (B) Apraxia.
Apraxia is the acquired inability to perform a complex or skilled motor act in the absence of impairments of arousal, attention, language, comprehension, motivation, or sensorimotor function. *Praxis* is the Greek word for "action." More commonly described varieties include limb kinetic, buccofacial, ideomotor, and ideational apraxia. Limb kinetic apraxia is the loss of ability to make precise, coordinated fine motor movements. In buccofacial apraxia, patients are unable to perform (on request) complex acts involving the lips, mouth, and face (e.g., whistling, blowing out a match, sticking out the tongue, or coughing). Persons with ideomotor apraxia are unable to perform on command complex motor acts with one or all extremities. The patient may be unable to demonstrate on-command activities (such as saluting, waving goodbye, blowing a kiss, or pantomiming the brushing of teeth, combing of hair, hammering of a nail, or the use of scissors). They may incorrectly use their body parts as tools. Some of these patients are able to spontaneously perform these acts. The inability to perform an ideational plan consisting of a sequence of acts is referred to as an ideational apraxia.

Q3 The answer is: (A) Cranial nerve I.
Olfaction is an important sensory modality, as olfactory symptoms in psychiatric and neurologic patients are frequent. Unfortunately, psychiatrists rarely perform this portion of the examination, and neurologists uncommonly complete it. The olfactory bulbs and tracts run along the inferior surface of the frontal lobes and project to limbic areas, as well as to regions important for memory. Head trauma may be associated with loss of smell; disinhibition may result from orbital frontal injury. Tumors in the midline frontal region may cause a loss of smell, apathy, or abulia. When testing is necessary, non-irritating stimuli should be used. Alcohol and ammonia may stimulate the trigeminal nerve, and the response to this stimulation may be confused with olfaction. Bear in mind that the patient may not be able to name unfamiliar or less commonly encountered scents (such as clove or nutmeg); therefore, coffee, peppermint, wintergreen, or vanilla should be used. Each nostril should be tested individually. Abnormalities may include anosmia or misidentification of a smell.

Q4 The answer is: (C) Cranial nerves III, IV, and VI.
Eye movements and lid elevation are controlled by cranial nerves III, IV, and VI. During the examination, any spontaneous eye movements in primary resting forward gaze should be observed. The range of conjugate gaze (tested by holding your finger about 2 feet away) should be assessed next. The finger should be moved slowly to allow for assessment of voluntary smooth pursuits in the up, down, oblique, left, and right directions. Patients with Parkinson disease manifest "jerky" smooth pursuits. Ask the patient to hold his or her head still. At the limits of conjugate gaze in each direction the examiner should hold gaze for several seconds and then observe for nystagmus. When present, this is referred to as *gaze-evoked nystagmus*. Barbiturates, tranquilizers, ethanol, and anticonvulsants commonly cause gaze-evoked nystagmus in both directions of gaze. Normal saccades are involuntary, fast, conjugate changes of eye position between fixations. Saccades are tested by having the patient fixate on your nose and then look quickly toward your finger and then back to your nose. Your finger should be held in the up, down, left, and then right positions. The accuracy of saccades should be assessed. One should observe if the patient overshoots (hypermetric saccades) and then saccades back to the target. Hypermetric saccades may be seen in conditions with cerebellar involvement (such as the cerebellar presentation of multisystem atrophy). One should also

observe if the patient undershoots (hypometric saccades) with several saccades toward the target. Patients with Parkinson disease manifest hypometric saccades. One should determine if the saccades slow. Slow saccades can be seen in a number of conditions that include Wilson disease, progressive supranuclear palsy, Huntington disease, and anticonvulsant toxicity. These are just a few examples of neurologic conditions with associated eye movement abnormalities. Ptosis of the eyelids should also be noted.

Q5 The answer is: (D) Myoclonus.

Myoclonus is characterized by involuntary, non-rhythmic, brief, sometimes repetitive muscle contractions that are irregular in frequency and amplitude. They are often asynchronous and asymmetric. They may be symmetric in spinal myoclonus. They may be cortical, subcortical, or spinal in origin.

Clonus is characterized by involuntary, monophasic, rhythmic contractions and relaxations of a group of muscles.

Chorea is manifest by involuntary, non-rhythmic, jerky, rapid movements of muscle groups.

Asterixis is also known as "liver flap" or negative myoclonus. This movement is characterized by an abrupt loss of voluntary muscle tone. It is commonly elicited by asking the patient to hold his or her arms outstretched with the wrists extended. When present, the hands, with or without the arms, may suddenly drop downward and then quickly recover, which causes an irregular and slow flapping motion.

Athetosis is manifest by involuntary slow, irregular, sinuous, snake-like writhing movements.

Dystonia is an involuntary movement or sustained posture that results from abnormal tonicity of muscle. Movements may be characterized as having prolonged or repetitive muscle contractions that may result in twisting or jerking movements of the body or a body part.

Tics are defined in several ways. They are characterized by simple or complex coordinated movements or vocalizations that are repetitive, impulsive, often abrupt, and which the patient feels he or she has little or no control over. Tics are experienced as almost irresistible impulses to perform an activity. Some tics can be suppressed.

Fasciculations are brief, irregular twitches of a muscle. They may be localized to a muscle or limb or be diffuse, depending on the etiology. Fasciculations occur as a benign phenomenon, as well as a manifestation of various neuropathies (for example, amyotrophic lateral sclerosis or diabetic peripheral neuropathy), radiculopathies, thyrotoxicosis, and in association with anticholinesterase use.

Tremor is usually an involuntary, rhythmic oscillation produced by rhythmic contractions of agonist and antagonist muscles. They may be present at rest or not.

Q6 The answer is: (C) Plantar.

The plantar reflex is the most important of the cutaneous reflexes for the psychiatrist to incorporate into the examination. It is useful for detecting corticospinal tract dysfunction. One should stroke the bottom of the foot from the heel forward. The normal response is plantarflexion of the foot and toes after the first 12 to 18 months of life. Disease of the corticospinal system may be associated with extension of the toes that has been described as upgoing. The upgoing great toe with fanning of the other four toes is referred to as the Babinski sign. This may also be referred to as the extensor plantar response. Some authorities recommend stroking the lateral aspect of the plantar surface rather than the medial one, so as to avoid a plantar grasp response. Patients who are very ticklish may voluntarily withdraw from the stimulus and demonstrate flexion of the hip and knee (usually with plantarflexion of the foot and toes). A triple-flexion response is a spinal reflex characterized by hip, knee, and ankle dorsiflexion.

Primitive reflexes or atavistic reflexes (mistakenly called frontal release signs) are present at birth and disappear in most people in early infancy. There is a large portion of the normal population in which a single primitive reflex persists. This is less concerning when it is a single reflex (such as a snout, glabellar, or palmomental reflex). A grasp or suck reflex is considered more worrisome. Asymmetry or multiple primitive reflexes are considered abnormal. Primitive reflexes are not thought to be useful for localization purposes. If they reappear in later life, they may be suggestive of diffuse cerebral, subcortical, or bilateral frontal lobe pathology.

The snout reflex can be assessed by gently tapping over the patient's upper lip. If this reflex is present, a puckering of the lips will be seen. The snout reflex is present in 30% to 50% of healthy adults over age 60 years.

A suck reflex may also be elicited and is considered a more worrisome reflex. When present, the suck reflex is elicited by stimulation of the lips; this is followed by sucking movements of the lips, tongue, and jaw.

The palmomental reflex is an ipsilateral contraction of the mentalis and orbicularis oris after stimulation of the thenar region of the hand. This reflex is present in 20% to 25% of healthy adults in their 30s and 40s. The glabellar reflex is assessed by tapping the patient's glabellar ridge between the eyes with your finger. It is best to stand to the side or from behind a seated patient to not cause a visual threat response. The patient should be asked not to blink. The reflex is present if there is persistence of blinking with gentle tapping.

The grasp reflex is elicited by stroking the palm of the patient's hand. The reflex is present if the patient's fingers flex or the hand closes.

Q7 The answer is: (C) Neurosyphilis.
The Argyll Robertson pupil (that accommodates but does not react) is found in neurosyphillis.

Unilateral pupillary dilation is detected in brain herniation.

Vertical gaze palsy is noted in progressive supranuclear palsy.

Ipsilateral pupillary dilation is but one of the features of Horner syndrome.

Wilson disease is often associated with Kayser-Fleischer rings in the cornea.

Neuropsychiatric Principles and Differential Diagnosis

Multiple-Choice Questions

Select the appropriate answer.

Q1 True or False. Any disease, toxin, drug, or process that affects a particular region can be expected to show changes in behavior that are mediated by the circuits within that region.

    A. *True*

    B. *False*

Q2 Which of the following syndromes is manifest by placidity, apathy, visual and auditory agnosia, hyperorality, and hypersexuality?

    A. *Anton syndrome*

    B. *Capgras syndrome*

    C. *Cotard syndrome*

    D. *Klüver-Bucy syndrome*

    E. *Ganser syndrome*

Q3 Which of the following conditions is MOST closely associated with the orbital or medial frontal cortex, the caudate nucleus, and the globus pallidus?

    A. *Depression*

    B. *Mania*

    C. *Obsessive-compulsive disorder*

    D. *Paraphilias*

    E. *Psychosis*

Q4 Which of the following neurologic disorders is MOST closely linked with fluctuating confusion, hallucinations, delusions, depression, and an REM behavior disorder (RBD)?

    A. *Amyotrophic lateral sclerosis*

    B. *Lewy body dementia*

    C. *Multiple sclerosis*

    D. *Progressive supranuclear palsy*

    E. *Traumatic brain injury*

Q5   Which of the following statements is LEAST likely to be accurate?

A.   *Affective and psychotic disorders may occur as a result of neurologic disease and be indistinguishable from idiopathic forms*

B.   *Cortical processing of sensory information proceeds from its point of entry through association areas (with progressively more complex interconnections with other regions having sensory, memory, cognitive, emotional, and autonomic information) resulting, ultimately, in perceptual recognition and emotional meaning for experiences*

C.   *Features of the patient's clinical history and examination can be suggestive of a medical or neurologic cause of psychiatric symptoms*

D.   *Spinothalamic circuits are heavily involved in cognitive and behavioral function; disruption of them can be associated with neuropsychiatric symptoms*

E.   *Many medical and neurologic conditions are associated with neuropsychiatric symptoms. Each condition may carry unique implications for prognosis, treatment, and long-term management*

Chapter 74

Answers

Q1 The answer is: (A) True.
Neuropsychiatric dysfunction can be correlated with altered function in anatomic regions. Any disease, toxin, drug, or process that affects a region can be expected to show changes in behavior that are mediated by the circuits within that region. The limbic system and the frontal-subcortical circuits are the ones most commonly involved in neuropsychiatric dysfunction. Understanding this neuroanatomic conceptual framework can guide lesion localization and creation of a differential diagnosis. Brain trauma, ischemic disease, demyelination, abscesses, or tumors, as well as degenerative dementias, can result in behavioral disinhibition. Damage to any portion of the circuit (between the orbital frontal cortex, ventral caudate, anterior globus pallidus, or medial dorsal thalamus) can also result in disinhibition.

Q2 The answer is: (D) Klüver-Bucy syndrome.
The Klüver-Bucy syndrome (manifest by placidity, apathy, visual and auditory agnosia, hyperorality, and hypersexuality) involves injury to bilateral medial temporal-amygdalar regions. Common causes of this syndrome include herpes encephalitis, traumatic brain injury, frontotemporal dementias, and late-onset or severe Alzheimer disease.

Q3 The answer is: (C) Obsessive-compulsive disorder.
Neuropsychiatric symptoms frequently correlate with neuroanatomic territories.

Depression is associated with the frontal lobes, the left anterior frontal cortex, the anterior cingulate gyrus, the subgenu of the corpus callosum, the basal ganglia, and the left caudate.

Mania is linked with the inferomedial and ventromedial frontal cortex, the right inferomedial frontal cortex, the anterior cingulate, the caudate nucleus, the thalamus, and temporal-thalamic projections.

Apathy is associated with the anterior cingulate gyrus, the nucleus accumbens, the globus pallidus, and the thalamus.

Obsessive-compulsive disorder is linked with the orbital or medial frontal cortex, the caudate nucleus, and the globus pallidus.

Disinhibition is associated with the orbitofrontal cortex, the hypothalamus, and the septum.

Paraphilias are associated with the medial temporal cortex, the hypothalamus, the septum, and the rostral brainstem.

Hallucinations are linked with the unimodal association cortex, the orbitofrontal cortex, the paralimbic cortex, the limbic cortex, the striatum, the thalamus, and the midbrain.

Delusions are associated with the orbitofrontal cortex, the amygdala, the striatum, and the thalamus.

Psychosis is associated with the frontal lobes and the left temporal cortex.

Q4 The answer is: (B) Lewy body dementia.
Neurologic disorders are frequently associated with prominent behavioral features.

Alzheimer disease is linked with depression, irritability, anxiety, apathy, delusions, paranoia, and psychosis.

Lewy body dementia is associated with fluctuating confusion, hallucinations, delusions, depression, and an REM behavior disorder (RBD).

Vascular dementia is linked with depression, apathy, and psychosis.

Parkinson disease is associated with depression, anxiety, drug-associated hallucinations and psychosis, and an RBD.

Frontotemporal dementia is linked with early impaired judgment, disinhibition, apathy, depression, delusions, and psychosis.

Progressive supranuclear palsy is linked with disinhibition and apathy.

Traumatic brain injury is associated with depression, disinhibition, apathy, and irritability; however, psychosis is uncommon.

Huntington disease is linked with depression, irritability, delusions, mania, apathy, obsessive-compulsive disorder, and psychosis.

Corticobasal ganglionic degeneration is linked with depression, irritability, RBD, and alien-hand syndrome.

Epilepsy is associated with depression and psychosis.

HIV infection is often manifested by apathy, depression, mania, and psychosis.

Multiple sclerosis is often manifested by depression, irritability, anxiety, euphoria, and psychosis.

Amyotrophic lateral sclerosis often manifests with depression, disinhibition, apathy, and impaired judgment.

Q5 The answer is: (D) Spinothalamic circuits are heavily involved in cognitive and behavioral function; disruption of them can be associated with neuropsychiatric symptoms.

Affective and psychotic disorders may occur as a result of neurologic disease and be indistinguishable from idiopathic forms.

Cortical processing of sensory information proceeds from its point of entry through association areas (with progressively more complex interconnections with other regions having sensory, memory, cognitive, emotional, and autonomic information) resulting, ultimately, in perceptual recognition and emotional meaning for experiences.

Features of the patient's clinical history and examination can be suggestive of a medical or neurologic cause of psychiatric symptoms.

Frontal-subcortical circuits are heavily involved in cognitive and behavioral function; disruption of frontal circuits at the cortical or subcortical level by various processes can be associated with neuropsychiatric symptoms.

Many medical and neurologic conditions are associated with neuropsychiatric symptoms. Each condition may carry unique implications for prognosis, treatment, and long-term management.

Chapter 75

Neuroimaging in Psychiatry

Multiple-Choice Questions

Select the appropriate answer.

Q1 Which of the following tests uses multiple serially acquired X-rays that are attenuated to varying degrees depending on the material through which they pass?

    A. *Computed tomography (CT)*

    B. *Functional magnetic resonance imaging*

    C. *Magnetic resonance imaging (MRI)*

    D. *Positron emission tomography (PET)*

    E. *Single-photon emission computed tomography (SPECT)*

Q2 True or False. With ionic contrast, idiosyncratic reactions (including nausea, flushing, hypotension, urticaria, and sometimes frank anaphylaxis) occur in approximately 5% of cases.

    A. *True*

    B. *False*

Q3 True or False. Because computed tomography (CT) scanning is readily available, it is commonly used to detect bleeding in pregnancy.

    A. *True*

    B. *False*

Q4 When using magnetic resonance imaging (MRI) scans, which of the following images are BEST for the detection of pathology?

    A. *Axial images*

    B. *Coronal images*

    C. *Sagittal images*

    D. *T1-weighted images*

    E. *T2-weighted images*

Q5 Which of the following tests relies on use of isotopes that are created via particle acceleration in a cyclotron?

    A. *Computed tomography (CT)*

    B. *Magnetic resonance imaging (MRI)*

    C. *Positron emission tomography (PET)*

    D. *Single-photon emission computed tomography (SPECT)*

    E. *X-rays*

Q6 Which of the following tests measures cerebral blood flow (CBF) and primarily cortical function?

    A. *Computed tomography (CT)*

    B. *Magnetic resonance imaging (MRI)*

    C. *Positron emission tomography (PET)*

    D. *Single-photon emission computed tomography (SPECT)*

    E. *X-rays*

Q1 The answer is: (A) Computed tomography (CT).

Computed tomography (CT) uses multiple serially acquired X-rays that are attenuated to varying degrees depending on the material through which they pass. For example, low-attenuation materials (such as air or fluid) appear dark on a CT image, whereas high-attenuation materials (such as bone) appear white. Gradations within the spectrum of attenuation allow for the visual differentiation of brain tissue. The serially acquired X-rays are acquired in a rotating axial manner, and these data are then reconstructed using computerized algorithms. The resulting CT image is therefore always an axial image (i.e., sagittal and coronal image reconstruction is not possible). The spatial resolution of CT has improved over the years and is as low as 1 mm.

Q2 The answer is: (A) True.

CT contrast is typically (but not always) ionic contrast that is radiopaque (i.e., it has very high X-ray attenuation, meaning that it appears white on the CT image). The CT contrast is introduced intravenously. Therefore, CT contrast is especially useful for visualization of lesions that compromise the integrity of the blood–brain barrier (e.g., cerebrovascular accidents, tumors, and inflammation).

Non-ionic contrast is also available but is many times more expensive than is ionic contrast.

However, ionic contrast is associated with a greater risk of side effects. With ionic contrast, idiosyncratic reactions (including nausea, flushing, hypotension, urticaria, and sometimes frank anaphylaxis) occur in approximately 5% of cases. Those at highest risk for idiosyncratic reactions include the young and the old (less than age 1 year or greater than age 60 years), and those with a history of cerebrovascular disease, asthma, allergies, and, of course, prior contrast reactions. Ionic contrast is also associated with chemotoxic reactions that can occur in the kidney and the brain. Chemotoxic reactions in the kidney include impaired renal function and renal failure. The main risk factor for renal chemotoxic reactions to ionic contrast is pre-existing renal insufficiency. Chemotoxic reactions in the brain typically manifest as seizures. These usually only occur in 1 in every 10,000 cases but may occur in up to 10% of cases in which gross disruption of the blood–brain barrier exists.

Q3 The answer is: (B) False.

CT is particularly useful for the detection of acute bleeding (less than 24 to 72 hours old) or acute trauma, but it is not the modality of choice for subacute bleeding (more than 72 hours old), or for patients who are markedly anemic (i.e., with a hemoglobin less than approximately 10 g/dL). Magnetic resonance imaging (MRI) (described later) is superior to CT for most other clinical situations.

However, because CT uses ionizing radiation, it is strongly contraindicated in pregnancy and is relatively contraindicated in children.

Q4 The answer is: (E) T2-weighted images.

MRI does not use radiation; instead, it uses strong magnetic fields and the magnetic properties of hydrogen atoms to create structural images. Hydrogen atoms in water act as small magnets when introduced into a magnetic field. In other words, the molecules align themselves in the same direction when introduced to the magnetic field. This alignment requires energy; when the magnetic field is removed, the atoms relax, giving off energy that is used to construct the images. This relaxation can occur at different rates with each relaxation rate resulting in imaging data that may be optimal for different clinical circumstances. For example, T1-weighted and T2-weighted images are two commonly used MRI parameters that differ in relaxation rates. T1-weighted images are best for visualizing normal anatomy, whereas T2-weighted images are better for detecting pathology. In contrast to CT images (which can only be viewed in the axial plane), MRI images can be reconstructed in multiple planes (i.e., axial, sagittal, and coronal) for more comprehensive viewing.

Q5 The answer is: (C) Positron emission tomography (PET).

As its name suggests, positron emission tomography (PET) uses the energy emitted by positrons from radionuclides to measure brain function. Positron-emitting radionuclides are unstable isotopes that are created via particle acceleration in cyclotrons. Although isotopes can be created for many atoms, because PET is used to study biological systems, isotopes for hydrogen (^{18}F), carbon (^{11}C), oxygen (^{15}O), and nitrogen (^{13}N) are typically used.

As the positively charged positrons are emitted from these unstable isotopes, they quickly contact negatively charged electrons. The resulting collision, termed an *annihilation event,* results in the emission of gamma rays. It is these gamma rays that the PET camera detects and uses to construct functional images. Fortunately, following an annihilation event, these gamma rays are emitted at exactly 180° from each other at a specific energy. Therefore, each annihilation event results in a line of coincidence. The time differential between gamma rays reaching detectors 180° from one another allows for accurate assessment of where the annihilation event took place within the brain.

In the clinical setting, PET is typically used to assess cerebral blood flow (CBF) (using ^{15}O) or cerebral glucose metabolism (using ^{18}F fluorodeoxyglucose). Both CBF and cerebral glucose are tightly coupled to neuronal activity, and thus serve as powerful measures of brain function. PET is the gold standard for clinical functional neuroimaging studies, as it has excellent spatial resolution (4 to 8 mm). However, PET is also very expensive because it requires proximity to a cyclotron.

Q6 The answer is: (D) Single-photon emission computed tomography (SPECT).

Single-photon emission computed tomography (SPECT) uses radionuclides for functional brain imaging. However, SPECT cannot measure cerebral glucose metabolism. Instead, radionuclides such as 99mTc-HMPAO are used to measure CBF. Instead of an annihilation event resulting in detection of dual photons (as is the case with PET), the radionuclides used for SPECT studies emit only a single photon. Therefore, lines of coincidence cannot be used to localize function within brain tissue as accurately as can be achieved with PET. The spatial resolution of SPECT is somewhat inferior (less than 8 mm) to that of PET. In addition, single-photon emission results in particularly inferior spatial resolution within deep brain structures. SPECT is most useful for assessing cortical brain function. Nonetheless, SPECT does have some advantages over PET. It is more widely available, is typically less expensive, and does not require an on-site cyclotron.

Clinical Neurophysiology and Electroencephalography

Multiple-Choice Questions

Select the appropriate answer.

Q1 In which year did the German neuropsychiatrist Hans Berger first demonstrate the *Elektrenkephalogramm* as a graphic representation of electrical activity in the human brain?

    A. *1712*

    B. *1857*

    C. *1929*

    D. *1935*

    E. *1972*

Q2 True or False. The electroencephalogram (EEG) has excellent temporal resolution but relatively poor spatial resolution; it can detect rapid changes in function, but it has difficulty localizing abnormalities.

    A. *True*

    B. *False*

Q3 True or False. Although the precise origin of the electrical activity is unknown, EEG activity recorded from the scalp is believed to originate from the postsynaptic potential of the neurons of the cortical pyramidal layer of the cortex.

    A. *True*

    B. *False*

Q4 Which of the following Greek letters is associated with a frequency of 8 to 13 Hz?

    A. *Alpha*

    B. *Beta*

    C. *Delta*

    D. *Gamma*

    E. *Theta*

Q5 Which of the following stages of sleep is MOST closely associated with sleep spindles?

    A. *Stage I*

    B. *Stage II*

    C. *Stage III*

    D. *Stage IV*

    E. *Rapid eye movement*

Q6   True or False. A spike on the EEG is a single wave that stands out from the background activity and has a duration of between 70 and 200 ms.

A. *True*

B. *False*

Q7   True or False. A normal EEG excludes the diagnosis of epilepsy.

A. *True*

B. *False*

Q8   True or False. The MOST common use of evoked potentials is to test the speed of conduction in a particular pathway.

A. *True*

B. *False*

Q9   True or False. The cell bodies of sensory neurons are located in the skin.

A. *True*

B. *False*

Chapter 76

Answers

Q1 The answer is: (C) 1929.

The history of the electroencephalogram (EEG) may be traced back to the 1700s when Luigi Galvani demonstrated that electrical stimulation of a peripheral nerve in a frog caused contraction. In the mid-19th century, Carlo Matteucci and Emil du Bois-Reymond established the field of electrophysiology. In 1929, the German neuropsychiatrist Hans Berger demonstrated the *Elektrenkephalogramm* as a graphic representation of electrical activity in the human brain. In 1935, Frederic and Erna Gibbs with William Lennox recorded the EEG in patients with epilepsy and demonstrated its clinical utility. The synaptic origin of the EEG was demonstrated by Renshaw in the 1940s. Starting in the 1950s, intracranial implantation of EEG electrodes was used for evaluation of epilepsy surgery. During this period, systematic description of sleep architecture with the EEG was also described. Computerized EEG acquisition and analysis have been possible since the 1970s. Long-term recording of simultaneous video and EEG tracings revolutionized the evaluation of epilepsy on many fronts.

Q2 The answer is: (A) True.

The EEG records low-voltage electrical activity produced by the brain. Recordings are often characteristic of certain ages and states of consciousness. Although primarily used to detect epileptic abnormalities, it is possible to recognize generalized malfunction of the brain, sleep disturbances, and other localized or paroxysmal abnormalities. The EEG has excellent temporal resolution but relatively poor spatial resolution; it can detect rapid changes in function, but it has difficulty localizing abnormalities.

Most commonly, the EEG is recorded from the scalp with small surface electrodes. However, other electrodes are sometimes used under special circumstances. Intracranial electrodes may be placed in the subdural or epidural space, or deep in the brain (as depth electrodes in patients with epilepsy). These are used to record electrical signals with much greater spatial resolution and sensitivity than can be achieved with surface electrodes; in addition, electrical signals may be applied to the electrodes to perform brain mapping.

Q3 The answer is: (A) True.

Although the precise origin of the electrical activity is unknown, EEG activity recorded from the scalp is believed to originate from the postsynaptic potential of the neurons of the cortical pyramidal layer of the cortex. These charges form an electrical dipole, with a positive charge on one end and a negative charge on the other; this creates an electrical field. The summation of the electrical fields may be recorded by surface electrodes.

The EEG records differences in electric fields, rather than a single action potential. As such, the voltage difference between two electrodes is measured by an amplifier; it is impossible to record from a single electrode. Each pair of electrodes outputs the difference between their potentials through a single channel, which may be graphically displayed on paper or on a computer monitor. The typical EEG machine connects a minimum of 21 electrodes and can display 16 (or more) channels. Electrical activity is recorded from a variety of standard sites on the scalp, according to a standard layout scheme (called the 10-20 International System of Electrode Placement) that can be easily replicated in all laboratories. Careful calibration of the signal intensity needs to be performed before each recording.

Q4 The answer is: (A) Alpha.

The electrical activity from any electrode pair on the EEG can be described in terms of amplitude and frequency. Amplitude ranges from 5 to 200 uV. The frequency of EEG activity ranges from 0 Hz to about 20 Hz. The frequencies are described by Greek letters: delta (0 to 3 Hz), theta (4 to 7 Hz), alpha (8 to 13 Hz), and beta (more than 13 Hz).

Q5 The answer is: (B) Stage II.

Drowsiness is stage I sleep. As sleep becomes deeper, high-voltage single or complex theta or delta waves, called vertex sharp waves, appear centrally. Stage II sleep is characterized by increased numbers of vertex sharp waves and runs of sinusoidal 12 to 14 Hz beta activity, called sleep spindles, occur. Deeper sleep (stage III, "slow wave" sleep), characterized by progressively more and higher-voltage delta activity, is not usually seen in routine EEG recordings.

Q6 The answer is: (B) False.

Paroxysmal abnormalities include the spike and the sharp wave. A spike is a single wave that stands out from the background activity and lasts less than 70 ms. A sharp wave is similar but lasts between 70 and 200 ms. A spike or sharp wave has an asymmetric up and down phase and is often followed by a slow wave. The existence of a spike or sharp wave is highly specific; a single sharp wave in the proper clinical context may be sufficient to confirm a seizure disorder. However, such findings are insensitive; the EEG is frequently normal and devoid of such discharges even in patients known to have epilepsy. Multiple recordings may be required to capture an abnormality and to make a diagnosis.

Q7 The answer is: (B) False.

A normal EEG does not exclude epilepsy because the EEG may be normal during a focal seizure that is observed clinically.

Q8 The answer is: (A) True.

Evoked potentials can be used to test the integrity of a pathway in the central nervous system. A sensory stimulus in any modality (e.g., visual, auditory, or somatosensory) will produce a change in the EEG. The change is usually small compared with the background EEG; the exact configuration of the change depends on the nature of the stimulus and the site of the recording on the scalp. The evoked potential is the change in the EEG, which is dependent on, and time-locked to, the stimulus; to see it, the stimulus must be repeated many times and the EEG averaged.

The most common use of evoked potentials is to test the speed of conduction in a particular pathway. Multiple sclerosis is a disease of central myelin; if myelin is damaged, conduction is slowed, and the evoked potentials will be delayed. Although many multiple sclerosis plaques are clinically silent, they often show themselves with this electrical test. Therefore, evoked potentials are quite useful in making the diagnosis of multiple sclerosis.

Visual evoked potentials were the first to become popular. They are ordinarily obtained with a checkerboard stimulus that alternates black and white squares repetitively. Each eye is stimulated individually and then responses are measured from the occipital area of the scalp. The major wave measured is a large positive wave at a latency of about 100 ms (P100). In multiple sclerosis or optic neuritis, the wave is delayed. Delayed or absent visual evoked potentials can be seen in many other conditions, including ocular conditions (e.g., glaucoma), compressive lesions of the optic nerve (e.g., pituitary lesions), and pathological conditions of the optic radiations or the occipital cortex.

Auditory stimulation produces complex waveforms. Stimulation with brief clicks produces six small waves in the first 10 ms. Quite surprisingly, the sources of this electrical activity are in serial ascending structures in the brainstem. It becomes possible to study the integrity of the brainstem with these waves, and the test has also been used to assess "brainstem death" in cases suspected of "brain death." The waves are also delayed in multiple sclerosis.

Somatosensory evoked potentials (SEPs) are the averaged electrical responses in the central nervous system to somatosensory stimulation. Like sensory nerve action potentials in the peripheral nervous system, most components of SEPs represent activity carried in the large sensory fibers of the dorsal column (medial lemniscus primary sensorimotor cortex pathway). SEPs can be used to test the integrity of the pathway and to test the speed of conduction in the pathway. SEPs from the upper extremity are commonly produced by stimulation of the median nerve at the wrist. The cerebral SEP to this type of stimulation was the first evoked potential to be discovered. The cerebral SEP to median nerve stimulation is best recorded from a site approximately 2 cm posterior to the contralateral central electrode. SEPs from the lower extremity are produced by stimulation of the posterior tibial nerve at the ankle or the peroneal nerve at the fibular head and are recorded best at the vertex of the head.

Q9 The answer is: (B) False.

The cell bodies of sensory neurons are located in the dorsal root ganglia. Each neuron has a central process entering the spinal cord through the dorsal horn and a peripheral process connecting to a sensory receptor in the skin or deep tissues of the limb. The receptors transduce somatosensory stimuli into electrical potentials, which eventually give rise to action potentials in the axons that are transmitted along the peripheral process to the central process. This is called the sensory nerve action potential. There are a variety of sensory neurons, each with a characteristic spectrum of axonal diameters. Some neurons are myelinated, whereas some are unmyelinated; in routine studies the unmyelinated fibers cannot be measured. Many sensory axons with differing function and size run together with motor axons.

Psychiatric Manifestations and Treatment of Seizure Disorders

Multiple-Choice Questions

Select the appropriate answer.

Q1 Which of the following is LEAST likely to be associated with the development of seizures and epilepsy?

A. *Alcohol use and abuse*

B. *Brain tumor*

C. *Cerebrovascular disease*

D. *Dementia*

E. *Marijuana use*

Q2 True or False. Cryptogenic epilepsies are associated with epileptic seizures without other neurologic or structural abnormalities of the brain.

A. *True*

B. *False*

Q3 True or False. Petit mal seizures are a form of generalized seizures.

A. *True*

B. *False*

Q4 True or False. Simple partial seizures are the MOST common type of seizures seen in adult medicine.

A. *True*

B. *False*

Q5 True or False. Psychomotor symptoms of complex partial seizures may take the form of complex actions, such as disrobing.

A. *True*

B. *False*

Q6 Which of the following BEST describes the sensation of insects crawling under the skin?

A. *Akathisia*

B. *An automatism*

C. *Chorea*

D. *Formication*

E. *Fornication*

Q7   Which of the following BEST describes the feeling of unfamiliarity as part of a complex partial seizure?

   A.   *Déjà vu*

   B.   *Derealization*

   C.   *Dissociation*

   D.   *Formication*

   E.   *Jamais vu*

Q8   Which of the following is the MOST common affective symptom associated with complex partial seizures?

   A.   *Anger*

   B.   *Depression*

   C.   *Fear*

   D.   *Irritation*

   E.   *Joy*

Q9   True or False. In a simple partial seizure, consciousness is maintained.

   A.   *True*

   B.   *False*

Q10 Which of the following is the name of the anterior transverse temporal gyrus from which auditory seizures are produced by discharges associated with partial seizures?

   A.   *Broca convolution*

   B.   *Geschwind gyrus*

   C.   *Hecker gyrus*

   D.   *Heschl convolution*

   E.   *Nauta niche*

Q11 Which of the following is the sensitivity of a single electroencephalogram (EEG) for the detection of epilepsy?

   A.   *Less than 5%*

   B.   *5% to 25%*

   C.   *30% to 50%*

   D.   *55% to 75%*

   E.   *More than 90%*

Q12 True or False. Patients with nonepileptic psychogenic seizures frequently have an antecedent history of sexual or other psychological trauma, and they are much more likely to be women.

   A.   *True*

   B.   *False*

Q13 Which type of epilepsy is MOST closely associated with a set of interictal personality changes?

   A.   *Complex partial seizures*

   B.   *Jacksonian seizures*

   C.   *Petit mal seizures*

   D.   *Pseudoseizures*

   E.   *Simple partial seizures*

Answers

Q1 The answer is: (E) Marijuana use.

Epilepsy is the most common neurologic disorder after strokes. Its incidence varies widely from country to country but is estimated to be between 40 and 70 per 100,000 person-years in developed countries. The incidence of epilepsy is high during infancy, decreases in adulthood, but increases with advancing age.

Most structural brain lesions increase the risk for seizures and epilepsy. Known risk factors for epilepsy include head trauma, cerebrovascular diseases, brain tumors, congenital or genetic abnormalities, infectious diseases, alcohol/drug use, and dementia. The relationship of marijuana use and seizure disorders is unclear.

Q2 The answer is: (B) False.

Idiopathic epilepsies are associated with epileptic seizures without other neurologic or structural abnormalities of the brain. They tend to have a genetic predisposition, an age-related onset, and are generally benign. Symptomatic epilepsies are secondary to a specific cerebral abnormality, either genetic (e.g., tuberous sclerosis), or acquired (e.g., trauma). A third category, the cryptogenic group, refers to epilepsies that are not idiopathic, but in which the underlying condition causing the symptomatic epilepsy cannot be detected.

Q3 The answer is: (A) True.

Absence ("petit mal") seizures are a form of generalized seizures. Absence seizures occur mainly during childhood and are less frequent after puberty. They are characterized by the arrest or suspension of consciousness for 5 to 10 seconds. Parents may not notice the typical brief seizures in an otherwise healthy child, but teachers will report that the child stares absently for short intervals throughout the day. Without treatment, absence seizures may occur up to 70 to 100 times a day, and such frequent blackouts can seriously impair a child's school performance. The physician can usually confirm the diagnosis by asking the child to hyperventilate because this maneuver will precipitate an attack. Other signs include rhythmic blinking (at a rate of 3 blinks/second) and rudimentary motor behaviors, called automatisms, which also occur in adult temporal lobe epilepsy (TLE). Absence seizures are the easiest seizure disorder to diagnose because of its pathognomic electroencephalogram (EEG) (a spike-and-wave pattern that occurs at a frequency of 3 cycles/second), especially when the child hyperventilates.

Q4 The answer is: (B) False.

Complex partial seizures are the most common type of seizures seen in adult medicine. They are characterized by an alteration of consciousness, as well as by other complex manifestations; they are also the most difficult to diagnose and to treat. Patients may experience any or all of four symptom types: psychomotor, psychosensory, cognitive, and affective.

Q5 The answer is: (A) True.

Psychomotor symptoms or "automatisms" may take the form of simple vegetative movements or complex actions, such as disrobing. The most common automatisms are oral and buccal movements (e.g., lip smacking, licking, or chewing), and the picking behaviors that are sometimes seen in patients with dementia. In some cases, these individuals may pick at their skin to the point of maceration. Walking is one of the most interesting automatisms that may occur during a complex partial seizure. The physician should not attempt to prevent such behavior during a seizure because the patient may become violent if restrained. When questioned about their behavior, patients often say they have the urge to leave their present location, and some may drive off or go to the bus station or airport out of a desire to travel. Psychomotor symptomatology also includes staring behavior similar to that seen in absence epilepsy. However, unlike absence seizures that last only about 6 seconds, staring episodes in complex partial seizures typically last about 1 to 3 minutes, long enough to be recognized.

Q6 The answer is: (D) Formication.

Psychosensory symptoms of complex partial seizures include visual, auditory, and other sensory symptoms. Although psychosensory symptoms are most often owing to a lesion in the temporal lobe, a parietal lobe lesion may also cause them. Patients generally describe their psychosensory symptoms as being similar to some other sensation or experience. For example, the patient may describe the sensation of insects crawling under the skin, a common paresthesia called formication. This may at least partially explain the scratching or picking automatisms seen in some patients. The visual phenomenon is not merely flashes of lights, but true hallucinations, such as the detonation of a bomb or a display of "fireworks." Olfactory or uncinate fits are also common and usually take the form of a noxious smell (e.g., burning rubber) or a metallic taste. It is important to question patients about olfactory or gustatory symptoms because they generally do not mention these sensations unless asked directly.

Q7 The answer is: (E) Jamais vu.

Cognitive symptoms of complex partial seizures may be simple or take the form of hallucinatory experiences similar to those reported by patients with psychosis. Unlike psychotic hallucinations, which may take various forms in an individual patient, the hallucinations that occur as part of a complex partial seizure are stereotypical and repetitive. Patients commonly envision scenes involving water. The perception that objects are getting bigger (macropsia) or smaller (micropsia) may also be reported.

Other cognitive symptoms include the feeling of familiarity known as *déjà vu* (French for "already seen") and, more commonly, the feeling of unfamiliarity referred to as *jamais vu* (French for "never seen"). Children generally find it easy to describe *jamais vu*, whereas adults find the sensation confusing and disturbing.

Q8 The answer is: (C) Fear.

Affective symptoms, or ictal emotions, are another characteristic of complex partial seizures. In some cases, patients with affective symptoms do not realize they are having a seizure. Because fear and anxiety are the most common affective symptoms reported in TLE, it is always important to rule out this possibility while considering the differential diagnosis of panic disorder. The diagnosis of complex partial seizures is further complicated by the fact that depression is a common affective symptom in the general population. However, unlike other types of depression, depression related to seizures begins and ends abruptly. Pleasant ictal feelings may also occur, but they are very rare. Some women may experience orgasms; the corresponding feeling in the male genitalia is generally an uncomfortable penile sensation. Although rage reactions and aggression are sometimes associated with TLE, these behaviors are extremely rare.

Q9 The answer is: (A) True.

In a simple partial seizure, consciousness is maintained. Because much of the motor cortex is devoted to controlling the face and hands, focal motor seizures most commonly affect these parts of the body. Motor movements may spread along the body, usually starting in the hands and then affecting other areas, such as the face and the upper half of the body. This is known as the "Jacksonian march." There is almost never movement of the hip or trunk. Motor seizures may also occur when the lesion (particularly a tumor) affects the frontal lobe. Turning of the head and eyes away from the side of the focus is an aversive seizure. In what is sometimes called a "fencing seizure," the arm also flexes ipsilateral to the focus and extends contralateral to the focus.

Simple partial seizures also include a large subgroup of sensory seizures that can be difficult to diagnose. The vertiginous seizure, originating in the temporal lobe, is probably the most common type of sensory seizure; as dizziness has a broad differential diagnosis, evaluation of this seizure can be challenging. Somatosensory seizures are usually described as a tingling feeling (paresthesia) or by a sensation of heat or water running over the affected area; this sensation may spread rapidly from one body part to another. Rarely, a patient will report pain or a burning sensation, as well as various auras. Somatosensory seizures may mimic transient ischemic attacks of the middle cerebral artery or migraines. However, with careful evaluation of the patient's history, it is possible to distinguish the three conditions clinically.

Q10 The answer is: (D) Heschl convolution.

Auditory seizures are produced by discharges in the anterior transverse temporal gyrus (Heschl convolution) and the superior temporal convolution. The patient reports tinnitus typically in the form of hissing, buzzing, or roaring sounds. Visual seizures, produced by discharges from the occipital focus, take the form of flickering lights or flashing colors (usually red or white), and are distinct from the "zig-zag" pattern of light sometimes reported by patients experiencing migraine. It is worth noting that nearly all epileptic patients have migrainous headaches and many migraine sufferers have abnormal EEGs. Despite the overlap between these two conditions, the visual features just described can help one distinguish migraines from simple partial seizures due to epilepsy.

Q11 The answer is: (C) 30% to 50%.
All patients with a new seizure or suspected seizure disorder should obtain an EEG. The sensitivity of a single EEG is relatively low (ranging from 30% to 50%) in the detection of epileptiform abnormalities, but the yield may be increased (to 80% to 90%) by obtaining multiple EEGs, an ambulatory 24-hour EEG, or a sleep-deprived EEG. Hyperventilation and photic stimulation (flashing lights) during the EEG may further increase the yield of the EEG in limited circumstances.

Q12 The answer is: (A) True.
Non-epileptic psychogenic seizures ("pseudoseizures" or "psychogenic seizures") represent a large and challenging subgroup of patients evaluated for a seizure disorder. They may represent up to 30% of patients with seizures refractory to traditional antiseizure medications. Most frequently, these seizures are a form of conversion disorder in which the patient produces these seizures without conscious effort and without an obvious secondary gain. Patients with non-epileptic psychogenic seizures frequently have an antecedent history of sexual or other psychological trauma, and they are much more likely to be women.

Although pre-existing risk factors and description of seizures (such as pelvic thrusting) can be helpful in raising suspicion of non-epileptic psychogenic seizures, conclusive diagnosis usually requires the use of video-EEG monitoring during which a typical episode is captured. Hyperkinetic frontal lobe seizures may mimic non-epileptic psychomotor seizures, leading to substantial difficulties in reaching the correct diagnosis in a small portion of patients.

Although excellent outcomes have anecdotally been reported if an underlying psychiatric conflict can be identified and resolved, these are often difficult to identify, and no definitive treatment exists for this condition. More than 70% of patients continue to have seizures chronically, a considerably higher rate than with patients with epileptic seizures. Unlike prevailing beliefs, the number of patients with non-epileptic psychogenic seizures and epileptic seizures is low.

Q13 The answer is: (A) Complex partial seizures.
Norman Geschwind described the following five personality changes associated with complex partial seizures: hypergraphia, hyperreligiosity, hyposexuality, aggressivity, and viscosity.

Some patients with epilepsy are deeply interested in religion, although not necessarily one of the world's major religions. In some adult patients, the onset of seizures coincides with a sudden loss of an interest in sex. Considering that patients rarely volunteer this information, the physician should make a point of asking whether the patient has noticed any change in sexual desire. Some patients with TLE also report a change in their sexual preference.

Aggressivity, the fourth type of personality change associated with epilepsy, is distinct from the automatic aggressive behavior occasionally seen during seizures. Again, patients often do not volunteer information about this type of personality change. If patients are asked about their temper, they may become defensive or evasive. On further questioning, one might learn that they engage in aggressive behavior (such as breaking dishes or throwing objects out of a window).

Finally, some patients with epilepsy develop a personality trait Geschwind called viscosity, meaning that the patients tend to be "sticky." Some patients with TLE may call the physician every night, and once they start talking they will not stop. These five characteristic personality disturbances provide evidence that brain lesions can cause long-term changes in behavior.

Differential Diagnosis and Treatment of Headaches

Multiple-Choice Questions

Select the appropriate answer.

Q1 Which of the following types of headaches is the MOST common?

    A. *Cluster headache*

    B. *Medication overuse headache*

    C. *Migraine headache*

    D. *Primary exertional headache*

    E. *Tension-type headache*

Q2 In which of the following types of headaches do the headaches occur more commonly in women, usually present with a unilateral pulsatile pain in the frontotemporal region or around the eye, frequently present with photophobia, phonophobia, nausea, and vomiting, and begin after ingestion of certain foods?

    A. *Cluster headache*

    B. *Medication overuse headache*

    C. *Migraine headache*

    D. *Primary exertional headache*

    E. *Tension-type headache*

Q3 True or False. Classic migraines occur in a minority of migraine sufferers.

    A. *True*

    B. *False*

Q4 Which of the following conditions is MOST likely to manifest with a "thunderclap headache"?

    A. *Cluster headache*

    B. *Meningitis*

    C. *Migraine headache*

    D. *Subarachnoid hemorrhage (SAH)*

    E. *Tension-type headache*

Q5   Which of the following causes of headache is MOST closely associated with an erythrocyte sedimentation rate above 40 in over 90% of cases?

A.   *Cluster headache*

B.   *Migraine headache*

C.   *Temporal arteritis*

D.   *Tension-type headache*

E.   *Trigeminal neuralgia*

Chapter 78
Answers

Q1 The answer is: (E) Tension-type headache.

The lifetime prevalence of the most common of headaches, the tension-type headache, is estimated at 30% to 78%, although most everyone has had this type of headache at one time or another.

Tension-type headache may result from persistent peripheral nociceptive hyperstimulation and may share many of the pathophysiological features of migraine. Whether tension-type headache is ultimately viewed as a variation of migraine or as a separate pathological condition remains unsettled. Recent information suggests a central, possibly hypothalamic cause for cluster headaches with important peripheral trigeminovascular activation as well.

Tension-type headache is somewhat more common in women than in men. Pain is generally the main complaint; there is little associated photophobia, phonophobia, or hyperacusis. Nausea may be a complaint as well, but vomiting is rare. Patients usually describe the pain as bilateral, bandlike, steady, and mild to moderate in intensity. Increased tenderness in the muscles of the head, the frontal, temporal, masseter, pterygoid, sternocleidomastoid, splenius, and trapezius, can sometimes be demonstrated with palpation using the second and third digits, but its absence does not rule out the disorder. Researchers may use a palpometer to measure muscle tenderness. Most patients can continue to function with tension-type headaches.

Q2 The answer is: (C) Migraine headache.

Migraine headaches have been classified as vascular headaches, although recent evidence suggests that dysfunction of neurotransmitter systems (e.g., substance P, neurokinin A, and serotonin) are involved in the pathophysiology. Migraines are more common in women (occurring in up to 20% of women). The female-to-male ratio for migraines is 3:2. These headaches tend to run in the families, with 70% of patients having a family history of migraines. Migraine symptomatology may be complex, but for an individual patient, headache occurs in a recurrent stereotyped manner.

Migraines usually manifest with a unilateral pulsatile pain in the frontotemporal region or around the eye. In half of patients, the pain eventually spreads to both sides of the head. The pain may become dull and symmetrical like that of a tension-type headache. Photophobia and phonophobia are common features. Autonomic dysfunction arises and includes slowed gastric emptying, nausea, and vomiting that can cause severe disability. The length of the headache can vary, but it usually lasts from 4 to 24 hours. Migraines may be precipitated by ingestion of certain foods (e.g., aged cheese, red wine, chocolate, and nuts), by skipping meals, by too little sleep, by too much sleep, and by psychological stress. Often, the weekends or the start of a vacation can precipitate a migraine. In women, migraines often begin at menarche and recur premenstrually. Contraceptive medication may worsen migraines in some women, whereas in others it may improve symptoms. Pregnancy offers relief from migraines in about three-fourths of women. Migraine symptoms often improve when patients reach their 30s and 40s. Nocturnal migraines arise during rapid eye movement sleep.

Q3 The answer is: (A) True.

Classic migraines (that occur in only about 15% of migraine sufferers) are preceded by an aura, usually a visual change (such as a field cut or scotoma), or flashing zig-zag lines (scintillations). Auras (any transient neurologic alteration) typically evolve over several minutes and can last up to an hour. Hallucinations (e.g., visual, olfactory, auditory, or gustatory), motor deficits (e.g., hemiparesis or hemiplegia), paresthesias (e.g., of the lips and hands especially), aphasia, perceptual impairments, anxiety, and depression are varieties of migraine auras. On rare occasions an aura may not be followed by a headache, and it can mimic other neurologic disorders (e.g., stroke, psychosis, or intoxication). By contrast, common migraines are those without an aura.

Patients who suffer from migraines are often debilitated by them and attempt to avoid sensory input to soothe sensory hypersensitivity (allodynia). They seek out dark, quiet rooms and prefer to be alone.

Q4 The answer is: (D) Subarachnoid hemorrhage (SAH).

A "thunderclap headache" is the classic description of the presentation of subarachnoid hemorrhage (SAH), but there are other causes of an excruciating and sudden headache (e.g., arterial dissection, cerebral venous thrombosis, unruptured vascular malformation, pituitary apoplexy, central nervous system hypotension, acute sinusitis, and a colloid cyst of the third ventricle).

SAH is caused by rupture of a cerebral artery or of a cerebrovascular malformation. The fatality rate with SAH is nearly 50%, and half of the survivors have severe deficits. The most common site of such a rupture is the circle of Willis. The sudden onset (reaching its peak within a minute) of a severe headache is the most common presentation, and it is often associated with nuchal rigidity. SAH often occurs during exertion (e.g., exercise, sexual intercourse, or straining on the toilet). Initially, there may be fever, nausea, vomiting, seizures, lethargy, and even coma. Focal neurologic deficits and retinal hemorrhages point toward SAH. A head computed tomography scan is needed to rule out an ischemic stroke. Diagnosis can usually be made on seeing blood on a non-contrast computed tomography scan or in the cerebrospinal fluid during a lumbar puncture.

Occasionally, SAH may be the result of vascular leaks, or sentinel bleeds, and the presentation is not quite as dramatic. Risk factors for SAH include head trauma, thrombocytopenia, use of Coumadin or heparin, clotting factor deficiency, cocaine use, and ingestion of tyramine while taking a monoamine oxidase inhibitor.

Q5 The answer is: (C) Temporal arteritis.

Temporal arteritis occurs almost exclusively in patients over age 55 years with a constant but dull headache over one or both temples. Jaw claudication (increasing jaw pain on chewing) is rare, but it was once considered pathognomic for the condition. In advanced cases, the temporal arteries can be red and tender.

Often there are systemic signs (such as low-grade fever, malaise, and weight loss), and there may be joint pain or other signs of rheumatic disease and visual loss including *amaurosis fugax*. Blindness as a result of ophthalmic artery occlusion and ischemia from cerebral artery occlusion can lead to serious and permanent complications.

An erythrocyte sedimentation rate above 40 is present in over 90% of cases. A biopsy of the temporal artery that shows a focal granulomatous arteritis with giant cells is the definitive test, but is often unnecessary.

Risk factors for temporal arteritis include age greater than 55 years and a history of polymyalgia rheumatica. Although the cause is unknown, in temporal cell arteritis the temporal and other cerebral arteries become inflamed. Histologically, a focal granulomatous arteritis with giant cells is seen. Temporal cell arteritis is treated with high-dose steroids to prevent blindness and other stroke syndromes.

Pathophysiology, Psychiatric Comorbidity, and Treatment of Pain

Multiple-Choice Questions

Select the appropriate answer.

Q1 Which of the following types of axons involved in the transmission of pain from the skin to the dorsal horn are the largest and most heavily myelinated fibers?

A. *A-beta*

B. *A-delta*

C. *C*

D. *A-gamma*

E. *C-delta*

Q2 Which of the following terms BEST defines pain from a stimulus that is not normally painful (e.g., light touch or cool air)?

A. *Allodynia*

B. *Hyperalgesia*

C. *Hyperesthesia*

D. *Hyperpathia*

E. *Psychogenic pain*

Q3 Which of the following diagnostic categories BEST describes a syndrome in which the focus of the clinical presentation is pain that causes significant impairment in occupational or social function, induces marked distress, or both?

A. *Conversion disorder*

B. *Factitious disorder with physical symptoms*

C. *Hypochondriasis*

D. *Pain disorder*

E. *Somatic symptom disorder*

Q4 Which of the following orally administered narcotics is the LEAST potent (milligram for milligram)?

A. *Codeine*

B. *Hydromorphone*

C. *Methadone*

D. *Morphine*

E. *Oxycodone*

Q5 Which of the following narcotics has the LONGEST duration of analgesic efficacy?

A. *Codeine*

B. *Fentanyl patch*

C. *Meperidine*

D. *Morphine*

E. *Oxycodone*

Chapter 79

Answers

Q1 The answer is: (A) A-beta.

Three different types of axons are involved in the transmission of pain from the skin to the dorsal horn. A-beta fibers are the largest and most heavily myelinated fibers that transmit awareness of light touch. A-delta fibers and C fibers are the primary nociceptive afferents. A-delta fibers are 2 to 5 μm in diameter and are thinly myelinated. They conduct "first pain," which is immediate, rapid, and sharp with a velocity of 20 m/sec. C fibers are 0.2 to 1.5 μm in diameter and are unmyelinated. They conduct "second pain," which is prolonged, burning, and unpleasant at a speed of 0.5 m/sec.

A-delta and C fibers enter the dorsal root and ascend or descend one to three segments before synapsing with neurons in the lateral spinothalamic tract (in the substantia gelatinosa in the gray matter).

Q2 The answer is: (A) Allodynia.

Qualities of neuropathic pain include hyperalgesia (an increased response to a stimulus that is normally painful), hyperesthesia (an exaggerated pain response to a noxious stimulus [e.g., pressure or heat]), allodynia (pain from a stimulus that is not normally painful [e.g., light touch or cool air]), and hyperpathia (pain from a painful stimulus with a delay and a persistence that is distributed beyond the area of stimulation).

Idiopathic pain, previously referred to as *psychogenic pain,* is poorly understood. The presence of pain does not imply or exclude a psychological component. Typically, there is no evidence of an associated organic etiology or an anatomic pattern consistent with symptoms that are often grossly out of proportion to an identifiable organic pathology.

Q3 The answer is: (D) Pain disorder.

Somatic symptom disorders comprise a group of disorders in which complaints and anxiety about physical symptoms are the dominant features. These complaints exist in the absence of sufficient organic findings to explain the extent of a person's pain. Most often there is a physical basis (including functional pathology, such as neuropathic pain) for at least a portion of the pain complaints, in which symptom reporting is magnified by somatizing. Pain-related psychological symptoms amplify pain perception and disability. Therefore there is a tremendous overlap between the somatoform component of a chronic pain syndrome and other psychiatric comorbidities.

Pain disorder is a syndrome in which the focus of the clinical presentation is pain that causes significant impairment in occupational or social function, induces marked distress, or both. Organic pathology, if present, does not explain the extent of pain complaints or the degree of associated social and occupational impairment. Pain disorder has three subtypes: psychological (in which psychological factors play the primary role in the onset, severity, exacerbation, or maintenance of the pain); non-psychiatric pain associated with a general medical condition; and combined type (pain associated with psychological factors and a general medical condition). Pain disorder has been variously called psychogenic pain disorder, somatoform pain disorder, and pain behavior.

Conversion disorder may be manifest as a pain syndrome with a significant loss of or alteration in physical function that mimics a physical disorder. Conversion symptoms may include paresthesia, numbness, dysphonia, dizziness, seizures, globus hystericus, limb weakness, sexual dysfunction, or pain. If pain or sexual symptoms are the sole complaints, the diagnosis is pain disorder or sexual pain disorder rather than conversion disorder. Pain, numbness, and weakness often form a conversion triad.

Factitious disorder with physical symptoms involves the intentional production or feigning of physical symptoms. The cause is a psychological need to assume the sick role, and as such, the intentional production of painful symptoms distinguishes factitious disorder from somatic symptom disorders.

Hypochondriasis involves the persistent belief that one has a serious illness, despite extensive medical evaluation to the contrary. Head and orofacial pains, cardiac and gastrointestinal pains, and feelings of pressure, burning, and numbness are common hypochondriacal concerns.

Q4 The answer is: (A) Codeine.

Dose equivalents for orally administered narcotics are as follows: codeine, 200 mg; hydromorphone, 8 mg; methadone, 10 mg; morphine, 30 mg; and oxycodone, 30 mg.

Dose equivalents for parenterally administered narcotics are as follows: codeine, 120 mg; hydromorphone, 2 mg; methadone, 5 mg; morphine, 10 mg; and oxycodone, 4.5 mg.

Q5 The answer is: (B) Fentanyl patch.

Each fentanyl patch needs to be reapplied every 72 hours (and a 50 μm patch is the equivalent of 30 mg/day of parenteral morphine).

The duration of effect for codeine is 4 hours, for meperidine it is 3 hours, for morphine it is 4 hours (but a controlled-release preparation lasts 12 hours), and for oxycodone it is 4 hours (but a slow-release preparation lasts 12 hours).

Psychiatric Aspects of Stroke Syndromes

Multiple-Choice Questions

Select the appropriate answer.

Q1   Which of the following statements is LEAST accurate?

    A.   *A transient ischemic attack (TIA) involves no permanent tissue damage*

    B.   *Hemorrhagic strokes, in addition to causing focal deficits, can cause more diffuse symptoms because of cerebral edema and an increase in intracranial pressure*

    C.   *Hemorrhagic strokes occur roughly four times as often as ischemic strokes*

    D.   *Ischemic strokes usually produce focal neurologic deficits, owing to the cessation of blood flow to a specific territory of the brain*

    E.   *Recognition of TIAs is essential, as they may be a harbinger of stroke*

Q2   Which of the following statements is LEAST accurate?

    A.   *Embolism accounts for more strokes than lacunar infarcts*

    B.   *Ischemic stroke may be caused by thrombosis, whereby a clot forms within an artery and blocks it*

    C.   *Ischemic stroke may be caused by an embolism, whereby a clot travels from a remote origin and lodges within an arterial vessel*

    D.   *Stroke may be caused by lipohyalinosis, whereby concentric narrowing of small penetrating arteries results in lacunar infarction*

    E.   *Thrombotic mechanisms cause approximately 20% of ischemic strokes*

Q3   Which of the following statements is LEAST accurate?

    A.   *Arterial dissection is a less common vascular cause of ischemic stroke, but it should be considered in younger patients with stroke, especially in those with a predisposing condition (e.g., Marfan syndrome or recent trauma to the head or neck)*

    B.   *Atherosclerosis of a large intracranial or extracranial artery can result in a thrombotic stroke*

    C.   *Lacunar strokes are of vascular origin, but they only affect the small branch vessels*

    D.   *One of the most common causes of embolic strokes is paradoxical embolus through a patent foramen ovale*

    E.   *Use of cocaine or methamphetamine may cause stroke, secondary to arterial vasospasm or acute atrial dysrhythmias*

Q4   Which of the following statements is LEAST accurate?

A.   *The hallmark presentation of ischemic stroke is the abrupt onset of a focal neurologic deficit*

B.   *Embolic strokes are more likely to produce a maximal deficit at the outset*

C.   *Few stroke physicians use a standardized scale (such as the National Institutes of Health Stroke Scale) that forms the basis of a rapid and focused evaluation and establishes standardized values for comparisons among stroke patients for treatment and research purposes*

D.   *The exact time of onset, to the minute if possible, is an essential data point, as some therapies for the management of acute stroke (such as thrombolysis) are only available within strict time frames*

E.   *Thrombotic and lacunar strokes are more likely to present with a stuttering course of waxing and waning neurologic symptoms that eventually result in a complete deficit*

Q5   Which of the following statements is LEAST accurate?

A.   *Antiplatelet therapy is a key component of secondary prevention*

B.   *Control of hypertension is a crucial factor in the reduction of the incidence of stroke*

C.   *Computed tomography (CT) is widely available and is quite accurate in differentiating intracerebral hemorrhage from ischemic stroke*

D.   *CT is superior to magnetic resonance imaging (MRI) for the detection of early ischemic lesions and for improved visualization of lesions of the brainstem and the cerebellum*

E.   *In the acute setting, intravenous thrombolytic therapy with recombinant tissue plasminogen activator (rt-PA) may significantly reduce both the short- and long-term sequelae of stroke*

Q6   Which of the following statements is LEAST accurate?

A.   *Approximately 60% of subarachnoid hemorrhages (SAHs) will go undetected by computed tomography (CT), due to technical limitations*

B.   *For SAH due to aneurysm rupture, current management includes neurosurgical clipping or endovascular coiling of the aneurysm to prevent rebleeding*

C.   *Intracranial hemorrhage may present with severe headache, nausea, and vomiting*

D.   *SAH most often presents as the abrupt onset of a severe headache, classically described by the patient as the "worst headache of my life"*

E.   *SAH may be preceded by the presence of multiple "harbinger" headaches in the days to weeks leading up to the event*

Chapter 80

Answers

Q1 The answer is: (C) Hemorrhagic strokes occur roughly four times as often as ischemic strokes.
Just the opposite is true; ischemic strokes occur roughly four times as often as hemorrhagic strokes.

Stroke is defined as the acute onset of a neurologic deficit due to a cerebrovascular cause. Strokes may be categorized as ischemic (in which the deficit is caused by blockage of an arterial-feeding vessel, which results in a lack of oxygen and metabolic nutrients to the affected territory) or hemorrhagic (in which the deficit is caused by vessel rupture).

Ischemic strokes usually produce focal neurologic deficits owing to the cessation of blood flow to a specific territory of the brain. In contrast, hemorrhagic strokes, in addition to causing focal deficits, can cause more diffuse symptoms as a result of cerebral edema and an increase in intracranial pressure.

By convention, a stroke is said to have occurred if the clinical deficit persists for greater than 24 hours. However, if a permanent deficit is seen on neuroimaging that directly correlates with the patient's syndrome, then a stroke has occurred. A transient ischemic attack (TIA), in contrast, involves no permanent tissue damage. Classically, it has been described as a focal deficit that lasts less than 24 hours. However, most patients with a TIA have symptoms for a shorter duration of time, typically less than 45 minutes. Recognition of TIAs is essential, as they may be a harbinger of stroke. In one study, 10.5% of patients sustained a stroke within the 3 months following the diagnosis of a TIA.

Q2 The answer is: (A) Embolism accounts for more strokes than lacunar infarcts.
Thrombotic mechanisms cause approximately 20% of ischemic strokes, embolism causes approximately 20% of cases, and lacunar infarcts comprise an additional 25%. The remainder is caused by more rare conditions or by an undetermined etiology (i. e., "cryptogenic stroke").

Several pathophysiological mechanisms lead to ischemic stroke: thrombosis, whereby a clot forms within an artery and blocks it; embolism, whereby a clot travels from a remote origin and lodges within an arterial vessel; or lipohyalinosis, whereby concentric narrowing of small penetrating arteries results in lacunar infarction.

Q3 The answer is: (D) One of the most common causes of embolic strokes is paradoxical embolus through a patent foramen ovale.
The most frequent cause of cardioembolic stroke is embolism of left atrial clot formed as a result of atrial fibrillation. Other, less common causes include cardiac mural thrombus, clot formed at the site of a prosthetic heart valve, paradoxical embolus through a patent foramen ovale, and endocarditis.

The most common cause of cerebrovascular stroke is atherosclerosis of a large intracranial or extra-cranial artery, resulting in thrombotic stroke. Lacunar strokes are also vascular in origin, but they only affect the small branch vessels. Arterial dissection is a less common vascular cause of ischemic stroke, but it should be considered in younger patients with stroke, especially in those with a predisposing condition (such as Marfan syndrome or recent trauma to the head or neck). Use of cocaine or methamphetamine may cause stroke, likely secondary to arterial vasospasm or acute atrial dysrhythmias.

Other vascular causes of stroke are rare, but include migraine, fibromuscular dysplasia, inflammation (e.g., with cerebral vasculitis), infection, and venous sinus thrombosis. There are also strokes related to cardiac causes, which most often result in embolic strokes. Strokes may be caused by blood-related disorders (such as hypercoagulability, sickle cell crisis, or elevations in blood cell counts resulting from polycythemia, leukocytosis, or thrombocytosis).

Q4 The answer is: (C) Few stroke physicians use a standardized scale (such as the National Institutes of Health Stroke Scale) that forms the basis of a rapid and focused evaluation and establishes standardized values for comparisons among stroke patients for treatment and research purposes.
Just the opposite is true; most stroke physicians use a standardized scale (such as the National Institutes of Health Stroke Scale), which establishes a method of performing a rapid and focused evaluation and establishes standardized values for comparisons among patients with stroke for treatment and research purposes.

The hallmark presentation of ischemic stroke is the abrupt onset of a focal neurologic deficit. Associated symptoms, such as a seizure or headache, may occur but are less common. Thrombotic and lacunar strokes are more likely to present with a stuttering course of waxing and waning neurologic symptoms that eventually result in a complete deficit, whereas embolic strokes are more likely to produce a maximal deficit at the outset.

The classic signs and symptoms of acute ischemic stroke are usually recognizable by physicians. However, a differential diagnosis should always be created, especially in cases with atypical features, such as a non-focal neurologic examination or an impaired level of consciousness. The differential diagnosis includes intracerebral or subarachnoid hemorrhage (SAH), epidural or subdural hematoma, TIA, mass lesions (such as a tumor or abscess), seizures, migraine headaches, and metabolic causes, such as hypoglycemia.

A careful history is a crucial first step in the management of a suspected acute ischemic stroke. The exact time of onset, to the minute if possible, is an essential data point, as some therapies for the management of acute stroke (such as thrombolysis) are only available within strict time frames. If the exact time of onset is not known, or if the patient was not witnessed at the time of symptom development, then the time of onset by default becomes the time at which the patient was last seen to be neurologically normal. A history of similar symptoms, which may suggest a recent TIA or even recent stroke, should also be ascertained. Essential components of the medical history include a history of cardiac problems, hypertension, diabetes mellitus, hypercholesterolemia, and use of tobacco or drugs. The medication list should be reviewed, especially if the patient is taking anticoagulants or antiplatelet agents. A thorough physical examination should follow, which should include the careful assessment of vital signs (including blood pressure measured in both arms). The examiner should also auscultate the carotid arteries to assess for the presence of carotid bruits. Of note, a lack of a bruit may accompany a complete or impending occlusion. Most important, a focused neurologic assessment should be done with the aim of localizing the lesion supplied by the suspected vessel.

Q5 The answer is: (D) CT is superior to magnetic resonance imaging (MRI) for the detection of early ischemic lesions and for improved visualization of lesions of the brainstem and the cerebellum.
It is MRI, not computed tomography (CT), that provides superior detection of early ischemic lesions and improved visualization of lesions of the brainstem and the cerebellum. However, to identify pathology within the target vessel, imaging with CT angiography or magnetic resonance angiography is required.

Antiplatelet therapy is a key component of secondary prevention. A recent meta-analysis demonstrated that the use of aspirin and other antiplatelet agents (such as clopidogrel) reduced the odds of recurrent non-fatal stroke by 31%.

Control of hypertension is a crucial factor in the reduction of the incidence of stroke. A recent meta-analysis determined that beta-blockers and diuretics were both effective in the prevention of stroke. Tight glucose control in diabetes mellitus is also recommended. Smoking cessation should be strongly encouraged. Unless contraindicated, anticoagulation for chronic conditions (such as atrial fibrillation with a history of thromboembolism) should be continued on a lifelong basis.

CT is widely available and is quite accurate in differentiating intracerebral hemorrhage from ischemic stroke. Thus, it is the first choice of imaging in most centers. It must be performed before the administration of a thrombolytic agent to rule out an underlying condition (such as a hemorrhage, abscess, or tumor) that would preclude its use.

In the acute setting, intravenous thrombolytic therapy with recombinant tissue plasminogen activator (rt-PA) may significantly reduce both the short- and long-term sequelae of stroke. Rt-PA exerts its action by converting plasminogen to plasmin, which helps to dissolve fibrin-containing clots. This therapy, approved in 1996 by the US Food and Drug Administration after a landmark 1995 trial by the National Institute of Neurologic Disorders and Stroke, demonstrated a benefit to patients administered rt-PA with acute stroke less than 3 hours old.

Q6 The answer is: (A) Approximately 60% of subarachnoid hemorrhages (SAHs) will go undetected by computed tomography (CT), due to technical limitations.
Approximately 5% to 10% of SAHs will be undetectable by CT due to technical limitations. In this case, if SAH is suggested by clinical history, a lumbar puncture should be performed to detect the presence of hemoglobin breakdown products (xanthochromia), which will appear within 12 hours after the hemorrhage. Further imaging modalities include CT angiography or cerebral angiography, which may help to

identify the aneurysm or other vascular abnormality, and Doppler ultrasound, which can monitor for the later development of cerebral vasospasm, which typically develops 5 to 14 days after the SAH.

For SAH due to aneurysm rupture, current management includes neurosurgical clipping or endovascular coiling of the aneurysm to prevent rebleeding. The optimal approach remains under study.

Intracranial hemorrhage may present with severe headache, nausea, and vomiting. The combination of an expanding hematoma, worsening edema, and compression of brainstem structures often leads to a progressive decline in the level of consciousness. The blood pressure may be markedly elevated on presentation, and it may either be the cause of the hemorrhage or the effect of the concomitant massive catecholamine release.

SAH most often presents as the abrupt onset of a severe headache, classically described by the patient as the "worst headache of my life." This severe pain is thought to be because of an elevation in intracranial pressure, leading to distortion of pain-sensitive structures. A progressive decline in mental status often follows, which may be due to decreased cerebral blood flow in the setting of elevated intracranial pressure. These symptoms are often accompanied by nausea, vomiting, and meningismus. As free-flowing blood traverses functional territories, SAH tends to produce more diffuse neurologic deficits than do ischemic strokes. Ischemia or even infarction from cerebral vasospasm may occur later in the course of SAH, resulting in more focal neurologic deficits.

SAH in particular may be preceded by the presence of multiple "harbinger" headaches in the days to weeks leading up to the event. These may be due to aneurysmal stretching before rupture or even sentinel hemorrhages.

Movement Disorders

Multiple-Choice Questions

Select the appropriate answer.

Q1 True or False. Basal ganglia disorders disrupt self-generated actions more than environmentally cued ones.

    A. *True*

    B. *False*

Q2 True or False. D_3 and D_4 dopamine receptors are found MOSTLY in the striatum.

    A. *True*

    B. *False*

Q3 Which of the following terms BEST describes a sudden inability to move that most often occurs when the patient tries to initiate a movement?

    A. *Bradykinesia*

    B. *Catatonia*

    C. *Freezing*

    D. *Rigidity*

    E. *Spasticity*

Q4 Which of the following is BEST characterized by abnormal trunk or limb postures?

    A. *Akathisia*

    B. *Asterixis*

    C. *Dystonia*

    D. *Hemiballism*

    E. *Myoclonus*

Q5 Which of the following terms BEST describes slow, writhing, nearly dystonic movements?

    A. *Athetosis*

    B. *Chorea*

    C. *Myoclonus*

    D. *Tics*

    E. *Tremor*

Q6 Which of the following is a prototypical genetic psychiatric disorder (autosomal dominant, characterized by a CAG triplet repeat expansion), notable for its adult onset?

A. *Fragile X syndrome*

B. *Huntington disease*

C. *Parkinson disease*

D. *Tourette syndrome*

E. *Wilson disease*

Q7 Which of the following disorders is an autosomal recessive disorder that causes copper deposition?

A. *Fragile X syndrome*

B. *Huntington disease*

C. *Parkinson disease*

D. *Tourette syndrome*

E. *Wilson disease*

Chapter 81

Answers

Q1 The answer is: (A) True.
Basal ganglia disorders disrupt self-generated actions more than environmentally cued ones.

Disorders of the basal ganglia broadly affect the motivation to act, both to start and to stop. When damage spreads to affective circuits, it creates disorders of motivation there too—depression and apathy on the one hand or excessively goal-directed, manic disinhibition on the other. When dysfunction spreads to cognitive circuits, thoughts can be slowed (bradyphrenia) and deficits in executive function may appear without the characteristic aphasia or agnosia of cortical dementias (such as Alzheimer disease). Conversely, it can cause wild, unregulated thought manifest by hallucinations and delusions.

Q2 The answer is: (B) False.
Dopamine is the best understood neurotransmitter related to basal ganglia function. Its receptors fall into two classes: the D_1 class, of which D_1 is mostly found in the striatum and D_5 extrastriatal, and the D_2 class, of which D_2 is primarily striatal, whereas D_3 and D_4 are mostly extrastriatal. Its release in the motor control areas of the striatum seems to facilitate limb movement via D_2 receptors, and to inhibit movement via D_1 receptors.

Q3 The answer is: (C) Freezing.
Rigidity is the cardinal hypokinetic sign. Although rigidity is characteristic of parkinsonism, it is sometimes present even in hyperkinetic conditions (such as Tourette syndrome). Rigidity produces a constant "lead pipe" resistance to movement along the whole range of the joint. It can quickly be assessed without touching the patient, by asking the patient to rapidly rotate the wrist back and forth, as if trying to screw in a lightbulb.

Cogwheel rigidity is simply a tremor superimposed on rigidity, although the tremor is not always apparent visually. Patients sometimes complain of an inner tremor not visible to others. Their complaint may be mistaken for somatization or a delusion, but it is more commonly evidence for parkinsonism. Rigidity makes movements low amplitude, and they rapidly decrease in size. Handwriting almost always demonstrates this.

Rigidity is different from spasticity, the jerky "clasp-knife" phenomenon seen after stroke-induced paralysis or paresis. The presence of hyperreflexia, muscle atrophy, flexor spasms, and toe-walking help distinguish spasticity from rigidity.

Patients with hypokinetic movement disorders often say they feel weak, but usually they have normal muscle bulk and can exert considerable strength if given enough time to fully engage their muscles. Basal ganglia movement disorders differ notably from the paralytic weakness of cortical strokes or peripheral nerve injuries.

Bradykinesia (slower movements) and akinesia (fewer movements) may culminate in freezing, a sudden inability to move that most often occurs when the patient tries to initiate a movement. Freezing is related to the psychiatric syndrome of catatonia.

Freezing, like many basal ganglia symptoms, is more a problem with internally motivated behaviors than with ones that are responses to environmental cues. Thus, it can sometimes be broken by odd sensory tricks (such as stepping over a line on the floor or hearing marching music).

Q4 The answer is: (C) Dystonia.
Dystonia is characterized by abnormal trunk or limb postures. It exists on a spectrum of abnormal muscle tensions and speeds that extend from rigidity through dystonia, then athetosis to chorea and dyskinesia. Dystonia is occasionally very painful, especially in acute drug reactions. Such acute reactions are usually treated with diphenhydramine; presence of this symptom suggests that the patient is at much higher risk for the later development of other extrapyramidal complications, including tardive dyskinesia.

Akathisia may also be caused by use of dopamine antagonists, and it usually occurs acutely rather than after chronic exposure. Its movements both feel and look voluntary—they are low amplitude and look restless. It is similar in look and feel to the fidgetiness of mania, or of boredom. It is of great clinical importance because it is triggered by a highly uncomfortable desire to move constantly, a desire that may even drive violent action. Treating akathisia often requires discontinuation of the neuroleptic. Although akathisia in some ways resembles restless legs syndrome, the latter is usually not drug-induced, happens primarily when the patient relaxes before sleep, and has a more distinctly sensory trigger, such as a feeling of limb "creepiness."

Myoclonus is an intermittent, ballistic jerk caused by a single muscle group, which promptly relaxes; it is involuntary. Myoclonus during sleep is normal and may be generated from a source outside the basal ganglia.

Asterixis is negative myoclonus, that is, a sudden lapse of tone with quick recovery. Both can be seen in encephalopathy, drug intoxication (especially with opiates), and neurodegenerative diseases.

Hemiballism (a repetitive flinging movement of a limb) is quite rare; it usually arises after a subthalamic nucleus lesion.

Q5 The answer is: (A) Athetosis.

Apart from the briefest, most ballistic movements, most hyperkinetic movements feel semipurposive, and the patient can usually suppress them for brief periods. For this reason they may be mistakenly considered psychogenic.

Athetosis, a slow, writhing, nearly dystonic movement, rarely needs to be distinguished from the quicker movements of chorea and dyskinesias, as their causes and treatment are similar. Choreoathetosis is often described as dance-like but is rarely so. Rhythmic chorea was common in Charcot's day, when the most common cause was tertiary syphilis or the hysterical chorea that imitated it. Common modern causes include lupus, pregnancy, Huntington disease, Wilson disease, and use of oral contraceptives or neuroleptics. Typical neuroleptics (such as haloperidol) generally suppress choreoathetosis but may eventually cause a tardive worsening of the hyperkinesis.

Action tremor is brought on by voluntary movement of the same limb. Both rest and action tremors are worsened by stress and often by caffeine. Action tremors classically improve with alcohol but rebound afterward.

Enhanced physiological tremor, a high-frequency low-amplitude action tremor, can be present in any situation that increases adrenaline (including hyperthyroidism and use of stimulants); it rarely interferes with tasks.

Essential tremor, also called hereditary tremor, is coarser: lower frequency and higher amplitude.

Drug tremors (e.g., from lithium or valproate) may be similarly coarse when severe.

The most important disorder to distinguish from action tremor is dysmetria—incoordination from cerebellar damage. Dysmetria, sometimes rather unhelpfully called an *intention tremor,* gets worse the closer the hand gets to a target, and is associated with other cerebellar signs (such as ataxia or ocular nystagmus).

Tics are intermittent, multifocal, usually stereotyped, and repetitive. They are typically driven by a conscious urge to move or by a premonitory sensation and can often be suppressed briefly. Complex tics include gestures and vocalizations that may feel meaningful and goal-directed. Complex tics exist on a continuum with the compulsive behaviors of obsessive-compulsive disorder, but people with tics often report a drive toward some sensory satisfaction rather than a drive away from a feared event. Simple tics (such as winks, sniffs, and shrugs) are common in the general population. The simplest tics (e.g., arm jerks) may feel involuntary and look myoclonic.

Q6 The answer is: (B) Huntington disease.

Huntington disease is a rare (approximately 8 per 100,000 of the population) but conceptually important condition because it is the prototypical hyperkinetic movement disorder. It often manifests with psychiatric changes, followed by the classic chorea. Dementia is a late phenomenon. Its symptoms are in many ways opposite to those of untreated Parkinson, and include prominent problems with early agitation, impulse control, and hallucinations. It is also a prototypical genetic psychiatric disorder, notable for its adult onset. It is autosomal dominant, characterized by a CAG triplet repeat expansion. Similar gene expansions have been found in other neuropsychiatric genetic disorders (such as fragile X syndrome). The longer the expansion, the earlier and worse the symptoms. Cell death in this disorder is prominent in the striatum and the cortex. Early in the disease, psychosis and chorea respond well to typical antipsychotics (such as haloperidol)—their extrapyramidal effects are in this situation desirable. Late in the disease, dystonia and rigidity may arise, and quetiapine or clozapine are better choices. Selective serotonin reuptake inhibitors are well tolerated for treatment of depression.

Tourette syndrome is defined by multiple motor tics and at least one vocal tic, lasting more than one year, starting before age 18 years. Tic disorders without vocalizations probably have very similar causes and treatments. Many children meet diagnostic criteria, especially between ages 6 and 9 years, but symptoms usually resolve by adulthood. The tics may reflect maturation of brain systems that control ballistic action. Tourette has a male-female predominance of 3:1 and a significant genetic component. Tourette is very often accompanied by obsessive-compulsive disorder and by depression—in fact, families of boys with Tourette syndrome often have girls with obsessive-compulsive symptoms but no tics. Tourette may also be associated with attention-deficit/hyperactivity disorder, impulsivity, and mild learning disabilities. Social phobia and an exaggerated fear of having tics are common.

Q7 The answer is: (E) Wilson disease.

Wilson disease causes a protean mix of psychiatric, neurologic, and hepatic problems, often beginning in early adulthood. It is an autosomal recessive disorder that causes copper deposition. The most common psychiatric symptoms are personality change and odd behavior; the most common neurologic symptoms are incoordination and slurred speech. Although Wilson disease is rare (with a prevalence of 0.25 per 100,000), it is clinically important because if it is detected early, it is highly treatable with copper chelation therapy and with dietary copper restriction. Diagnosis is confirmed by low serum ceruloplasmin, by a high 24-hour urinary copper level, by liver biopsy, or by a slit-lamp examination by an ophthalmologist (looking for Kayser-Fleischer rings). The latter are only rarely detectable by non-ophthalmologists, especially when at a psychotherapeutic distance from the patient. Magnetic resonance imaging scans may show an increased striatal T2 signal. The presence of bronze skin is generally a late sign.

Chapter 82

Psychiatric Aspects of Traumatic Brain Disorder

Multiple-Choice Questions

Select the appropriate answer.

Q1   Which of the following is the MOST common cause of traumatic brain injury (TBI)?

    A.   *An unknown cause*

    B.   *Being assaulted*

    C.   *Being struck in the head (or against an object)*

    D.   *Falls*

    E.   *Motor vehicle accidents*

Q2   What is the term that BEST describes the hematomas in the brain that develop at the point of contact and at a point contralateral to the point of contact?

    A.   *Coup-contrecoup contusions*

    B.   *Intracerebral hematomas*

    C.   *Extradural hematomas*

    D.   *Subarachnoid hemorrhages*

    E.   *Subdural hematomas*

Q3   Which of the following tests, in addition to assessment of the duration of disrupted memory, BEST assesses the severity of traumatic brain injury (TBI)?

    A.   *Beck Depression Inventory*

    B.   *CAGE*

    C.   *Glasgow Coma Scale (GCS)*

    D.   *Michigan Alcohol Screening Test*

    E.   *SCID*

Q4   Which of the following is the BEST type of testing to use to determine cognitive dysfunction that accompanies traumatic brain injury (TBI)?

    A.   *Computed tomography*

    B.   *Magnetic resonance imaging*

    C.   *Neuropsychological testing*

    D.   *Positron emission tomography*

    E.   *Single-photon emission computed tomography*

Q5 Which of the following statements is LEAST likely to be accurate about traumatic brain injury (TBI)?

A. *No single path or pattern of recovery follows a brain injury*

B. *Procedural memory involves the recall of specific facts*

C. *The duration of posttraumatic amnesia, the inability to recall information presented after the accident, correlates with the severity of one's injury*

D. *The Rancho Los Amigos Levels of Cognitive Functioning Scale is widely used in delineating the stages of recovery*

E. *Although neurologic damage can occur without loss of consciousness, it is considered a hallmark of most TBI*

Chapter 82

Answers

Q1 The answer is: (D) Falls.

Among the most common causes of traumatic brain injury (TBI) are falls (28%) and motor vehicle accidents (20%). Having the head struck by, or against, an object (19%), being assaulted (11%), and experiencing other (13%) or unknown (9%) problems make up the remaining cases.

Men sustain a TBI at a rate 1.5 times higher than that of women and are hospitalized almost twice as frequently. TBI occurs most frequently in children ages 0 to 4 years, followed by older adolescents (ages 15 to 19 years). The highest rates of hospitalization and death following TBI are found in adults over age 75 years. Falls produce the most injuries for children younger than age 15 years and for adults over age 55 years. Motor vehicle accidents account for the most injuries among adolescents ages 15 to 19 years and adults ages 20 to 55 years.

Earlier research has found that 56% of adults identified as having brain injuries had elevated blood alcohol levels at the time of injury; 49% had a blood alcohol level at or above the legal level. Recurrent brain injury is common; the risk of a second injury is three times higher than it is for those in the general (non-injured) population. Following a second injury, the risk for a third injury becomes nearly 10 times higher than the risk for an initial injury. Finally, review of data from the United States National Health Interview, a national database used to estimate the incidence and features of persons with brain injury, found that the highest rates of injury occurred in families with the lowest income levels.

Q2 The answer is: (A) Coup-contrecoup contusions.

Hematomas may develop at the point of contact and at a point contralateral to the point of contact (known as *coup-contrecoup contusions*). Contusions are seen more frequently in the poles of the frontal lobes, the inferior aspects of the frontal lobes, the cortex above and below the operculum of the Sylvian fissures, the temporal poles, and the lateral and inferior aspects of the temporal lobes. They may develop quickly within minutes of the injury or evolve slowly over several hours or days. The presence of these contusions contributes to neuronal necrosis and to elevated intracranial pressure. In addition to contusions, contact forces can result in small or complete tears at the pontomedullary junction, damage to any of the cranial nerves, damage to the hypothalamus or pituitary gland, and damage to blood vessels. Moreover, there can be multiple areas of focal damage.

TBI is a spectrum disorder; injury can be focal, diffuse, or both. Damage can occur as a result of forces exerted on the brain at the time of injury, known as the primary injury, and from subsequent physiological processes (such as swelling or hypoxia) triggered by the initial insult; these are classified as secondary injuries. Focal damage typically is the result of contusions or mass lesions. Most often they arise from contact injuries (such as falls or blows to the head) and result in skull fractures and hematomas (extradural, subarachnoid, subdural, or intracerebral hematomas).

Q3 The answer is: (C) Glasgow Coma Scale (GCS).

TBI is typically classified as mild, moderate, or severe based primarily on the duration of altered mental status (including the degree of responsiveness, as measured by the Glasgow Coma Scale [GCS], and the duration of disrupted memory). These terms can be misleading, as they reflect the degree of damage the brain has sustained; they do not necessarily reflect the severity of the disruption in the patient's daily function.

Individuals with a severe injury can essentially make a full recovery, whereas others with mild to moderate injuries can remain significantly disabled for many years. The GCS, developed by Teasdale and Jennett, assigns points for increasingly complex levels of response to three dimensions (verbal and motor response and eye opening); the ratings in each domain are totaled to produce an overall score that can range from 3 to 15. Ratings can also be done serially to provide a measure of recovery. GCS scores have been predictive of ultimate outcome, with lower initial scores being associated with more severe injury and worse recovery.

The Beck Depression Inventory (a screening test for depression), the CAGE (a screening test for alcohol abuse), the Michigan Alcohol Screening Test, and the Structured Clinical Interview for *Diagnostic and*

Statistical Manual of Mental Disorders, Fourth Edition (SCID) do not adequately assess cognitive function or predict its outcome.

Q4 The answer is: (C) Neuropsychological testing.

Mild TBI may not show up on a computed tomography scan, on magnetic resonance imaging, or on an electroencephalogram. When there are positive radiologic findings, the injury is classified as a complicated mild TBI. Performance on a routine neurologic examination, which tends to focus on sensorimotor function, may be essentially normal, although performance may represent a decline relative to preinjury performance. Acute symptoms may persist for varying lengths of time. Physical symptoms often encompass nausea, vomiting, dizziness, headaches, blurred vision, an increased sensitivity to noise and light, diminished libido, sleep disturbance, quickness to fatigue, lethargy, or sensory loss.

Cognitive deficits typically involve attention, concentration, perception, memory, speech/language, or executive functions. These cognitive deficits are best identified through an in-depth neuropsychological evaluation. Behavioral changes (such as irritability, quickness to anger, disinhibition, or emotional lability) may follow.

Q5 The answer is: (B) Procedural memory involves the recall of specific facts.

Declarative memory (i.e., the ability to recall events [episodic memory] and specific facts [semantic memory]) is more vulnerable to damage because of the active processes and neural structures involved.

No single path or pattern of recovery follows a brain injury, as there are so many variables involved (e.g., the location and extent of injury, the patient's age and overall health, the presence of alcohol, the medical and psychological history, concurrent processes [such as infections or seizures], and availability of appropriate rehabilitation services and supports).

The duration of posttraumatic amnesia, the inability to recall information presented after the accident, correlates with the severity of one's injury. Although some patients have a period of retrograde amnesia (i.e., the inability to recall information acquired before the trauma), problems acquiring, storing, and retrieving new information are more common. Memory is not a unitary construct; there are different forms of memory that may be affected to differing degrees depending on the nature and the location of the injury. Because different neuroanatomic structures are involved with these various forms, there is typically sparing of some forms of memory. Procedural memory (i.e., memory for motor sequences that occur outside of conscious awareness) is typically less affected than is memory for more language-based or visual information. This also means that there is not a specific profile of memory deficit associated with TBI.

The Rancho Los Amigos Levels of Cognitive Functioning Scale is widely used in delineating the stages of recovery. It is an 8-point scale describing stages of cognitive and behavioral change used to track improvement following a TBI. Although the scale provides a useful way of identifying a patient's level of recovery, it has not been able to predict the ultimate rate or level of recovery. It has less relevance beyond level IV, as patients show increasingly varied patterns of recovery beyond this level. Patients do not progress through the levels at a uniform or predictable rate. Individuals may progress through different levels at different rates. Progress in various domains is not universal; some levels of function (such as motor function) progress more rapidly and recover more fully than do language or memory.

Although neurologic damage can occur without loss of consciousness, it is considered a hallmark of most TBI. The depth and duration of lost consciousness generally reflect the severity of injury. The longer the duration, the more severe the injury and the more guarded the prognosis for recovery.

SECTION 19
LAW AND PSYCHIATRY

Chapter 83

Intimate Partner Violence

Multiple-Choice Questions

Select the appropriate answer.

Q1 Which of the following statements is LEAST accurate?

  A. *A victim who discloses domestic violence and leaves the relationship has a lower risk (than those who stay) of being murdered by her batterer*

  B. *Despite improved provider awareness, attitudes, stereotypes, time constraints, a sense of futility, and perceived lack of resources remain barriers to detection of domestic violence*

  C. *Domestic violence has grave and extensive public health implications, not the least of which are physical injury, physical and mental disability, and possible death of the abused*

  D. *The societal costs of domestic violence include health care expense, lost wages, and decreased or lost productivity, as well as the generational implications of, and the long-term effects on, children who witness such violence*

  E. *Victims of domestic violence live with shame, fear, limited (and often highly controlled) resources, and a perpetrator-distorted sense of reality, which serve as deterrents to disclosure*

Q2 Which of the following statements is LEAST accurate?

  A. *An estimated 10% to 15% of married couples experience some instance of physical violence from domestic violence*

  B. *Domestic violence in the United States affects women six times more often than men*

  C. *Most episodes of domestic violence involve men who abuse their female partners*

  D. *Same-sex couples appear to have rates of violence similar to their heterosexual counterparts*

  E. *Women are more likely to be assaulted, raped, or murdered by a current or previous male partner than by a stranger*

Q3 Which of the following statements is LEAST accurate?

  A. *Abused women account for one-fourth of all women who present to emergency psychiatric services*

  B. *Among women seen emergently for non–motor vehicle trauma, the prevalence of intimate partner abuse is as high as 40%*

  C. *Approximately 2% of women seen in the emergency department present for abuse-related acute trauma*

  D. *Domestic violence is more common among those of lower socioeconomic status and lower educational backgrounds*

  E. *In the pediatric setting, more than half of the mothers of abused children are being abused themselves*

Q4 Which of the following statements is LEAST accurate regarding domestic violence?

  A. *Abused women often turn to drugs or to alcohol (for an escape, and to tolerate or numb their experience of abuse)*

  B. *Certain personality types have been defined or identified to predispose a person to be abused*

  C. *Drug or alcohol use by a woman's partner may also increase her risk, as his irritability, irrationality, and disinhibition increase*

  D. *Filing a restraining order, especially a temporary restraining order, further increases the risk of domestic violence*

  E. *Young women (age teens and 20s), especially if single (divorced or separated) or pregnant, are more likely to be abused by a current or former partner*

Q5   Which of the following statements is LEAST accurate regarding domestic violence?

A.   *It is often some major life event for the couple (such as marriage, pregnancy, or birth) that triggers the first violent episode of domestic abuse*

B.   *Perpetrators of domestic violence have family histories that frequently reveal violence in which the perpetrator is experienced as either a witness or a victim*

C.   *Perpetrators of domestic violence tend to not be assertive in direct and positive ways, but feel intensely inadequate, and thus jealous and untrusting of their partners*

D.   *Perpetrators of domestic violence often blame the victim for provoking or deserving the abuse*

E.   *The victim of domestic abuse rarely feels sorry for the perpetrator's pain and does not believe that she has provoked him*

Q6   Which of the following statements is LEAST accurate regarding domestic violence?

A.   *Chronically mentally ill or cognitively limited victims may not have the vocabulary or experience to describe their abusive situations to providers or to otherwise protect themselves*

B.   *Direct questions about domestic violence should be asked in front of the suspected perpetrator*

C.   *Most states have mandatory reporting requirements for physicians who suspect child abuse or neglect; this includes the witnessing of partner abuse*

D.   *Persistent battering and emotional torment are correlated with shame, fear, worthlessness, hopelessness, depression, anxiety, dissociation, or numbness*

E.   *The patient who has a record full of unscheduled visits, emergency department encounters, frequent accidents, unusual traumatic injuries, or multiple somatic complaints should be carefully and privately questioned about domestic violence*

Chapter 83

Answers

Q1 The answer is: (A) A victim who discloses domestic violence and leaves the relationship has a lower risk (than those who stay) of being murdered by her batterer.
If not handled well, disclosure and detection of domestic violence may seriously increase the victim's risk: a victim who leaves has a 75% greater risk (than those who stay) of being murdered by her batterer.

Despite improved provider awareness, attitudes, stereotypes, time constraints, a sense of futility, and perceived lack of resources remain barriers to detection of domestic violence. This domestic violence has grave and extensive public health implications, not the least of which are the physical injury, physical and mental disability, and possible death of the abused. The societal costs of domestic violence include health care expense, lost wages, and decreased or lost productivity, as well as the generational implications of, and the long-term effects on, children who witness such violence.

Victims of domestic violence live with shame, fear, limited (and often highly controlled) resources, and a perpetrator-distorted sense of reality, which serve as deterrents to disclosure.

Q2 The answer is: (A) An estimated 10% to 15% of married couples experience some instance of physical violence from domestic violence.
In fact, an estimated 30% to 50% of married couples experience some instance of physical violence.

Although controversy exists, a large national survey demonstrated that domestic violence in the United States affects women six times more often than men, with 4.5 million annual episodes of abuse perpetrated against women by an intimate partner or a former partner. Female victims experience a mean of 3.4 assaults per year, which translates to 1.5 million American women assaulted by an intimate partner yearly, or a victimization rate of 44.2 per 1000 women.

Most (85%) episodes of domestic violence involve men who abuse their female partners. In fact, women are more likely to be assaulted, raped, or murdered by a current or previous male partner than by a stranger (72.1% vs. 10.6%).

Same-sex couples appear to have rates of violence similar to their heterosexual counterparts.

Q3 The answer is: (D) Domestic violence is more common among those of lower socioeconomic status and lower educational backgrounds.
Psychiatrists, and other health care providers, should maintain a high level of suspicion regardless of the patient's socioeconomic, educational, professional, ethnic, racial, or religious affiliation. Domestic violence is the great equalizer; it respects no such boundaries.

Among women seen emergently for non-motor vehicle trauma, the prevalence of intimate partner abuse is as high as 40%. In the emergency department, 11% of women seen for any cause are in abusive relationships, although only 2% of women seen in the emergency department present for abuse-related acute trauma.

In the pediatric setting, more than half of the mothers of abused children are being abused themselves.

Psychiatrists have an even greater opportunity and challenge to ascertain and to address the needs of abused women, who account for one-fourth of all women who present for emergency psychiatric services, one-third of all women who attempt suicide, one-half of all women in outpatient psychiatric care, and almost two-thirds of women on inpatient psychiatric units.

Q4 The answer is: (B) Certain personality types have been defined or identified to predispose a person to be abused.
The only unifying feature of victims of domestic violence is the existence of a partner who is violent. All segments of the population are represented. No previctimization personality type has been defined or identified to predispose a person to be abused.

However, the repeated abuse experience often leads to a pattern of behavior that appears character-disordered. Persistent emotional badgering, physical abuse, and/or sexual assault result in intense shame and an overwhelming sense of worthlessness and incompetence. When such women present for medical attention, especially when accompanied by their batterer, they often seem dependent and overly passive. They frequently do not *look* abused, or present with injuries or obvious evidence of battering. They may have vague physical or behavioral complaints. They may be seen as "somatic" and emotionally unstable.

Abused women often turn to drugs or to alcohol (for an escape, and to tolerate or numb their experience of abuse). Drug or alcohol use by a woman's partner may also increase her risk, as his irritability, irrationality, and disinhibition increase.

Filing a restraining order, especially a temporary restraining order, further increases the risk. This act of independence may fuel the abuser's need to assert his dominance and control.

Young women (age teens and 20s), especially if single (divorced or separated) or pregnant, are more likely to be abused by a current or former partner.

Q5 The answer is: (E) The victim of domestic abuse rarely feels sorry for the perpetrator's pain and does not believe that she has provoked him.
A pattern of repetitive, predictable, and escalating domestic violence often develops. Extreme remorse and reconciliation typically follow each act of violence. The perpetrator demonstrates his profuse contrition with outpourings of gifts and professions of love and affection. The victim is often sorry for the perpetrator's pain and feels guilty for having provoked him. Both insist, and often believe, it will never happen again. This phase of reconciliation is followed by a period of growing tension that ultimately concludes in another violent eruption.

It is often some major life event for the couple (such as marriage, pregnancy, or birth) that triggers the first violent episode of domestic abuse.

Perpetrators of domestic violence have family histories that frequently reveal violence in which the perpetrator is experienced as either a witness or a victim.

Perpetrators of domestic violence tend to not be assertive in direct and positive ways, but feel intensely inadequate, and thus jealous and untrusting of their partners. Any suggestion of autonomy is seen as an affront and as intolerable.

With the victim of domestic violence, the perpetrator will often downplay the extent, frequency, or damage of the abuse. The perpetrator may blame the effects of intoxication (a form of abuse in and of itself) and blame the victim for provoking or deserving the abuse.

Q6 The answer is: (B) Direct questions about domestic violence should be asked in front of the suspected perpetrator.
Questioning about domestic violence should be carried out in a straightforward, non-judgmental fashion, in a private setting. Asking such questions in front of the perpetrator not only inhibits an honest response but endangers the victim. In the case of non-English-speaking patients, intimates, family, or friends should never serve as interpreters.

Chronically mentally ill or cognitively limited victims may not have the vocabulary or experience to describe their abusive situations to providers or to otherwise protect themselves.

Most states have mandatory reporting requirements for physicians who suspect child abuse or neglect; this includes the witnessing of partner abuse.

Persistent battering and emotional torment are correlated with shame, fear, worthlessness, hopelessness, depression, anxiety, dissociation, or numbness. She may also fear the abuser will be more violent, more persuasive, provide counter-accusations, or be jailed, leaving her destitute and homeless.

The patient who has a record full of unscheduled visits, emergency department encounters, frequent accidents, unusual traumatic injuries, or multiple somatic complaints should be carefully and privately questioned about domestic violence.

Psychiatric Correlates and Consequences of Abuse and Neglect

Multiple-Choice Questions

Select the appropriate answer.

Q1   Which of the following provides federal funding for the prevention and treatment of child abuse?

   A. *AMA*

   B. *APA*

   C. *CAPTA*

   D. *NCEA*

   E. *UNICEF*

Q.2   True or False. Each state can determine the grounds for intervention to protect a child, but there are common trends among states.

   A. *True*

   B. *False*

Q3   True or False. More children suffer from neglect than from physical and sexual abuse combined.

   A. *True*

   B. *False*

Q4   True or False. Like emotional abuse, neglect is MORE difficult to identify than is physical abuse because the more easily identified stigmata of scars, marks, or bruises are often not present.

   A. *True*

   B. *False*

Q5   True or False. Parents who have been victims of abuse are no more at risk of being an abuser than are parents who have never suffered abuse.

   A. *True*

   B. *False*

Chapter 84

Answers

Q1 The answer is: (C) CAPTA.

Both federal and state laws address the abuse and neglect of children and the elderly. In 1974, Congress passed landmark legislation to provide federal support to aid in the battle against child mistreatment. In the federal Child Abuse Prevention and Treatment Act (CAPTA), the federal government provided states with federal funding for the prevention and treatment of child abuse. This funding was conditional on the states adopting mandatory reporting laws. Currently, all states have mandatory reporting statutes for child abuse and neglect that require certain groups of professionals (such as physicians, day care providers, and teachers) to notify authorities when they become aware that a child may be the victim of abuse or neglect. However, each state provides its own definition of child abuse and neglect and states have differences as to who must report and the circumstances under which the report must be made.

The American Medical Association's (AMA) Diagnostic and Treatment Guidelines on Elder Abuse and Neglect provide reference criteria to assist physicians in the recognition, diagnosis, and response to cases of elder mistreatment; however, it does not provide for federal funding. Similarly, the American Psychiatric Association (APA) provides educational materials, but not federal funding for the recognition and treatment of abuse.

In 1998, the National Center on Elder Abuse (NCEA) was established. State agencies and national professional organizations have established numerous guidelines and reference sources to assist in the detection, intervention, monitoring, and treatment of both child and elder abuse and neglect.

In 2003, the United Nations Children's Fund (UNICEF) published a report on child deaths due to mistreatment in industrialized countries. The UNICEF report found that 3500 children under age 15 years die each year from abuse or neglect in 27 wealthy nations.

Q2 The answer is: (A) True.

Each state can determine the grounds for intervention to protect a child, but there are common trends among states.

For example, a "child" is generally defined as a person who is under age 18 years and not an emancipated minor. Emancipation status is not available in every state, but in the majority of states in which it is, emancipation is a legal status that allows minors to attain the rights of legal adulthood, provided certain criteria are met, before the age at which they would normally be considered adults.

Twenty-eight states provide emancipation status and 22 states do not.

Q3 The answer is: (A) True.

According to the most recent data report from the National Child Abuse and Neglect Data System (NCANDS), neglect is the most common form of child maltreatment reported to state protective services. More children suffer from neglect than from physical and sexual abuse combined.

Even though neglect comprises approximately one-half of all reported cases of child mistreatment in the United States, it receives less consideration in the literature and the media as compared with physical and sexual abuse. Part of the reason that child neglect receives disproportionately less attention than abuse may be related to difficulties in defining what constitutes neglect.

Neglect is generally defined as deprivation of adequate clothing, food, medical attention, or shelter, or a failure to provide other needed age-appropriate care. Although the federal government, through CAPTA, provides minimum standards for child neglect, as in the case of child abuse, states have operationalized the federal standard by implementing definitions that vary widely. Neglect is generally considered as an act of omission rather than one of commission, and most definitions incorporate the concept of non-provision of, or inability to provide, adequate care.

Q4 The answer is: (A) True.

Like emotional abuse, neglect is more difficult to identify than is physical abuse because the more easily identified stigmata of scars, marks, or bruises are often not present.

In the absence of demonstrable evidence of harm in settings of neglect, it is often difficult for child protective services to intervene because intervention requires such evidence. Neglect is typically broken down into five main categories: emotional neglect, physical neglect, medical neglect, failure to thrive, and educational neglect.

Q5 The answer is: (B) False.
Studies and case reports have enumerated criteria associated with abuse and neglect. Some of the most frequently cited risk factors include child morbidity, cultural background, family violence, low socioeconomic status, parental mental or physical illness, parents who themselves were victims of abuse, and social isolation and/or family breakdown. These risk factors are often grouped into three main categories: child-associated risk factors, family-associated risk factors, and environmental characteristics.

Legal and Ethical Issues in Psychiatry I: Informed Consent, Competency, Treatment Refusal, and Civil Commitment

Multiple-Choice Questions

Select the appropriate answer.

Q1 Which of the following matters are BEST defined as those in which a party has committed an act in violation of a statute, and for which the penalty may be a monetary fine, incarceration, or both?

    A. *Civil matters*

    B. *Criminal matters*

    C. *Ethical matters*

    D. *Malpractice matters*

    E. *Medical matters*

Q2 True or False. A fact witness may offer opinion testimony and is generally allowed to use hearsay evidence.

    A. *True*

    B. *False*

Q3 Which of the following is NOT considered to be one of the four core ethical principle of clinical care?

    A. *Autonomy*

    B. *Beneficence*

    C. *Competence*

    D. *Justice*

    E. *Non-malfeasance*

Q4 True or False. The patient's signature on a consent form constitutes informed consent.

    A. *True*

    B. *False*

Q5 True or False. Psychiatrists can declare an individual to be legally incompetent.

    A. *True*

    B. *False*

Q6 Which of the following questions is NOT a core element of a clinical assessment to determine a person's capacity to make treatment decisions?

A. *Does the patient express a preference or choice?*

B. *Does the patient have a factual understanding, at the level of a layperson, of the basic relevant information concerning the medical condition and the proposed treatment, risks, and benefits?*

C. *Does the patient have an appreciation of the significance of the information to the situation at hand?*

D. *Does the patient arrive at a decision in a logical manner that considers the information provided in the context of other personal factors (i.e., is the patient rational)?*

E. *Does the patient agree with the clinical assessment and clinical recommendations of the caregiver?*

Answers

Q1 The answer is: (B) Criminal matters.

Criminal matters are those in which a party has committed an act in violation of a statute, and for which the penalty may be a monetary fine, incarceration, or both.

Civil matters are those in which a dispute arises in which one party claims to have been injured by another, or some other transgression has occurred, that can be remedied by the payment of money (damages) or performance or cessation of certain activities (injunctive relief).

Q2 The answer is: (B) False.

There are two basic types of witnesses: fact witnesses and expert witnesses. Psychiatrists may be called on to serve in either role. Anyone who has firsthand knowledge of events and facts relevant to the case can be asked to serve as a fact witness. Fact witnesses may testify only as to the information they have obtained firsthand; they may not introduce hearsay evidence, that is, information they have heard from others, except under certain limited circumstances. Most importantly, fact witnesses may not give opinion testimony. Thus, a treating clinician testifying as a fact witness for a patient may testify about his or her observations obtained in treatment but may not offer an opinion regarding negligence by a previous treater.

When evidence is to be introduced on a subject that is outside the realm of knowledge of the average juror or judge, testimony by an expert witness may be allowed or required to meet the burden of proof. To qualify as an expert, a witness must have knowledge of the subject in question beyond that of the average layperson by education, training, and experience. Unlike fact witnesses, expert witnesses may offer opinion testimony and are generally allowed to use hearsay evidence.

From time to time, psychiatrists may be asked to serve as either fact witnesses or expert witnesses in litigation matters in which their patients are involved. Although a patient can generally insist that the treating clinician provide copies of records and testify as a fact witness, the psychiatrist need not, and should not, serve as an expert witness. It is generally accepted that treating clinicians should not serve as expert witnesses on behalf of their own patients as the two roles are incompatible. For example, clinicians have a fiduciary duty to act in the best interests of their patients, whereas expert witnesses have an ethical obligation to be objective, regardless of the impact on the litigant's position. In addition, in forming an objective opinion, experts must assess the litigant's claims against information obtained from collateral sources and be prepared to reject the litigant's claims. In other words, a treating clinician serving as an expert witness must challenge his or her patient's version of events, an activity that poses great risk for the therapeutic relationship. Clinicians who agree to serve as experts but who do not follow the proper methodology for conducting forensic evaluations may find their testimony excluded under the rules of evidence.

Q3 The answer is: (C) Competence.

The four ethical principles that form the foundation of clinical care are autonomy, beneficence, justice, and non-malfeasance.

According to Judge Benjamin Cardozo's opinion in the Schloendorff decision in 1914, "Every human being of adult years and sound mind has a right to determine what shall be done with his body"; this is the essence of the principle of autonomy.

Q4 The answer is: (B) False.

Informed consent is best described as a process in which one person, the patient, agrees to allow another person, the treater, to do something to, or for, him or her. The emphasis in this definition of informed consent is on the *process*, that is, the interactions between the patient and the clinician, during which there is an exchange of information and acceptance or rejection of the proposed treatment. The role of forms in the informed consent process is commonly misunderstood. The patient's signature on a consent form does not constitute informed consent itself; it is merely evidence that the informed consent process occurred.

Informed consent evolved from simple consent, which was one of the two basic defenses to a common-law claim of battery. Simple consent required only that the would-be patient explicitly or implicitly agreed to treatment by the physician; little or no explanation was required. The move toward requiring more substantive consent was fueled by a number of forces, including increased professionalization of medicine, a decline in religious fatalism, and an increased belief that health could be improved through individual effort and through science and technology. Informed consent was a logical result of the civil liberties movement and the shift toward autonomy in medical ethics.

Q5 The answer is: (B) False.
Only a court (and not a psychiatrist) can declare an individual to be legally incompetent. Although evaluation of a patient's decision-making capacity by a physician or mental health professional is commonly referred to as a "competency evaluation," the evaluating clinician has no authority to change the patient's legal status.

Q6 The answer is: (E) Does the patient agree with the clinical assessment and clinical recommendations of the caregiver?
In conducting a clinical assessment of a person's capacity to make treatment decisions, four elements should be examined: (1) Does the patient express a preference or choice? (2) Does the patient have a factual understanding, at the level of a layperson, of the basic relevant information concerning the medical condition and the proposed treatment, risks, and benefits? (3) Does the patient have an appreciation of the significance of the information to the situation at hand? (4) Does the patient arrive at a decision in a logical manner that considers the information provided in the context of other personal factors (i.e., is the patient rational)?

It should be noted that the patient's decision may still be rational, even if it is contrary to what most individuals, and the caregivers, might choose. Competent people are entitled to make choices that others may deem inadvisable or irrational. Such is the essential nature of individual autonomy.

The Role of Psychiatrists in the Criminal Justice System

Multiple-Choice Questions

Select the appropriate answer.

Q1   True or False. In the United States, the trial of an incompetent individual is incompatible with justice and violates the Constitutional guarantee of due process under law.

A.   *True*

B.   *False*

Q2   In the United States, which of the following cases established the standard for competency to stand trial?

A.   *Dusky v. United States*

B.   *Perry v. Louisiana*

C.   *Sell v. United States*

D.   *United States v. Charters*

E.   *Washington v. Harper*

Q3   True or False. If a defendant is found incompetent to stand trial (IST), the proceedings are suspended so that the defendant can be "restored to competency" as determined on subsequent assessment.

A.   *True*

B.   *False*

Q4   In which of the following cases did the Supreme Court hold that in order for a state to impose antipsychotic medication on an objecting defendant for the purpose of rendering the defendant competent to stand trial (CST), the state must show that the treatment is both medically necessary and appropriate?

A.   *Dusky v. United States*

B.   *Godinez v. Moran*

C.   *Perry v. Louisiana*

D.   *Riggins v. Nevada*

E.   *Washington v. Harper*

Q5   True or False. A fundamental principle of criminal justice is that individuals with severe mental illness or developmental disabilities are not to be held responsible for their otherwise criminal acts.

A.   *True*

B.   *False*

Q6   True or False. Evaluations of criminal responsibility are, by necessity, retrospective mental status examinations.

A.   *True*

B.   *False*

Chapter 86
Answers

Q1 The answer is: (A) True.
It is now well established in the United States that the trial of an incompetent individual is incompatible with justice and violates the Constitutional guarantee of due process under law. Requiring that the defendant be competent to stand trial (CST) serves several purposes, which include the following: (1) the fact-finding portion of the proceedings can only be accurate if the defendant can work with his or her attorney with an understanding of the proceedings; (2) only a competent defendant can exercise the Constitutional rights to a fair trial and to confront his or her accuser in a meaningful way; (3) the integrity and dignity of the legal process are preserved by ensuring that the defendant is CST; and (4) the purposes of retribution and individual deterrence are served only if the convicted defendant is CST.

Q2 The answer is: (A) Dusky v. United States.
In the United States, the standard for competency to stand trial was established in Dusky v. United States. Under the Dusky standard, the relevant inquiry is whether the defendant "has sufficient present ability to consult with his lawyer with a reasonable degree of rational understanding, and whether he has a rational as well as a factual understanding of the proceedings against him." When the issue of competency to stand trial is raised, the trial judge must conclude that the defendant is competent by a preponderance of the evidence, that is, that it is more likely than not that he or she meets the Dusky criteria.

There have been numerous efforts to define the characteristics that distinguish defendants who are CST from those who are not. A federal district court specified the following components of CST as meeting the Dusky criteria and indicating that a defendant is CST:

"(1) that he has mental capacity to appreciate his presence in relation to time, place, and things; (2) that his elementary mental processes are such that he apprehends (i.e., seizes and grasps with what mind he has) that he is in a Court of Justice, charged with a criminal offense; (3) that there is a Judge on the Bench; (4) a Prosecutor present who will try to convict him of a criminal charge; (5) that he has a lawyer (self-employed or Court-appointed) who will undertake to defend him against that charge; (6) that he will be expected to tell his lawyer the circumstances, to the best of his mental ability (whether colored or not by mental aberration) the facts surrounding him at the time and place where the law violation is alleged to have been committed; (7) that there is, or will be, a jury present to pass on evidence adduced as to his guilt or innocence of such charge; and (8) he has memory sufficient to relate those things in his own personal manner."

Q3 The answer is: (A) True.
If a defendant is found incompetent to stand trial (IST), the proceedings are suspended so that the defendant can be "restored to competency" as determined on subsequent assessment. The restoration process may involve both treatment of the incapacitating illness and educational efforts aimed specifically at participation in the trial process. Programs aimed at "restoring" the competency of mentally ill and cognitively impaired defendants have been instituted. Depending on the severity of the crime and the nature of the underlying illness, the charges may be dropped at this point. For example, in practice, charges of misdemeanor or non-violent offenses may be dropped when the individual has a mental illness and is committed for further treatment.

In cases involving more serious crimes, the defendant might be committed to an inpatient psychiatric facility for treatment and restoration of competency if the defendant has a treatable mental illness that impairs his or her competence to stand trial. The defendant will be reassessed for competence to stand trial periodically, as required according to the statute in that jurisdiction. In Jackson v. Indiana, the Supreme Court held that defendants who have no hope of restoration of competency cannot be committed indefinitely to state psychiatric facilities unless they meet the usual civil commitment criteria and standard procedures are followed.

Q4 The answer is: (D) Riggins v. Nevada.

In United States v. Charters, a US Court of Appeals in 1988 addressed the issue of what procedures were necessary to protect the rights of a defendant who had been found IST and was refusing treatment with antipsychotic medication. The court held that even though the involuntary treatment would constitute a deprivation of certain liberty interests, the defendant's rights could be adequately protected through a process that left the decision about whether involuntary medication should be administered "to appropriate professionals exercising their specialized professional judgments rather than to traditional judicial or administrative-type adjudicative processes."

Four years later in 1992, the Supreme Court addressed the circumstances under which an IST defendant could be involuntarily medicated to restore his competency to stand trial in Riggins v. Nevada. The Supreme Court held that for a state to impose antipsychotic medication on an objecting defendant for the purpose of rendering the defendant CST, the state must show that the treatment is both medically necessary and appropriate. In deciding the case, the Court looked to its earlier opinion in Washington v. Harper, in which it held that a state may treat an inmate with antipsychotic medication against his will if the inmate has a serious mental illness and "is dangerous to himself or others and the treatment is in his medical interest."

The Supreme Court in 2003 refined its holding regarding involuntary medication of IST defendants in Sell v. United States. Dr. Sell, a dentist accused of insurance fraud and attempting to have witnesses murdered, was found IST. The government sought to treat him with antipsychotic medication, which he refused, claiming that he had an absolute right to refuse treatment. The Court held that when a defendant is charged with non-violent crimes, the Constitution permits the government to administer antipsychotic drugs against the defendant's will to render the defendant CST only under limited circumstances. The Court held that involuntary administration of psychotropic medication to a non-violent IST defendant can occur only when a court determines that (1) important governmental interests are at stake; (2) the forced medication will significantly further those important-to-government interests—that is, the medication is "substantially likely to render the defendant CST and substantially unlikely to have side effects that will interfere significantly with the defendant's ability to assist counsel in conducting a defense"; (3) the involuntary treatment with medication is "necessary to further those interests and find that alternative, less intrusive treatments are unlikely to achieve substantially the same results"; and (4) that administering the drugs is medically appropriate.

Q5 The answer is: (A) True.

A fundamental principle of criminal justice is that individuals with severe mental illness or developmental disabilities are not to be held responsible for their otherwise criminal acts. The concept itself, and the derivative question of what to do with individuals who are found not guilty by reason of insanity, have been the subject of much debate and have generated fluctuating standards. Few activities of mental health professionals get as much media and public attention and spark as much controversy as testimony on these matters.

The history of the insanity defense is the product of society's struggles over moral responsibility, ecclesiastical influences, historical events, the nature and level of understanding of mental illness from a scientific standpoint, and public attitudes about the mentally ill. For example, the episodic mental illness of King George III is believed to have had a major influence on the attitudes of the public, and therefore the jurors of the time may have benefited some criminal defendants of the period. There are numerous examples of the criminal responsibility standard being tightened after the perpetrator of a notorious crime is found not guilty by reason of insanity, for example, James Hadfield, Daniel M'Naghten, and John Hinckley. The modifications are such that these infamous defendants would have been found criminally responsible under the new standard.

For an individual to be convicted of a crime, there must be a guilty act (*actus reus*) and guilty intent (*mens rea*). *Mens rea* is considered in both a general and a specific form. In its general form, it refers to the overall capacity of an individual to form the intent to commit the crime in question, and thus his or her blameworthiness or legal liability. For example, an individual who takes someone else's automobile for his own use when directed to do so by auditory hallucinations or is not even aware that he is stealing a vehicle is unlikely to be found to have had the necessary intent to be found blameworthy. In its specific or narrow form, *mens rea* is an element of a group of crimes referred to as specific intent crimes, for example, larceny of a motor vehicle (knowingly taking possession of property that is not your own, for your own use, and with the intent to deprive the true owner of its use) or murder.

Q6 The answer is: (A) True.

Evaluations of criminal responsibility are, by necessity, retrospective mental status examinations. The focus of criminal responsibility evaluations is assessment of the individual's mental state at the time of using the current examination, a review of medical and criminal records, and information from collateral sources and a conclusion regarding that status relative to the jurisdictional standards for criminal responsibility. Under ideal conditions, the accused is evaluated by mental health professionals as close to the occurrence of the act as possible. In many cases, however, the forensic evaluator may not see the defendant until months or years after the crime.

Several clinical conditions can affect criminal responsibility, for example, delirium, depression, psychosis, delusions, panic and other anxiety disorders, sleep disorders, obsessive-compulsive disorder, seizures, and other neurologic disorders. In light of this, the clinical evaluation should be detailed and extensive, with a full review of systems. Medical records should be examined and laboratory studies ordered to assess for the presence of other illnesses and conditions, including intoxication.

Criminal responsibility evaluations are complicated not only by the retrospective nature of the analysis, often over time, but by the fact that the sources of information are often incomplete or biased. Police reports, statements from family members, victim statements, and the defendant's self-report are also essential parts of the evaluation. All of them are affected, to greater or lesser degrees, by their own inherent bias, which is often difficult to detect.

Legal and Ethical Issues in Psychiatry II: Malpractice and Boundary Violations

Multiple-Choice Questions

Select the appropriate answer.

Q1   Which of the following is BEST defined as an injury to another party that gives rise to a right on the part of the injured person to sue for damages?

A.   *Malfeasance*

B.   *Misdiagnosis*

C.   *Negligence*

D.   *Privilege*

E.   *Tort*

Q2   Which of the following is NOT considered a necessary element of a malpractice claim?

A.   *Damages*

B.   *Dereliction of duty*

C.   *Direct causation*

D.   *Duress*

E.   *Duty*

Q3   True or False. Expert witnesses who offer their opinions on any of the four elements in a malpractice case must testify to a "reasonable degree of medical certainty."

A.   *True*

B.   *False*

Q4   True or False. The psychiatrist or inpatient unit is liable if a suicidal patient is refused further insurance coverage for inpatient hospitalization, is discharged, and then commits suicide.

A.   *True*

B.   *False*

Q5   Which of the following is BEST considered as an unintentional tort?

   A.   *Assault*

   B.   *Battery*

   C.   *False imprisonment*

   D.   *Misdiagnosis*

   E.   *Undue familiarity*

Q6   True or False. Psychiatrists have an ethical and legal duty to maintain the confidentiality of information disclosed by patients during treatment, without exception.

   A.   *True*

   B.   *False*

Chapter 87

Answers

Q1 The answer is: (E) Tort.

A tort is an injury to another party that gives rise to a right on the part of the injured person to sue for damages. Personal injury or tort law embodies the principle that a person injured by the acts of another should receive compensation for the harm done. This concept dates back more than 2000 years.

Medical malpractice is a subset of tort law that is concerned with alleged negligence by medical professionals. Medical malpractice as a concept represents the application of tort principles to the actions of professionals and, like tort law itself, is an ancient phenomenon.

There are two types of torts: intentional and unintentional. Both may be the subject of malpractice claims in psychiatry. Intentional torts are injuries that result from some intentional action on the part of the actor, also referred to as the "tortfeasor," who will ultimately be the defendant if a lawsuit is pursued. In psychiatric malpractice claims, typical intentional torts are battery, assault, false imprisonment, abandonment, intentional infliction of emotional distress, and undue familiarity (i.e., sexual misconduct and other boundary violations). Unintentional torts arise out of negligent acts or omissions (e.g., misdiagnosis or failure to diagnose, failure to protect the patient from self-harm, or harm to others).

Tort law serves two purposes. First, it fulfills the long-established concept that individuals who are injured by the negligent actions of others should receive compensation for the damage they have suffered. Second, the threat of liability serves as a deterrent to negligent behavior.

Q2 The answer is: (D) Duress.

The four elements of a malpractice claim are often referred to as the four Ds: duty, dereliction of duty, direct causation, and damages. If the defendant convinces the jury, or the judge in a bench trial, that all four elements have been proved by a preponderance of the evidence, that is, that it is more likely than not to have occurred, the defendant will be required to compensate the victim for the harm suffered.

First, the plaintiff must prove that the defendant owed a duty to the injured party. All individuals owe a general duty of reasonable care, such that their ordinary behavior does not result in harm to others (e.g., drivers have a general obligation not to drive recklessly). The duty to behave in a non-negligent fashion toward a specific individual or group arises when there is a special relationship. Thus, although a physician does not have a specific duty to a person until a doctor–patient relationship is established, once that relationship begins, the physician has a duty to perform in accordance with the standard of care of the average physician practicing in that specialty. To prove the existence of a duty, the plaintiff must establish that a doctor–patient relationship existed. Simply put, a doctor–patient relationship is established when the physician accepts responsibility for the patient's care by becoming involved with the treatment. Curbside or informal consultations, or even more formal consultations, will not establish the existence of a relationship, so long as the consultant does not assume a treatment role.

The second element of a malpractice claim is dereliction of the duty or negligence. It can be characterized as a departure from the standard of care that results from failure to exercise the level of diligence or care exercised by other physicians of that specialty. An error or injury does not constitute malpractice if it occurs during treatment in which the physician has exercised due diligence. To establish this element, the plaintiff must introduce evidence of the applicable standard of care. This is perhaps the most critical element in malpractice claims, as the applicable standard varies according to the situation, the type of practitioner, and the jurisdiction. Specialists, or those who claim to have special expertise, are held to a higher standard of practice than general practitioners.

The third element (causation) and fourth element (damages) are closely tied to the first two: the plaintiff must show that the negligent behavior is the direct cause or proximate cause of actual damages. Causation in personal injury law is assessed in two ways. First, the "but-for" test is applied: "But-for the alleged negligence, would the injury have occurred?" Second, was there proximate or legal cause (i.e., was the injury foreseeable)? The test for foreseeability is whether the claimed harm was "a natural, probable, and foreseeable consequence" of negligence on the part of the actor.

Q3 The answer is: (A) True.

Expert witnesses who offer their opinions on any of the four elements must testify to a "reasonable degree of medical certainty," that is, they are confident that their opinions are more likely true than not.

Q4 The answer is: (A) True.

The psychiatrist or inpatient unit is liable if a suicidal patient is refused further insurance coverage for inpatient hospitalization, is discharged, and then commits suicide. A psychiatrist's duty to his or her patient continues, regardless of whether the patient's insurer will continue to pay for services.

Q5 The answer is: (D) Misdiagnosis.

In psychiatric malpractice claims, typical intentional torts are battery (the touching of another person without consent or justification), assault (an action that causes fear in the victim, owing to the reasonable apprehension that an unpermitted touching will occur), false imprisonment (which can occur with confinement to a locked ward, room seclusion, or restraints; it does not require actual physical restraint or physical confinement if the patient believes that the door to his room is locked), abandonment (the unilateral termination of the doctor–patient relationship without justification, leading to harm to the patient), intentional infliction of emotional distress, and undue familiarity (i.e., sexual misconduct and other boundary violations).

Unintentional torts arise out of negligent acts or omissions (e.g., misdiagnosis or failure to diagnose, failure to protect the patient from self-harm, or harm to others).

Q6 The answer is: (B) False.

Psychiatrists have an ongoing ethical and legal duty to maintain the confidentiality of information disclosed by patients during treatment and may be held liable for unauthorized disclosure. However, numerous ethical and legal exceptions exist to the requirement of confidentiality; all these exceptions represent a balancing of the relative harms that result from maintaining or breaching confidentiality in given situations. Ethical exceptions to confidentiality tend to be permissive, for example, "A psychiatrist may breach confidentiality if ..." These exceptions tend to be commonsense in nature but leave the discretion to the practitioner, without imposing obligations. The legal exceptions, found in case law, statutes, and regulations, tend to fall into two broad categories: immunity from liability for disclosure in good faith and required disclosures.

Whether a given exception falls into the immunity for disclosure or mandatory disclosure category depends on the nature of the exception and the jurisdiction. For example, all 50 states in the United States have statutes that designate a range of professionals as mandated reporters who are obligated to report suspected child abuse or neglect to state social service agencies. Many states also require reporting of known or suspected abuse or neglect of the elderly or disabled. In recent years, a number of states have also begun requiring physicians and others to report known or suspected cases of domestic violence to law enforcement or designated agencies.

Of all the exceptions to confidentiality, perhaps the best known involves the duty to protect third parties from the violent acts of patients. This duty exists in some but not all jurisdictions. The rationale for the duty to act to protect third parties was set forth in the California court's decision in Tarasoff v. Board of Regents, in which the court held that psychotherapists have a duty to act to protect third parties in which the therapist knows or should know that the patient poses a threat of serious risk of harm to the third party.

The variations among jurisdictions in the law regarding the duty to protect can lead to much confusion. Clinicians are advised, as a basic matter, to become familiar with the standards in the jurisdictions in which they practice. It is important to remember that the duty represents an exception to confidentially, which is recognized in all jurisdictions as being of paramount importance in clinical care, and that any breach of confidentiality must be justified and reasonable. It should be limited to disclosure of the minimum amount of information necessary to serve the purpose in question. Thus, even in jurisdictions in which there is a duty to protect third parties or efforts to protect are made permissible by statute, the clinician should first take steps that will protect the third party without disclosing confidential information, for example, arranging for hospitalization. Only when necessary to prevent harm should the patient's clinical information be disclosed to the intended victim or police.

Other exceptions to confidentiality include statutory provisions that allow disclosure of clinical information in pursuit of the civil commitment process, bill collection, and in defense of malpractice claims. It is also accepted that a reasonable amount of information may be disclosed when applying to admit or transfer a patient to a hospital.

SECTION 20
CARE IN SPECIAL SETTINGS

Chapter 88

Emergency Psychiatry

Multiple-Choice Questions

Select the appropriate answer.

Q1 Which of the following MOST often account for emergency mental health visits?

A. *Anxiety disorders*

B. *Mood disorders*

C. *Psychosis*

D. *Substance-related disorders*

E. *Suicide attempts*

Q2 True or False. A medical workup should be considered for any new onset of psychiatric symptomatology or any significant change or exacerbation of symptoms.

A. *True*

B. *False*

Q3 True or False. A plan for suicide with a low risk of medical consequences means that the patient does not have a strong desire to die.

A. *True*

B. *False*

Q4 Which of the following agents can treat opiate intoxication in the emergency department (ED)?

A. *Benztropine*

B. *Flumazenil*

C. *Hydrocodone*

D. *Naloxone*

E. *Physostigmine*

Q5 Which of the following signs or symptoms is LEAST likely to be present in a patient with opiate withdrawal?

A. *Abdominal cramping*

B. *Chills*

C. *Constricted pupils*

D. *Rhinorrhea*

E. *Yawning*

Q6   Which of the following drugs is also known as "angel dust"?

    A.   *Crack cocaine*

    B.   *Crystal methamphetamine*

    C.   *Heroin*

    D.   *LSD*

    E.   *Phencyclidine (PCP)*

Q7   True or False. Pressured or loud speech, invasion of someone else's personal space, clenching of the jaw, or tension of other muscles may each indicate escalating agitation.

    A.   *True*

    B.   *False*

Q1 The answer is: (D) Substance-related disorders.

In 2001, there were over 2 million visits to US emergency departments (EDs) for mental health–related chief complaints, accounting for more than 6% of all ED visits, and representing an increase in the percentage of all visits by 28% over the previous decade. Among emergency mental health visits, substance-related disorders (30%), mood disorders (23%), anxiety disorders (21%), psychosis (10%), and suicide attempts (7%) are the most common.

Q2 The answer is: (A) True.

For any patient who presents to an ED with an altered mental status (be it a change in cognition, emotional state, or behavior), it is crucial to rule out an underlying medical condition that causes or contributes to the presentation. A change in mental state may indicate a primary psychiatric condition, delirium (an acute and reversible condition secondary to a medical illness), or dementia (a chronic condition associated with long-term, irreversible brain pathology). Therefore, it is important to consider medical etiologies for any presentation that appears psychiatric in nature. A missed medical diagnosis in lieu of an assumed psychiatric diagnosis could result in dire consequences for the patient.

A medical workup should be considered for any new onset of psychiatric symptomatology or any significant change or exacerbation of symptoms. This initial medical workup is often referred to as medical clearance. The term *medical clearance* generally refers to a medical evaluation aimed at ruling out underlying medical conditions that cause or contribute to a psychiatric presentation. Although much attention has been paid to defining a standard for medical clearance, there is no clear consensus regarding the required elements of the medical evaluation.

Q3 The answer is: (B) False.

If a patient has a plan and/or the intent to commit suicide, the lethality of the plan, as well as the patient's perception of the risk, must be assessed. A medically low-risk plan may still coincide with a strong intent to die if the patient believes that the lethality of the attempt is high. Similarly, the possibility that the patient could have been rescued if he or she had followed through on the plan should be evaluated; an impulsive ingestion of pills in front of a family member after an argument conveys less risk than a similar attempt in a remote location. If a patient has attempted suicide previously, details of that attempt may facilitate an understanding of the current risk. In addition, the clinician should assess other risk factors for suicide.

Q4 The answer is: (D) Naloxone.

Opiate intoxication seen in the ED is commonly the result of heroin, oxycodone, methadone, hydrocodone, or fentanyl. Intoxication can be identified by drowsiness and by pupillary constriction; in addition, patients describe a sense of euphoria or calm. The greatest risk of opiate overdose is respiratory depression. Frequently, accidental overdose occurs when a patient either miscalculates his or her dose after a period of abstinence (due to decreased tolerance) or when the drug is found to be purer than is expected. Opiate intoxication can be treated in the emergency setting with naloxone, an opioid antagonist, although drowsiness and respiratory depression may return as the naloxone wears off. In addition, the naloxone will cause an acute and uncomfortable withdrawal syndrome that often leads to agitation on awakening.

Benztropine can treat dystonic reactions induced by dopamine blockers. Flumazenil can reverse benzodiazepine intoxication (but may induce benzodiazepine withdrawal and seizures in a benzodiazepine-dependent person). Hydrocodone is a narcotic that, if administered to a person already intoxicated by opiates, would further increase opiate intoxication. Physostigmine can reverse the peripheral and central manifestations of anticholinergic excess; bradyarrhythmias and seizures may result from rapid (high-dose) intravenous infusions.

Q5 The answer is: (C) Constricted pupils.

Early symptoms of opiate withdrawal include anxiety, yawning, diaphoresis, rhinorrhea, dilated pupils, abdominal and leg cramping, and chills. Elevated blood pressure, pulse, and temperature, as well as nausea and vomiting, will follow. A urine drug screen can usually confirm recent opiate use. In the emergency setting, symptomatic treatment consists of the use of clonidine for autonomic instability (monitor for hypotension), dicyclomine for abdominal cramps, and quinine sulfate for leg cramps (limited to once per day because of the risk of cardiovascular or renal toxicity). The patient can be referred to a licensed detoxification facility for methadone or buprenorphine detoxification.

Q6 The answer is: (E) Phencyclidine (PCP).

Phencyclidine (PCP) is also known as "angel dust." Intoxication with PCP is usually heralded in the emergency setting by agitation, paranoia, hallucinations, and violent or bizarre behavior.

Intoxication can cause nystagmus, ataxia, and slurred speech; at higher doses it may lead to seizures, a hypertensive crisis, coma, and death.

Treatment is supportive and should include management in a contained and quiet setting (because of the risk of violence). Antipsychotics, particularly high-potency neuroleptics (such as haloperidol), may be useful. PCP-induced psychosis can last from days to weeks; these patients may require hospitalization if symptoms do not improve within several hours. No withdrawal syndrome is associated with abstinence from PCP.

Q7 The answer is: (A) True.

Early signs of agitation include pacing, tapping of the fingers and feet, sighing, moaning, breathing heavily, fidgeting, staring intensely, or appearing distracted by internal stimuli. Physical signs (such as elevations in blood pressure, pulse, or respiratory rate) may be noted. Pressured or loud speech, invasion of others' personal space, clenching of the jaw, or tension of other muscles often indicate escalating agitation. Rapid movements, yelling, slamming doors, or throwing objects are important signals that the patient is out of control. Agitation can herald a psychiatric emergency; it jeopardizes the safety of the patient, as well as others in the treatment environment, and it impedes optimal evaluation and treatment.

If there is a risk of harm to the patient or to others, a physically safe environment, without access to objects that could be used as weapons, using the least restrictive means possible, should be arranged. Pharmacologic interventions to reduce agitation should also be considered. Agitation is best managed by attempting to prevent or treat it as early as possible. The agitated patient should be enlisted in this task (i.e., to monitor his or her own internal state, to report increases in anxiety or distress, and to consider effective means for the reduction of distress to avert any behavioral dyscontrol). Modulation of the environment (by decreasing interpersonal interactions and auditory or visual stimulation) is an important initial step in management. A safe environment (free from the risk of harm) should be created to reduce agitation for some patients. Staff or family members should be available to communicate with the patient. Offers of food and drink may also be helpful.

Rehabilitation Psychiatry

Multiple-Choice Questions

Select the appropriate answer.

Q1 During rehabilitation from which of the following conditions is depression MOST likely to be observed?

  A. *Colon cancer*

  B. *Lymphoma*

  C. *Lung cancer*

  D. *Multiple sclerosis*

  E. *Traumatic brain injury*

Q2 True or False. Fluent aphasia and expressive aprosodia are each strongly associated with left-sided brain lesions.

  A. *True*

  B. *False*

Q3 True or False. Men who have sustained spinal cord injuries are incapable of achieving an erection.

  A. *True*

  B. *False*

Q4 True or False. Patients who have had a history of a serious accident or physical impairment are more likely to experience a variety of social and physical health problems compared with other psychiatric patients, while experiencing comparable levels of mental health problems.

  A. *True*

  B. *False*

Chapter 89

Answers

Q1 The answer is: (E) Traumatic brain injury.

Many patients undergoing rehabilitation are at significant risk for the development of psychiatric complications. For example, in people with traumatic brain injury, the prevalence of depression may be as high as 40% to 50%. In those with cancer, rates of depression vary according to the type of cancer: higher rates are associated with cancer of the oropharynx (22% to 57%), pancreas (33% to 50%), and lung (11% to 44%), whereas colon cancer (13% to 25%) and lymphoma (8% to 19%) have lower rates. In those with multiple sclerosis, depression ranges from 22% to 46%.

In addition, thoughts of suicide are more common among those with chronic illnesses compared with those without such conditions.

Q2 The answer is: (B) False.

Expressive aprosodia is an underappreciated example of dysfunctional poststroke communication. It involves an impaired ability to convey affect through inflection, gesture, and facial expression. The damage is in the non-dominant frontotemporal region and is an analogue of aphasia, which is associated with the frontotemporal region on the dominant hemisphere.

Patients with expressive aprosodia sometimes have depressive cognitions but cannot convey their depressed mood; this leads to underdiagnosis of depression. However, a patient with an expressive aprosodia may be misdiagnosed as having depression when his or her unemotional apathetic speech is misinterpreted as a sign of a mood disorder.

Dominant hemisphere lesions generate confounds for psychiatric diagnosis as well. The most prominent of these are the aphasias. Fluent aphasia, such as Wernicke aphasia, presents with well-articulated incoherent speech and failure to comprehend without a motor or sensory deficit. This disordered, fluent speech can be confused with *loose associations*, a common characteristic of thought disorders and schizophrenia. History is the key to differentiating a fluent aphasia with sudden onset in a previously well-functioning patient from schizophrenia, in which an insidious onset and chronic course along with emotional and social impoverishment are evident.

Q3 The answer is: (B) False.

Managing changes in sexual function is a major concern following spinal cord injury. Complete spinal cord lesions can cause genital anesthesia, but some patients retain some genital sensation, response, and even orgasmic capability if the lesion is partial. Some men can ejaculate without pharmacologic assistance, although most cannot. Many women and men report the development of new areas of arousal above the level of the lesion, sometimes resulting in satisfying "phantom orgasms" with caressing or other tactile stimulation. An element of neuroplasticity appears to be present in this regard.

Men may be able to achieve reflex erections sufficient for intercourse, or may respond to treatment with PGE2 agents, but results are variable; the level and completeness of the injury, sacral sparing, and other individual factors likely contribute in this regard. Women are similarly affected but can use supplemental lubricants if vaginal lubrication is insufficient and intercourse is desired. Difficulties with positioning, bowel and bladder incontinence, autonomic dysreflexia, and spasticity during sexual activity can be problematic for both women and men. Some patients find that their preferences regarding specific sexual choices evolve in a manner that supports their remaining physical capabilities, such as increased interest in providing the partner with oral-genital stimulation and enjoying the shared sensual experiences that result from this.

Q4 The answer is: (A) True.

Patients who have had a history of a serious accident or physical impairment are more likely to experience a variety of social and physical health problems compared with other psychiatric patients, while experiencing comparable levels of mental health problems.

For example, such patients were much more likely to be separated or divorced (33.3% compared with 22.7%) and to have had conflict-laden or severed relationships (59.5% compared with 49.4%). In addition, they were almost twice as likely to have failed or dropped out of an educational program, and they were more likely to have disability insurance as an income source (27.8% compared with 16.1%).

Chapter 90

Military Psychiatry

Multiple-Choice Questions

Select the appropriate answer.

Q1 Which of the following is NOT a common psychiatric syndrome in the immediate aftermath of military operations or terrorist events?

    A. *Acute stress disorder*

    B. *Bipolar disorder*

    C. *Panic attacks and panic disorder*

    D. *Substance use disorder*

    E. *Unexplained physical symptoms*

Q2 Which of the following medications or treatments used in resuscitative efforts is LEAST likely to cause delirium?

    A. *Atropine*

    B. *Epinephrine*

    C. *Intravenous fluids leading to hyponatremia*

    D. *Lidocaine*

    E. *Morphine sulfate*

Q3 Which of the following is LEAST likely to protect servicemen and servicewomen exposed to combat or terrorist attack from development of a psychiatric disorder?

    A. *Physical injury*

    B. *Safety and security of the recovery environment*

    C. *Strong leadership*

    D. *Unit cohesion*

    E. *Unit loyalty and interpersonal trust*

Q4 Which of the following is LEAST likely to precipitate a psychiatric disorder in a serviceman or servicewoman exposed to combat or to a terrorist attack?

    A. *Deployments that disrupt families*

    B. *Exposure to simultaneous stressors*

    C. *Physical injury*

    D. *Strong leadership*

    E. *Witnessing a grotesque death, torture, or other atrocity*

Q5   Which of the following statements is LEAST accurate?

A.   *Each branch of the US military services has specialized rapid intervention teams to provide consultative assistance and acute treatment as necessary to units that have experienced traumatic events*

B.   *Mental health teams are now routinely assigned to US forces in combat and are deployed in operations other than war*

C.   *Neuropsychiatric symptoms may be manifest as an emotional response, as a consequence of a neurologic injury, and from the neurotoxic effects of specific chemical or biological agents*

D.   *Psychosocial interventions have an important role in secondary prevention in military trauma victims*

E.   *There is convincing evidence to show that group debriefings and critical incident stress debriefings reduce the incidence of posttraumatic stress disorder (PTSD)*

Chapter 90

Answers

Q1 The answer is: (B) Bipolar disorder.

In the theater of war, there is the terror of unanticipated injury, loss, and death. During military operations, psychological injury may occur in conjunction with physical injury, exposure to the injury and death of others, potential exposure to biological or chemical agents, disruption of one's physical environment, or because of the terror and helplessness that these events combine to evoke.

Negative effects of combat exposure can persist for decades. Combat exposure results in high prevalence rates of psychiatric diagnoses and psychosocial problems: 28% develop posttraumatic stress disorder (PTSD); 21% engage in spousal or partner abuse; 12% experience job loss; 9% are unemployed; 8% have substance abuse problems within 1 year; 8% get divorced or separated; and 7% sustain major depressive disorder. In addition, other conditions are common: delirium, depression, acute stress disorder, generalized anxiety, panic attacks/disorder, substance use disorder, hypochondriasis, unexplained physical symptoms, dissociation, dissociative disorders, battle fatigue, and operational stress.

However, there is no indication that bipolar disorder arises commonly in such situations.

Q2 The answer is: (B) Epinephrine.

Although each of the medications listed can be employed during resuscitative efforts, atropine (via its anticholinergic side effects), lidocaine, morphine sulfate, and intravenous fluids that lead to hyponatremia can result in mental status changes consistent with delirium. Epinephrine tends to cause anxiety, as well as elevations in heart rate and blood pressure (but not delirium).

Q3 The answer is: (A) Physical injury.

In groups (such that exist in the military, police or firefighters, and paramedics), certain factors may diminish the potential sequelae of trauma. Loyalty and interpersonal cohesion within such organizations provide ready access to social supports during the acute phase of a disaster and its aftermath. When organizations possess effective leaders, an environment embodied by strong loyalty, mutual trust, and respect is more likely to exist. Such an environment may facilitate voluntary participation in high-risk rescue/recovery or combat missions and facilitate the synchronization of individual efforts necessary for success in these types of operations.

Ongoing factors (including the security and safety of recovery environments, the extent of secondary traumatization, rotation schedules, the degree of recognition or compensation for efforts, and one's belief in the mission) all affect the rate and severity of psychiatric illness and symptoms of distress. Personal attributes or behaviors (such as "overdedication" to the task at hand) may further contribute to the development of dysfunction. Symptoms in civilian victims of war or the aftermath of disaster may be mitigated or exacerbated by several factors (e.g., by perceptions of community's leadership, preparedness for disaster, response to crisis, recognition of heroes, and provision of medical, financial, or emotional assistance) both immediately after the crisis, and over time.

Specific experiences, such as physical injury, or the witnessing of grotesque deaths, torture, or other atrocities, place individuals at increased risk for adverse mental health consequences.

Q4 The answer is: (D) Strong leadership.

The high intensity and long duration of a disaster or combat situation increases the likelihood of psychiatric casualties. Specific experiences, such as physical injury, or the witnessing of grotesque deaths, torture, or other atrocities, place individuals at increased risk for adverse mental health consequences. Deployments and peacekeeping missions disrupt families and are often poorly timed with regard to other life events. Exposure to multiple simultaneous stressors and to traumatic events increases the risk of pathological outcomes.

Q5 The answer is: (E) There is convincing evidence to show that group debriefings and critical incident stress debriefings reduce the incidence of posttraumatic stress disorder (PTSD).

Group debriefing techniques and critical incident stress debriefings have been used, although there is no convincing evidence that such debriefings reduce the incidence of PTSD; in fact, several studies suggest that these interventions may be harmful. However, ongoing and frank discussions among squad members after a critical incident (such as an ambush or a raid) can open lines of communication to coordinate and evaluate the efficacy of actions, while fostering cohesion and group understanding of an event. These discussions, termed "After Action Reports," "Lessons Learned," or "Historical Debriefings," may serve to sustain the performance of persons critical to the management of the mission, may decrease individual isolation, and help to identify team members who may require further psychiatric or other mental health attention.

Chapter 91
Disaster Psychiatry
Multiple-Choice Questions

Select the appropriate answer.

Q1 Which of the following people tracked responses to disaster (involving normal grief, abnormal grief, the response to stress and loss, and the effects of witnessing a disaster) in the study of the 1942 Cocoanut Grove fire?

A. *Erikson*

B. *Fullilove*

C. *Lindemann*

D. *Rousseau*

E. *Yalom*

Q2 In which edition of the *Diagnostic and Statistical Manual of Mental Disorders* (DSM) did the diagnosis of posttraumatic stress disorder first appear?

A. *DSM-I*

B. *DSM-II*

C. *DSM-III*

D. *DSM-IV*

E. *DSM-5*

Q3 Which of the following is NOT generally considered to be a reasonable short-term goal for disaster psychiatrists following a disaster?

A. *Engaging survivors in the context in which they can be found*

B. *Helping students in middle school plan out their educational plans for high school and college*

C. *Orienting mental health workers to the environment and to the function of the mental health team*

D. *Providing information to survivors, disaster workers, and the general public about normal and expected responses, concerning signs and symptoms, health and reliance-enhancing activities, and where to go for further help if symptoms emerge*

E. *Screening survivors for risk factors and for traumatic stress reactions that suggest the need for further services*

Q4 Which of the following terms BEST defines the individual's capacity for successful adaptation and competent function (despite experiencing chronic stress or adversity); good outcomes despite serious threats to adaptation or development; and the ability to maintain relatively stable healthy levels of psychological and physical function?

A. *Coping*

B. *Denial*

C. *Reaction formation*

D. *Resiliency*

E. *Sublimation*

Q5 Which of the following is NOT a standard component of psychological first aid in the early phases after a disaster?

    A. *Administering meperidine to reduce physiological arousal*

    B. *Keeping families together and facilitating reunions with loved ones*

    C. *Mobilizing support for those who are most distressed*

    D. *Protecting survivors from further harm*

    E. *Providing information and fostering communication and education*

Q6 Which of the following is NOT a predisaster factor associated with adverse mental health outcomes after a disaster?

    A. *Age between 20 and 40 years*

    B. *Female sex*

    C. *Minority background*

    D. *Psychiatric history*

    E. *Poverty or low socioeconomic status*

Answers

Q1 The answer is: (C) Lindemann.

The most well-known early attempt of a psychiatrist to track such responses to disaster was by Erich Lindemann in his study of the 1942 Cocoanut Grove fire. He attempted to define in psychiatric language responses of normal grief, abnormal grief, responses to stress and loss, and the effects of witnessing a disaster.

Kai Erikson described the "disaster syndrome" in his sociological study of the Buffalo Creek flood.

Rousseau described how the formation of disaster plans is often abandoned because of the overwhelming complexity of the task. Psychiatrists or mental health organizations interested in disaster psychiatry must therefore prepare for disasters by familiarizing themselves with existing systems of disaster response, by building relationships with other agencies around disaster preparedness, and by forming action plans that include defined relationships within a system of disaster response (in advance of a disaster).

Fullilove noted that in the face of overwhelming catastrophe, people react at first with shock and paralysis and seem to wander as if in a daze. They appear docile and eager to follow those with a plan. Later, anger and despair emerge. When people lose their homes and their community, they may lack a cognitive map and have little sense of how to move through space, therefore paralysis ensues.

Yalom described the relevant curative factors of trauma groups: universality, catharsis, instillation of hope, provision of information, and review of existential factors. Time-limited supportive educational groups are designed to help people manage the overwhelming impact of trauma, to decrease isolation, and alleviate alienation. Cognitive-behavioral groups provide an opportunity to share the trauma experience, develop a narrative, and teach coping skills to manage recurrences of posttraumatic stress disorder and other symptoms. Psychodynamic groups can help individuals integrate a traumatic experience into their general life experience, and help them to move forward in developing a comprehensive view of themselves as individuals, in personal and professional relationships, and as members of their community.

Q2 The answer is: (C) DSM-III.

Posttraumatic stress disorder first appeared as a diagnostic category under anxiety disorders in DSM-III, and as its own unique stress syndrome in DSM-IV, as a direct result of the Vietnam War.

Q3 The answer is: (B) Helping students in middle school plan out their educational plans for high school and college.

A variety of short-term goals for disaster psychiatrists have been described. Common themes include the following: orienting mental health workers to the environment and to the function of the mental health team (including finding the existing hierarchy, making introductions, asking for their observations about needs, and defining your teams' availability and capacity); engaging survivors in the context in which they can be found and encouraging the supportiveness of a given context (disaster psychiatry takes place in shelters, on the streets, in schools and hotels, in waiting rooms of housing, in health care systems, and in disaster-relief centers, as the outreach model appears to be the best way to engage a vulnerable population that may be resistant to mental health treatment, described as "therapy by walking around"); screening survivors for risk factors and for traumatic stress reactions that suggest they need further services (aside from attending to blatant stress reactions, attention to risk factors can guide clinicians to who may be in need of further assessment and services); and providing information to survivors, disaster workers, and the general public about normal and expected responses, concerning signs and symptoms, health and resilience-enhancing activities, and where to go for further help if symptoms emerge (this is best achieved by becoming familiarized with the system to ensure that information is consistent and easily accessible).

Although helping students in middle school plan out their educational plans for high school and college is important, it is not a short-term goal for disaster psychiatrists.

Mental health services are not limited to the survivors of the disaster.

Q4 The answer is: (D) Resiliency.

Psychological resiliency has been defined as the individual's capacity for successful adaptation and competent function (despite experiencing chronic stress or adversity); good outcomes in spite of serious threats to adaptation or development; and the ability to maintain relatively stable healthy levels of psychological and physical function.

Rebuilding, getting together with family and friends, and engaging in both spiritual/religious and recreational activities are considered coping tools that can facilitate recovery and resiliency. In addition, positive reframing, or seeing the good that can come from disaster, can strengthen a sense of community and help foster resiliency at the individual and community level.

Denial, reaction formation, and sublimation are psychological defenses that people use to cope, but they do not define resiliency.

Q5 The answer is: (A) Administering meperidine to reduce physiological arousal.

Administering meperidine to reduce physiological arousal is neither a tactic of psychological first aid nor a reasonable intervention, as use of short-lasting narcotics will do little to improve function following a disaster.

Other key components of early intervention after a disaster include the following: basic needs (providing survival, safety, and security; providing food and shelter; orienting survivors to the availability of services/support; communicating with family, friends, and community; and assessing the environment for ongoing threats); needs assessment (assessing the current status of individuals, groups, and/or populations and institutions/systems; asking how well needs are being addressed, what the recovery environment offers, and what additional interventions are needed); rescue and recovery environment observations (observing and listening to those most affected; monitoring the environment for toxins and stressors; monitoring past and ongoing threats; monitoring services that are being provided; and monitoring media coverage and rumors); outreach and information dissemination (offering information/education and "therapy by walking around"; using established community structures; distributing flyers; hosting websites; and conducting media interviews and programs and distributing media releases); technical assistance (improving the capacity of organizations and caregivers to provide what is needed to re-establish community structure; fostering family recovery and resilience; safeguarding the community; and providing assistance, consultation, and training to relevant organizations, other caregivers and responders, and leaders); fostering resilience and recovery (fostering, but not forcing, social interactions; provide coping skills training; providing risk-assessment skills training; provide education on stress responses, traumatic reminders, coping, normal vs. abnormal functioning, risk factors, and services; offering group and family interventions; fostering natural social supports; looking after the bereaved; and repairing the organizational fabric); triage (conducting clinical assessments, using valid and reliable methods; referring when indicated; identifying vulnerable, high-risk individuals and groups; and providing for emergency hospitalization); and treatment (reducing or ameliorating symptoms or improving function via individual, family, and group psychotherapy, pharmacotherapy, or short- or long-term hospitalization).

Q6 The answer is: (A) Age between 20 and 40 years.

Age between 40 and 60 years is a risk factor, as is the presence of exposed children in the home.

Within-disaster factors for adverse outcomes include bereavement, injury, and the severity of exposure, panic/horror, threat to life, and relocation or displacement.

Postdisaster factors linked with a worse outcome include resource deterioration, social support deterioration, marital distress, loss of home/property or finances, alienation and mistrust, peritraumatic reactions, and avoidance coping.

SECTION 21

PREPARING FOR THE FUTURE

Coping with the Rigors of Psychiatric Practice

Multiple-Choice Questions

Select the appropriate answer.

Q1　Which of the following statements is LEAST accurate?

　　A.　*Burnout is a pathological syndrome in which prolonged occupational stress leads to emotional and physical depletion, and ultimately to the development of maladaptive behaviors (e.g., cynicism, depersonalization, hostility, and detachment)*

　　B.　*The chronic and devastating nature of many psychiatric diseases decreases the emotional burden on the clinician*

　　C.　*The daily practice of psychiatry is filled by issues of transference and countertransference, which can lead to the development of intense emotions in the patient and in the clinician*

　　D.　*The daily stress of practicing medicine, when left unaddressed or unmanaged, can progress over time to burnout*

　　E.　*The very same character traits that make physicians successful (e.g., perfectionism, an exaggerated sense of responsibility, and selflessness) also make physicians vulnerable to stress*

Q2　Which of the following statements is LEAST accurate?

　　A.　*Less than one-fourth of all psychiatrists have had one (or more) of their patients commit suicide*

　　B.　*Psychiatrists may experience grief, guilt, inadequacy, anxiety, depression, shock, shame, betrayal, and anger in response to a patient's suicide*

　　C.　*Psychiatrists must consistently control their affect to do their jobs well*

　　D.　*Rules regarding confidentiality inhibit sharing the details of one's day with family and friends*

　　E.　*Vocational burnout for psychiatrists is associated with low satisfaction in relationships*

Q3　Which of the following statements is LEAST accurate?

　　A.　*Boundary crossings are often considered as harmless deviations from clinical practice or from the therapeutic frame*

　　B.　*Boundary violations are deviations that are harmful and exploitive of the patient's emotional, financial, or sexual needs*

　　C.　*Building an allied and collaborative relationship with a patient is a key component of effective treatment, and it may offer some protection against future litigation*

　　D.　*The most frequent malpractice claim against psychiatrists occurs in cases in which a patient has alleged sexual misconduct*

　　E.　*Warning signs of boundary violations include believing that the patient is deserving of special treatment, allowing the patient to maintain a large, unpaid bill, and being reluctant to discuss the case with colleagues or supervisors*

Q4   Which of the following statements is LEAST accurate?

A.   *Consultation is not a sign of weakness; rather, it is the sign of a wise physician who recognizes that to help patients, one must first help oneself*

B.   *Having responses in mind before a crisis makes it more likely that one will stay calm in a tense situation*

C.   *Residency training is seldom considered grueling or demanding*

D.   *Self-knowledge can be used to inform diagnoses and to minimize potentially harmful reactions to patients (e.g., managing hostility toward a patient so that it will not interfere with treatment)*

E.   *Signs of burnout include detachment from the meaning of one's work, open hostility, deep-rooted cynicism, and overwhelming occupational dissatisfaction*

Chapter 92

Answers

Q1 The answer is: (B) The chronic and devastating nature of many psychiatric diseases decreases the emotional burden on the clinician.

Just the opposite is true; the chronic and devastating nature of many psychiatric diseases increases the emotional burden on the clinician.

Burnout is a pathological syndrome in which prolonged occupational stress leads to emotional and physical depletion, and ultimately to the development of maladaptive behaviors (e.g., cynicism, depersonalization, hostility, and detachment).

The daily practice of psychiatry is filled by issues of transference and countertransference, which can lead to the development of intense emotions in the patient and in the clinician.

The daily stress of practicing medicine, when left unaddressed or unmanaged, can progress over time to burnout.

The very same character traits that make physicians successful (e.g., perfectionism, an exaggerated sense of responsibility, and selflessness) also make physicians vulnerable to stress.

Q2 The answer is: (A) Less than one-fourth of all psychiatrists have had one (or more) of their patients commit suicide.

Actually, half of all psychiatrists have had one (or more) of their patients commit suicide; approximately one-third of those psychiatrists experienced such a loss while they were still in residency training.

Psychiatrists may experience grief, guilt, inadequacy, anxiety, depression, shock, shame, betrayal, and anger in response to a patient's suicide. The experience of anger and hostility toward the patient who committed suicide may further trigger guilt and self-blame.

Despite the intensely emotional nature of psychiatric work, psychiatrists must consistently control their affect to do their jobs well. When patients are overwhelmed by sadness, despair, anger, or frustration, psychiatrists must keep their own reactions in check, sometimes bottled deep within. Although this control of affect is necessary for the practice of psychiatry, it can ultimately lead to the denial of emotions. If one denies the existence of an affect (even after the patient has left the office), it can lead to increased stress and to vulnerability to burnout.

Rules regarding confidentiality inhibit sharing the details of one's day with family and friends.

Vocational burnout for psychiatrists is associated with low satisfaction in relationships.

Q3 The answer is: (D) The most frequent malpractice claim against psychiatrists occurs in cases in which a patient has alleged sexual misconduct.

The most frequent malpractice claim against psychiatrists occurs in cases in which a patient has committed suicide; thus documentation of both the risks and the protective factors, in addition to the rationalizations behind clinical decisions, is crucial. Perhaps the most protective factor is a strong alliance with the patient.

Boundary crossings are often considered as harmless deviations from clinical practice or from the therapeutic frame.

Boundary violations are deviations that are harmful and exploitive of the patient's emotional, financial, or sexual needs.

Building an allied and collaborative relationship with a patient is a key component of effective treatment, and it may offer some protection against future litigation.

Warning signs of boundary violations include idealizing the patient and believing that the patient is deserving of special treatment, holding sessions at the end of the day or even "after hours," allowing sessions to go longer than the allotted time, allowing the patient to maintain a large, unpaid bill, and, most important, being reluctant to discuss the case with colleagues or supervisors. Any of these signs should immediately prompt the clinician to seek objective consultation to examine these issues in depth.

Q4 The answer is: (C) Residency training is seldom considered grueling or demanding.
Several factors make residency training especially demanding: a lack of control, sleep deprivation, responsibility without authority, and balancing autonomy with dependence.

Consultation is not a sign of weakness; rather, it is the sign of a wise physician who recognizes that to help patients, one must first help oneself. Consultation should be considered for a variety of problems: symptoms of depression, disabling anxiety, self-prescription, escalating use or abuse of alcohol, inappropriate expressions of anger, impulsive behavior, or impaired clinical judgment. Other signals that should prompt consultation include working longer hours, having trouble in significant relationships, and becoming socially isolated.

When a potentially difficult meeting or conversation is anticipated, it is helpful to rehearse statements and responses to questions. Having responses in mind before a crisis makes it more likely that one will stay calm in a tense situation. This technique also fosters a sense of control over the unexpected. One can also imagine expressing intense feelings (such as anger, sadness, or fear) as a means of decompression. Fantasizing in this way is most useful when one recognizes that the fantasy is distinct from real action; fantasies need not be enacted.

Self-knowledge (autognosis) allows psychiatrists to share common experiences and to identify individual reactions to clinical situations. This knowledge can then be used to inform diagnoses and to minimize potentially harmful reactions to patients (e.g., managing hostility toward a patient so that it will not interfere with treatment). Autognosis rounds have proven valuable for psychiatric resident groups at the Massachusetts General Hospital for the past five decades.

Signs of burnout include detachment from the meaning of one's work, open hostility, deep-rooted cynicism, and overwhelming occupational dissatisfaction.

Chapter 93

Psychiatry and the Media

Multiple-Choice Questions

Select the appropriate answer.

Q1 True or False. Media portrayals of electroconvulsive therapy have been particularly distorted.

   A. *True*

   B. *False*

Q2 True or False. A large body of multinational research demonstrates unequivocally that exposure to media reports of suicide can increase suicide attempts and deaths.

   A. *True*

   B. *False*

Q3 True or False. Researchers have concluded that the risk of learning aggressive behavior increases when the perpetrator of violence is attractive, the violence is seen as justified, the violence (and weapons used) is realistic, the violence is rewarded (or at least not punished), or the violence is portrayed as funny.

   A. *True*

   B. *False*

Q4 True or False. Most children aged 8 years and younger cannot reliably tell fantasy from reality and cannot comprehend complex motives and intentions.

   A. *True*

   B. *False*

Chapter 93

Answers

Q1 The answer is: (A) True.
Media portrayals of electroconvulsive therapy have been particularly distorted. Electroconvulsive therapy is routinely portrayed in films as brutal and punishing, even as a method of murder, with no therapeutic benefit.

Q2 The answer is: (A) True.
A large body of multinational research demonstrates unequivocally that exposure to media reports of suicide can increase suicide attempts and deaths. Reviews of research have found that stories of both fictional and real-life suicides can lead to imitation, but the effect of news stories tends to be greater. Several factors seem to increase the likelihood of imitation; these include stories of celebrities (entertainers or politicians) who commit suicide; extensive, prominent news coverage of the suicide; coverage that glamorizes or sensationalizes the suicide; and detailed descriptions of the suicide method. Imitation is decreased if the negative consequences of suicide (such as disfigurement of the body, a cult-related suicide, or suffering of and condemnation by the survivors) are portrayed. Adolescents and young adults may be particularly prone to imitate suicides that are portrayed in the media, especially when the stories are of victims in their age-group.

Q3 The answer is: (A) True.
Researchers have concluded that the risk of learning aggressive behavior increases when the perpetrator of violence is attractive, the violence is seen as justified, the violence (and weapons used) is realistic, the violence is rewarded (or at least not punished), or the violence is portrayed as funny. The risk is reduced when violence is punished, or when harmful consequences of violence (such as pain) are shown.

Q4 The answer is: (A) True.
Most children aged 8 years and younger cannot reliably tell fantasy from reality and cannot comprehend complex motives and intentions. They focus more on how something looks than what is said about it. Older children can begin to grasp more subtle aspects of program content (such as plots, themes, and historical or geographic setting), and how these combine with technical elements to affect how the program makes us feel. They can also start to question the motivations behind characters' behaviors (from sexuality to substance use) and aspects of their appearance (such as clothing or weight) and identify harmful stereotypes (such the portrayal of "crazy people").

Global Mental Health in the Twenty-First Century

Multiple-Choice Questions

Select the appropriate answer.

Q1 According to the World Health Organization, which of the following conditions causes the greatest global burden of disease?

    A. *Alcohol abuse*

    B. *Bipolar disorder*

    C. *Major depression*

    D. *Obsessive-compulsive disorder*

    E. *Schizophrenia*

Q2 True or False. Torture and degrading experiences are at least equal in their physical and mental impact on survivors.

    A. *True*

    B. *False*

Q3 True or False. In general, health and mental health providers should avoid specifically asking the patient about his or her torture experience.

    A. *True*

    B. *False*

Chapter 94

Answers

Q1 The answer is: (C) Major depression.

Mental illness confers extensive disability not only in wealthy countries but also in middle-income and poor countries. In addition, mental illness appears to be on the rise throughout the world. Thirteen percent of all disability-adjusted life years lost in 1998 were secondary to mental illness. This includes 23% of disability-adjusted life years in wealthy countries and 11% in poor countries. According to the World Health Organization, major depressive disorder is fifth on the list of the 10 leading disease causes of the global burden of disease; 5 of the 10 leading causes of the global burden of disease are mental illnesses (with alcohol abuse, bipolar disorder, schizophrenia, and obsessive-compulsive disorder following closely on the heels of major depressive disorder). In high-income countries, dementia is the third leading cause of neuropsychiatric burden. Moreover, mental illnesses are expected to rise to 15% of the global burden of disease by the year 2020. This would make them the second leading cause of global burden behind cardiovascular disorders.

Q2 The answer is: (A) True.

Recent studies have emphasized the importance of appreciating the psychological and physical suffering caused by torture; torture and degrading experiences are at least equal in their physical and mental impact on survivors.

Clinical case studies have documented chronic neuropsychiatric findings (including abnormal neurologic examination and cerebral atrophy) in torture survivors. Nearly two-thirds have neurologic impairments; two-thirds of those had experienced a head injury.

Q3 The answer is: (B) False.

At the core of the physical and psychological problems of torture survivors is the patient's "trauma story." Torture survivors readily tell their trauma story to their health and mental care practitioners regardless of their sex, ethnic background, or the severity of the torture—if they are asked about it by the health care provider. Not uncommonly, torture survivors do not tell their trauma story within the medical setting because they do not believe that their doctor's office is an appropriate place for the trauma story to be revealed. Therefore, health and mental health care providers must specifically ask the patient about his or her torture experience. Many health care providers are afraid of doing this because they are afraid of opening up a Pandora's box (filled with emotional upset) that cannot be closed within a brief doctor's visit. However, this fear is unfounded. Patients will use their time, no matter how limited it is, to give a brief account of their trauma experience, and in fact may benefit from a well-circumscribed medical visit because it places boundaries around their emotional distress. In other words, most patients believe that they cannot lose control during a brief medical visit. Medical practitioners do not need to collect the entire trauma story within a single visit. In fact, it is beneficial to the patient for the story to be collected over time.

The trauma history, when obtained, is an essential component of the history of the present illness. Knowing what actually happened to the patient allows the practitioner to discover the physical and mental sequelae associated with torture. The medical and psychiatric practitioner must distinguish between symptoms of emotional distress that are cultural expressions of suffering, and more specific symptoms of disease and illness.

Health care practitioners who do not have specialized training in psychiatry need to learn how to identify and refer to psychiatric professionals. If generic approaches to the treatment of torture survivors (such as psychotherapy and use of psychotropics) fail, the health care provider needs to consider a more specific treatment approach that brings the patient into remission.

Index